Musculoskeletal Diseases 2009-2012

Diagnostic Imaging

J. Hodler • G.K. von Schulthess • Ch.L. Zollikofer (Eds)

MUSCULOSKELETAL DISEASES 2009-2012

DIAGNOSTIC IMAGING

**41th International Diagnostic Course
in Davos (IDKD)**
Davos, March 29-April 3, 2009

including the
Nuclear Medicine Satellite Course "Diamond"
Davos, March 27-29, 2009

Pediatric Satellite Course "Kangaroo"
Davos, March 28-29, 2009

Second IDKD in Anavyssos (Greece), October 4-9, 2009

presented by the Foundation for the
Advancement of Education in Medical Radiology, Zurich

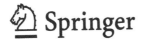 Springer

J. Hodler
Radiology, Orthopedic University
Hospital Balgrist,
Zurich, Switzerland

G. K. von Schulthess
Nuclear Medicine,
University Hospital,
Zurich, Switzerland

Ch. L. Zollikofer
Kilchberg/Zurich, Switzerland

Library of Congress Control Number: 2009923138

Springer is a part of Springer Science+Business Media

springer.com

© Springer-Verlag Italia 2009

ISBN: 978-88-470-1377-3   Springer Milan Berlin Heidelberg New York
e-ISBN: 978-88-470-1378-0

Cover design: Simona Colombo, Milan, Italy
Typesetting: C & G di Cerri e Galassi, Cremona, Italy
Printing and binding: Grafiche Porpora, Segrate (MI), Italy

Printed in Italy

Springer-Verlag Italia S.r.l., Via Decembrio 28, 20137 Milan

Preface

The International Diagnostic Course in Davos (IDKD) offers a unique learning experience for imaging specialists in training as well as for experienced radiologists and clinicians seeking state of the art knowledge and an update regarding the latest developments in the field of musculoskeletal imaging.

This syllabus is designed to provide IDKD course participants with the necessary background material so that they can fully concentrate on the workshops. However, this text is also a comprehensive overview of current musculoskeletal imaging. While it is aimed at general radiologists, radiology residents, rheumatologists, and orthopedic surgeons, it is also of relevance to clinicians in other specialties who wish to update their knowledge in this discipline.

The authors are internationally renowned experts in their fields. The chapters are disease-oriented and cover all the major imaging modalities, including magnetic resonance imaging, standard radiography, computed tomography, and ultrasound.

Additional information can be found on the IDKD website: www.idkd.org

J. Hodler
G.K. von Schulthess
Ch.L. Zollikofer

Table of Contents

Nuclear Medicine Satellite Course "Diamond"

Pediatric Satellite Course "Kangaroo"

List of Contributors

WORKSHOPS

Imaging of the Shoulder I

William E. Palmer

Musculoskeletal Imaging and Intervention Division, Department of Musculoskeletal Radiology, Massachusetts General Hospital, Boston, MA, USA

Rotator Cuff Disorders

In the patient with suspected rotator cuff disorder, the decision to perform conventional or arthrographic magnetic resonance (MR) imaging depends on the clinical need to identify and distinguish partial tears from small complete tears. Pre-operative assessment of the size and location of a cuff tear, the presence of intra-substance propagation, and the quality of the retracted tendon margin are other important aspects that must be considered as well. In older patients, in whom surgery would be performed only to repair complete cuff tears, conventional MR images are sufficient to differentiate torn, retracted tendons from normal tendons and to demonstrate bony abnormalities of the coracoacromial arch. In athletes and younger patients, in whom surgery would be performed to repair partial cuff tears, MR arthrography can optimize anatomical resolution and diagnostic confidence.

Rotator cuff disorders predominate in the older population and are often presumed to result from a lifetime of wear and tear combined with long-standing mechanical impingement by hypertrophic abnormalities of the coracoacromial arch, such as bony proliferation at the acromioclavicular joint, coracoacromial ligament, or acromial margin. In the athlete, overuse of the shoulder accelerates the cycle of inflammation in the subacromial-subdeltoid bursa, which leads to tendinosis followed by tendon degeneration and eventual tear. Overuse and cumulative injury may also promote hypertrophic changes in the coracoacromial arch, resulting in mechanical impingement at an earlier stage in life.

Both conventional (non-arthrographic) and arthrographic MR images can demonstrate the uniform thickness and hypointensity of a normal cuff tendon, or the retracted margin of a large cuff tear. The diagnostic challenge occurs in the early stages of cuff disease, when there may be subtle differences in the imaging appearances of tendinopathy versus partial-thickness tear, or in partial- versus full-thickness tear. Rim-rent tears are particularly difficult to identify when there is no tendon retraction.

In the older patient with impingement, full-thickness cuff tear often begins at the anterior margin of the supraspinatus tendon, adjacent to the rotator interval, and propagates posteriorly into the infraspinatus tendon. This usual pattern of propagation explains why tears always show a greater degree of tendon retraction anteriorly than posteriorly. To identify the smallest cuff tears, it is necessary to identify the most anterior aspect of the greater tuberosity adjacent to the bicipital tendon groove, and then scrutinize the attachment site of the supraspinatus tendon. This region may be difficult to evaluate on oblique coronal images when the shoulder is positioned in excessive internal rotation and therefore should also be inspected on axial and oblique sagittal images.

On conventional MR images, tendon retraction obviously indicates rotator cuff tear. The other primary, specific imaging finding in cuff tear is the presence of focal fluid interrupting the tendon at or near its osseous attachment site. To best identify this fluid, the MR protocol should include an oblique coronal pulse sequence that combines T2 weighting with adequate spatial resolution. At higher field strengths, an effective fast spin-echo sequence might prescribe an intermediate TE (40-50 ms) to gain sufficient T2-weighting while maintaining the signal-to-noise ratio. Fat-suppression is valuable because it enables the detection of marrow edema and smaller cysts at the site of tendon attachment to the greater tuberosity. Posterior cysts are seen in all age groups regardless of cuff pathology. Anterior cysts at the supraspinatus insertion site are closely related to rotator cuff tear, including partial-thickness tear, which may be difficult to identify on MR images. In the presence of equivocal cuff tear, anterior intraosseous cysts in the greater tuberosity should boost diagnostic confidence and lead to closer scrutiny of the supraspinatus tendon.

Secondary imaging findings, such as tendon thinning or thickening, contour irregularity, and signal heterogeneity, lack diagnostic specificity and can be misleading in image interpretation. They may be seen in abnormal tendons with tendinopathy or cuff tears, but may also be present in normal tendons that exhibit anatomical variation (interposed muscle slips) or imaging artifact (magic angle phenomenon, volume averaging).

MR Arthrography in Cuff Disorders

On arthrographic MR images, intra-articular contrast solution outlines the inferior cuff surface, fills partial cuff tears, and, in complete tears, leaks from the glenohumeral joint into the subacromial-subdeltoid space. The presence or absence of extra-articular contrast solution distinguishes partial and complete cuff tears. The sensitivity and specificity of arthrographic MR images in the diagnosis of full-thickness tear are comparable to those of conventional arthrography (i.e., nearly 100%).

Conventional and arthrographic MR images show equally well any atrophy or fatty replacement of cuff muscles. Arthrographic MR images may have an advantage in demonstrating other anatomical features that are useful in the prediction of cuff repairability and post-operative prognosis. They depict the location and size of the cuff tear, the degree of tendon retraction, and the contour of the torn tendon margin. This information adds value to the diagnostic report and may influence pre-operative planning. For example, the surgeon may elect to perform an open procedure rather than an arthroscopic repair, depending upon the size of the cuff tear and the leak of contrast material into a delaminated tendon.

Arthrographic MR images are particularly well suited to the diagnosis of partial-thickness tears, since they usually begin at the articular (inferior) surface of the supraspinatus tendon. In this location, high-signal contrast solution can fill focal cuff defects. Whenever partial-thickness tears involve the superior (bursal) surface or the intra-substance of tendon, they do not fill with contrast material and therefore may be overlooked on T1-weighted arthrographic MR images. For this reason, the arthrographic MR protocol should include T2-weighted oblique coronal images, which can reveal bursal collections and extra-articular fluid disrupting cuff fibers.

On arthrographic MR images, fat suppression aids in the differentiation of partial- and full-thickness tears and is especially valuable whenever cuff tendons show contrast solution that extends to the bursal surface, but not definitely through it. Contrast solution and normal fat in the subacromial-subdeltoid space both show increased signal intensities on T1-weighted images without fat-suppression and therefore may be indistinguishable. On fat-suppressed T1-weighted images, the signal from contrast solution remains increased, whereas the signal from normal fat is selectively decreased. When fat-suppression is used, persistent high signal intensity in the subacromial-subdeltoid space indicates a full-thickness cuff tear, whereas low signal intensity indicates a partial-thickness tear. This benefit is critical in assessment of the post-operative cuff.

Cuff delamination indicates poor tendon quality and is important to recognize for pre-operative planning. When delamination occurs, there is dehiscence of tendon fibers and dissociation of bursal and articular surfaces. As a result of this cleavage plane that develops within the cuff tendon, three secondary phenomena commonly occur. First, articular surface fibers can retract proximally more than bursal surface fibers. In both partial- and full-thickness tear, the visualization of asymmetric fiber retraction is strong evidence of tendon delamination. Second, the delaminating tear can propagate posteriorly within the cuff substance without disrupting either the bursal and articular surfaces or the tendon attachment to the greater tuberosity. In this situation, the size of a cuff tear can be easily underestimated. For example, the MR images may demonstrate a definite partial- or full-thickness tear of the supraspinatus tendon, but may show no evidence of the intrasubstance propagation extending posteriorly into the infraspinatus tendon. Diagnostic difficulty results because the delaminating tear represents a potential space that may not be filled with enough fluid to become visible. In shoulder adduction, the routine imaging position, fluid is squeezed out of the cleavage plane due to the increased tension that develops in the tendon when it is draped and stretched over the humeral head. The delaminating tear may be better seen on arthrographic MR images if contrast solution diffuses into the defect. The tear may be best seen in ABER (abduction - external rotation) images. In the ABER position, the delaminating tear widens due to laxity in the tendon, fills with fluid or contrast solution, and thus becomes obvious. Third, fluid in a delaminating tear can dissect into the myotendinous junction of the supra- or infraspinatus tendon and result in an intramuscular cyst or ganglion. The presence of an intramuscular cyst should raise the likelihood of a delaminating rotator cuff tear.

Imbibition suggests decreased quality of tendon tissue. Tendons that imbibe contrast solution have increased signal intensity on fat-suppressed T1-weighted images, indicating the diffusion of gadolinium into the tendon substance. At surgery, these tendons are swollen and friable due to inflammation or degeneration. They require debridement to expose healthy tissue for suturing, increasing the technical difficulty of cuff repair and decreasing the likelihood of operative success. Imbibition usually involves the torn tendon along its retracted margin, which can be thickened or attenuated. In severe tendinosis, imbibition may occur without the focal disruption of cuff fibers. If contrast diffuses across the full tendon thickness and leaks into the subacromial-subdeltoid space, it simulates complete cuff tear. At surgery, these tendons are diffusely boggy and severely degenerated, but they remain attached to the greater tuberosity.

Glenohumeral Instability

Anterior glenohumeral instability causes significant morbidity in young patients, particularly athletes, and often requires surgical reconstruction to restore shoulder function. The clinical spectrum of instability ranges from obvious recurrent dislocations to equivocal symptoms that may mimic other shoulder disorders, such as rotator cuff tear and biceps tendon dislocation. In patients with inconclusive clinical evaluations, imaging studies are commonly used to guide the selection of appropriate therapy and preoperative planning.

By demonstrating the inferior labral-ligamentous complex, MR imaging is a major contribution to the evaluation of patients with suspected glenohumeral instability. The anterior band of the inferior glenohumeral ligament is critical in maintaining passive anterior stability of the shoulder and functions as a unit with the glenoid labrum, which anchors the ligament to the glenoid rim. The origin of the inferior glenohumeral ligament creates a stress point on the labrum. During shoulder dislocation or abduction-external rotation, tension is transmitted through the inferior glenohumeral ligament to the labral attachment site. Excessive tension can avulse the labrum from the glenoid rim, rendering the ligament incompetent. Thus, the inferior glenohumeral ligament can appear normal but lose its stabilizing function if its labral anchor is partially or completed detached. Rupture of the inferior glenohumeral ligament is a much less common cause of anterior instability than avulsion of the glenolabral attachment site.

This functional anatomy of the inferior labral-ligamentous complex enables a biomechanical approach to the diagnosis of anterior shoulder instability. Specific MR criteria can be used in the differentiation of stable and unstable shoulders because these images can show the location and length of labral abnormalities relative to the origin of the inferior glenohumeral ligament. If the torn labral segment extends into the attachment site of the inferior glenohumeral ligament, there is a high likelihood of anterior instability. This information may guide the orthopedic surgeon in preoperative planning and in the selection of appropriate surgical or conservative treatments. Less commonly, patients develop trauma-related instability due to ligamentous stretching and laxity without an associated labral tear. Both MR imaging and MR arthrography are less valuable in these cases because the entire inferior labral-ligamentous complex appears intact. Currently, no accurate MR imaging criteria are recognized in the diagnosis of capsular laxity.

Capsular insertion sites have been used to evaluate joint stability. Type I capsule arises from the glenoid labrum, type II from the scapular neck within 1 cm of the labral base, and type III from the scapular neck more than 1 cm medial to the labral base. MR arthrography of the shoulder has helped to shift diagnostic emphasis onto the labral-ligamentous complex and away from the capsular insertion site. Appearances of the capsular insertion site are markedly variable in individuals and are heavily dependent upon both the position of the shoulder (e.g., internal vs. external rotation) as well as the degree of capsular distension due to effusion or injected contrast solution. The three types of capsular insertions represent normal variations in the size, morphology, and location of the subscapularis recess. Since the incidences of capsular insertion types are statistically similar in stable and un-

stable shoulders, type III capsular insertion cannot be used to predict anterior glenohumeral instability. Following an anterior stabilization procedure, however, it is most important to assess the integrity of the capsular reconstruction site, since the inferior labral-ligamentous complex has been surgically distorted.

The lexicon of glenohumeral instability has evolved into a complex collection of eponyms that refer to closely related abnormalities of the inferior labral-ligamentous complex. The Bankart lesion generally refers to a complete labral tear at the origin of the inferior glenohumeral ligament, resulting in disruption of the scapular periosteum and detachment of the labrum from the glenoid rim. A partial Bankart lesion is sometimes used to describe an incomplete labral tear in the same location. Osseous Bankart lesion indicates an osteochondral fracture of the glenoid rim at the inferior labral-ligamentous attachment site.

The Perthes lesion also refers to labral detachment from the glenoid rim, but the inferior labral-ligamentous complex remains attached to the scapular periosteum, which is stripped medially on the glenoid neck. If the Perthes lesion is nondisplaced, the tear may become synovialized or filled with granulation tissue, preventing the sublabral leak of contrast solution and leading to a false-negative diagnosis of labral tear. Although the Perthes lesion can appear deceptively normal on arthrographic MR images, the shoulder remains susceptible to anterior subluxation and recurrent instability.

Anterior labral-ligamentous periosteal sleeve avulsion (ALPSA) is similar to the Perthes lesion, except the inferior labral-ligamentous complex becomes bunched and retracted medially, resembling a rolled-up sleeve. Thus, the labrum is permanently displaced from the glenoid rim in the ALPSA lesion but may re-approximate its normal position in the Perthes lesion. Glenolabral articular disruption refers to a partial anteroinferior labral tear that is associated with an adjacent articular cartilage defect involving the glenoid fossa. This lesion may not always be associated with anterior instability, but may progress to rapid joint degeneration, with intra-articular loose bodies. The latter may also result from cartilage defects involving the humeral head. Humeral avulsion of the glenohumeral ligament is a rare cause of debilitating anterior instability. It results from anterior dislocation and may be associated with subscapularis tendon avulsions from the lesser tuberosity.

Although arthrographic MR images have demonstrated >90% accuracy in the detection of anteroinferior glenoid labral tears, diagnostic confidence may be further increased when the shoulder is imaged in ABER. The ABER position is achieved by flexing the elbow and placing the patient's hand posterior to the contralateral aspect of the head or neck. In this position, MR images of the shoulder are prescribed in an axial oblique plane from a coronal localizer image, parallel to the long axis of the humerus.

In unstable shoulders, the most important abnormality is a tear of the inferior labral-ligamentous complex at the glenoid attachment site. When shoulders are imaged in the ABER position, diagnostic confidence is increased because the anterior band of the inferior glenohumeral ligament is stretched, transmitting tension to the labrum. Thus, an anteroinferior glenoid labral tear that is nondisplaced when the shoulder is neutral in position has a greater likelihood of being displaced from the glenoid rim and becoming more conspicuous when the shoulder is in ABER. For the same reason, ABER images may demonstrate the degree of medial stripping of the scapular periosteum following anterior labral-ligamentous detachment from the glenoid rim. The ABER position may also be valuable in the detection of partially healed labral tears (e.g., Perthes lesion), in which the surface of the tear becomes re-synovialized although the labral-ligamentous anchor remains incompetent. These tears may not fill with contrast on arthrographic MR images obtained in the usual adducted position, but may become visible on ABER images because the labrum is more likely to become displaced from the glenoid rim.

There are, however, potential limitations in ABER imaging. Approximately 20% of patients may be unwilling or unable to assume the ABER position due to shoulder pain or apprehension. Even motivated, experienced technologists require substantial extra time for repeat patient positioning, coil placement, and ABER image acquisition. Therefore, the ABER technique can be time-consuming, adding at least 10 min to the routine MR protocol.

Suggested Reading

Chang D, Mohana-Borges A, Borso M, Chung CB (2008) SLAP lesions: anatomy, clinical presentation, MR imaging diagnosis and characterization. Eur J Radiol 68(1):72-87

Fritz LB, Ouellette HA, Fritz TA et al (2007) Cystic changes at the supraspinatus and infraspinatus insertion sites: association with age and rotator cuff disorders in 238 patients. Radiology 244(1):239-248

Kassarjian A, Torriani M, Onellette H, Palmer WE (2005) Intramuscular rotator cuff cysts: association with tendon tears on MRI and arthroscopy. AJR Am J Roentgenol 185(1):160-165

Tung GA, Hou DD (2003) MR arthrography of the posterior labrocapsular complex: relationship with glenohumeral joint alignment and clinical posterior instability. AJR Am J Roentgenol 180:369-375

Waldt S, Burkart A, Imhoff AB et al (2005) Anterior shoulder instability: accuracy of MR arthrography in the classification of anteroinferior labroligamentous injuries. Radiology 237:578-583

Walz DM, Miller IL Chen S, Hofman J (2007) MR imaging of delamination tears of the rotator cuff tendons. Skeletal Radiol 36:411-416

Imaging of the Shoulder II

Klaus Woertler

Department of Radiology, Technische Universität München, Munich, Germany

Introduction

This chapter focuses on articular pathologies of the shoulder, in particular, impingement and rotator cuff pathology, glenohumeral instability, and biceps tendon and rotator interval lesions. The magnetic resonance imaging (MRI) and MR arthrography (MRA) appearances of these conditions are described.

Impingement and Rotator Cuff Pathology

Impingement

Impingement syndromes in the shoulder can be classified as: (1) primary extrinsic (subacromial, subcoracoid), (2) secondary extrinsic (instability-related), and (3) secondary intrinsic (internal; anterosuperior, posterosuperior).

Primary extrinsic impingement is caused by entrapment of the anterior rotator cuff under the coracoacromial arch or, rarely, the coracoid process. The secondary forms of impingement are initiated by abnormal translation of the humeral head due to glenohumeral instability or microinstability and predominate in athletes who must execute overhead motions or throwing.

Subacromial ("outlet") impingement (Fig. 1) is by far the most common type of impingement in the shoulder.

It is typically seen in individuals older than 40 years of age with stable shoulders. The clinical syndrome results from a mismatch between the width of the supraspinatus outlet and the thickness of the anterior portion of the rotator cuff and subacromial bursa. Predisposing factors include variants of acromial shape (type III acromion, lateral downslope), subacromial spur formation, os acromiale, thickening of the coracoacromial ligament, acromioclavicular osteoarthritis (rare), and cuff hypertrophy. Subacromial impingement leads to chronic subacromial bursitis and tendinopathy, predominantly of the supraspinatus tendon, which progresses to partial and complete tearing.

Rotator Cuff Pathology

The majority of rotator cuff lesions result from degenerative changes in older individuals with subacromial impingement syndrome. "Traumatic" tears are commonly found with pre-existing degeneration or might be associated injuries in shoulder dislocation. True traumatic lesions of the rotator cuff are rare in younger individuals. Sports-related rotator cuff lesions most often represent articular-sided partial tears that develop due to overuse or secondary to (micro)instability.

Partial (partial-thickness) rotator cuff tears can be classified as articular-sided, bursal-sided, or intratendinous.

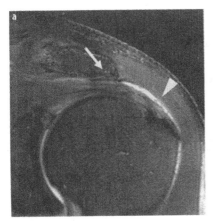 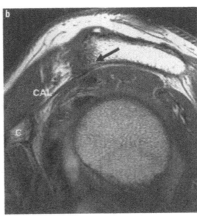

Fig. 1 a, b. Subacromial impingement. **a** Coronal intermediate-weighted turbo spin-echo (TSE) image with fat-suppression; **b** sagittal T1-weighted TSE image show subacromial spur (*arrows*) at the acromial insertion of the coracoacromial ligament (*CAL*), subacromial/subdeltoid bursitis, and bursal-sided partial tear of the supraspinatus tendon (*C* coracoid process)

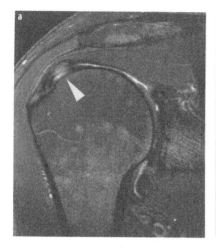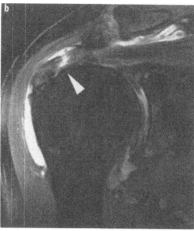

Fig. 2 a, b. Rotator cuff tears. **a** Coronal intermediate weighted TSE image with fat-suppression shows articular-sided partial tear (*arrowhead*) of the supraspinatus tendon. Note the articular cartilage defect of the humeral head (**b**) Coronal T2-weighted TSE image with fat-suppression reveals full-thickness tear (*arrowhead*) of the supraspinatus tendon and large bursal effusion in a patient with advanced degenerative changes of the glenohumeral joint

The term "rim rent tear" describes an articular-sided partial-thickness tear involving the insertional fibers ("footprint") of the tendon. It is virtually synonymous with the PASTA (partial articular surface tendon avulsion) lesion. Complete (full-thickness) tears are transtendinous in at least one portion of the involved tendon and lead to communication between the glenohumeral joint and the bursa. On conventional MRI (Fig. 2), fluid-like intratendinous signal intensity on images with T2 contrast represents the diagnostic criterion for diagnosis of a rotator cuff tear. In a partial tear, fluid signal traverses only a portion of the tendon; and in a complete tear, the entire thickness of the tendon (at least on one section). MRI shows a high sensitivity and specificity for the detection of complete tears, but has a limited sensitivity in the depiction of partial tears. MRA can increase the sensitivity of MRI in diagnosing partial tears to over 80%, mainly by improving the detection of articular-sided lesions.

In patients with rotator cuff tears, the following information, which can be derived from MRI, is essential for treatment planning: involved tendon(s), size of the tear, presence of tendon retraction, quality of muscles, and presence of associated lesions. The size of the tear should be measured in two dimensions on images with T2 contrast or on MRA. According to Patte and coworkers, tendon retraction in full-thickness tears can be quantified as follows:

Grade 1   Tendon retracted but lateral to humeral equator
Grade 2   Tendon medial to humeral equator but lateral to glenoid
Grade 3   Tendon medial to glenoid

Rotator cuff tears induce muscle atrophy and, with time, irreversible fatty degeneration of the muscle bellies (Fig. 3). Since the extent of muscle degeneration correlates with the clinical outcome of surgical repair procedures, muscular quality should routinely be evaluated by MRI. Fatty degeneration can be semiquantitatively assessed using the grading system proposed by Goutallier and coworkers, evaluating the most lateral sagittal oblique section of a T1- or T2-weighted sequence, which shows the scapular spine and coracoid process in continuity with the scapular body:

Grade 0   Normal muscle, no fat
Grade 1   Muscle contains some streaks of fat
Grade 2   Significant fatty infiltration, but still less fat than muscle
Grade 3   Fatty infiltration with equal amounts of fat and muscle
Grade 4   Fatty infiltration with more fat than muscle

Advanced muscular degeneration (>grade 2) is regarded as an exclusion criterion for anatomic rotator cuff repair in most cases.

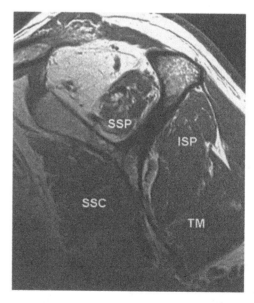

Fig. 3. Muscle degeneration consecutive to a supraspinatus tendon tear. Sagittal T1-weighted SE image shows marked atrophy and fatty degeneration of the supraspinatus muscle (grade 2-3) with the otherwise normal appearance of the muscle bellies. *SSC*, Subscapularis; *SSP*, supraspinatus; *ISP*, infraspinatus; *TM*, teres minor

Glenohumeral Instability

Traumatic Glenohumeral Instability

Traumatic glenohumeral instability is initiated by a single traumatic event of shoulder dislocation that leads to discontinuity of the labroligamentous complex (LLC), thus giving rise to further episodes of shoulder subluxation or dislocation. In the majority of patients, traumatic glenohumeral instability occurs in an anteroinferior direction. Posterior instability is far less common and is more often caused by violent muscle contraction in electrical accidents or seizures.

The MRI findings in traumatic anterior instability include lesions of the anteroinferior LLC (Fig. 4), compression injuries of the humeral head (Hill-Sachs defect), and associated injuries of the superior labrum, rotator cuff, and rotator interval. MRA provides high sensitivity and specificity for the detection of LLC lesions and has proved reliable in classification of these injuries. Images obtained in the ABER (abduction and external rotation) position can be helpful in depicting discontinuity of the anteroinferior LLC.

Whereas classic Bankart and Perthes lesions (Fig. 5) are most common in patients with acute instability, ALPSA (anterior labroligamentous periosteal sleeve avulsion) and "non-classifiable" lesions of the LLC are more often seen in patients with multiple episodes of shoulder dislocation. "Non-classifiable" lesions present with advanced destruction of the LLC and more or less extensive scar tissue formation, thus indicating a poor anatomic substrate for arthroscopic refixation. The HAGL (humeral avulsion of glenohumeral ligaments) lesion is a relatively rare capsular injury that does not involve the LLC at

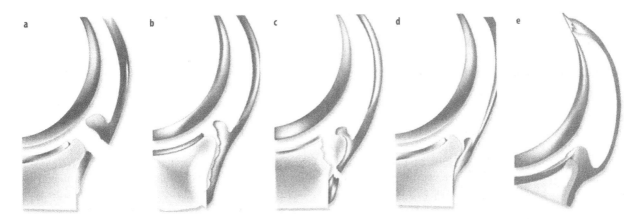

Fig. 4 a-e. Labroligamentous injuries in anterior glenohumeral instability. **a** Classic Bankart lesion: complete avulsion of the labroligamentous complex (LLC) from the glenoid, with torn scapular periosteum; **b** Perthes lesion: Bankart variant lesion with detached labrum and stripped but intact scapular periosteum; **c** bony Bankart lesion: osseous avulsion of the LLC from the anteroinferior glenoid; **d** ALPSA lesion: chronic variant of a Perthes lesion, with medial displacement and inferior rotation of the LLC; **e** HAGL lesion: avulsion of the inferior glenohumeral ligament (IGHL) from the humeral neck. (Modified from Woertler and Waldt, 2006)

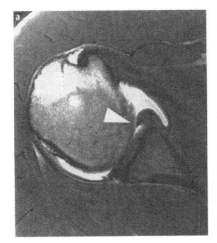
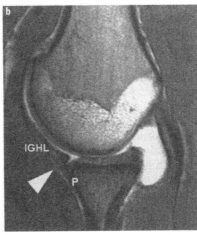

Fig. 5 a, b. Perthes lesion. **a** Transverse T1-weighted magnetic resonance arthrogram (MRA) shows contrast media undermining the anteroinferior labrum (*arrowhead*). **b** Corresponding T1-weighted image obtained in the abduction and external rotation (ABER) position demonstrates detachment of the labrum (*arrowhead*) but continuity of the scapular periosteum (*P*) and inferior glenohumeral ligament (*IGHL*)

the glenoid, but represents a tear of the inferior gleno-humeral ligament (IGHL) at its humeral insertion. The Hill-Sachs defect is typically located at the posterolateral circumference of the humeral head. On transverse images, it should be seen at or slightly above the level of the coracoid. Due to an adjacent zone of bone contusion, acute and subacute lesions are easy to detect on fat-suppressed images with T2 contrast. The following MRI findings are of particular relevance for therapeutic decisions in patients with anterior glenohumeral instability: quality of the LLC, presence of a HAGL lesion, presence and size of a bony glenoid defect (bony Bankart lesion or chronic wear), presence of a large Hill-Sachs defect, associated injuries, e.g., tears of the superior labrum, anterior to posterior (SLAP lesions).

A reverse pattern of injuries (posterior labral lesions, reverse Hill-Sachs defect) is seen in patients with traumatic posterior instability. If the initiating event was a seizure or electric shock, these findings can frequently be found bilaterally. Acute dislocations can remain locked with the arm in adduction and internal rotation.

Atraumatic Glenohumeral Instability

Atraumatic glenohumeral instability is typically bilateral, multidirectional, and particularly seen in patients with general laxity of the joints (congenital hypermobility syndrome). In atraumatic instability, MRI does not reveal a specific pattern of findings. MRA usually shows an increased capsular volume and a wide rotator interval, but no or little morphologic alterations of intra-articular structures. In athletes, laxity of the capsule is, however, often associated with labral or rotator cuff lesions.

Microtraumatic Glenohumeral Instability

The concept of microtraumatic instability in throwers and overhead athletes is controversially discussed in the literature. Repetitive capsular microtrauma due to overuse is thought to lead to increased anterior (repetitive abduction and external rotation) or posterior (repetitive abduction, flexion, and internal rotation) translation of the humeral head and, consecutively, to structural damage of the labrum and rotator cuff (secondary impingement). MRA is best-suited to depict structural alterations of the joint capsule, glenoid labrum, biceps anchor, and articular surface of the rotator cuff in these patients.

In this context, posterosuperior glenoid impingement (PSI) represents the most common form of internal impingement. PSI is caused by anterior microinstability and leads to repetitive and extensive contact between the undersurface of the rotator cuff (posterior portion of supraspinatus tendon and/or infraspinatus tendon) and the posterosuperior glenoid when the arm is in high abduction and external rotation. The condition can be diagnosed on MRA by identification of the "kissing lesions" pattern, with corresponding lesions of the undersurface of the rotator cuff, posterosuperior labrum, greater

tuberosity, and superior glenoid, often in association with lesions of the anterior capsule and tears of the superior labral-bicipital complex (SLAP lesions).

Biceps Tendon and Rotator Interval Lesions

SLAP Lesions

Tears of the superior glenoid labrum that extend in an anterior to posterior direction are referred to as SLAP (superior labral anterior to posterior) lesions. In arthroscopic series. the incidence of these injuries varies from 4 to 10%. Four different types of SLAP lesions were described in the original classification by Snyder: In type 1, there is degenerative fraying of the superior labrum. Type 2 represents avulsion of the superior labrum and biceps anchor from the glenoid. Type 3 is a bucket-handle tear of the superior labrum, with preservation of the biceps anchor. Type 4 is defined as bucket-handle tear of the superior labrum, involving the long head of biceps tendon.

In the etiology of SLAP lesions, three different mechanisms of injury have been described: acute compression of the biceps anchor during a fall onto an outstretched arm or flexed elbow, forced external rotation and abduction (anterior shoulder dislocation) with tearing of the anterior labrum from anteroinferior to superior, and repetitive torsion of the biceps anchor in throwers and overhead athletes ("peelback mechanism"). Associated lesions include ganglia (labral cysts), anteroinferior labroligamentous injuries (in patients with anterior glenohumeral instability), articular-sided rotator cuff tears, and the typical corresponding lesions in patients with PSI.

Standard MRI is of limited value for the detection of SLAP lesions due to its rather low sensitivity (13-65%). On MRA (Fig. 6), SLAP lesions can be diagnosed with a sensitivity of 84-92% and a specificity of 69-99%. Type 1 lesions are characterized by surface irregularity and increased signal intensity caused by degenerative alterations of the fibrocartilage. In type 2 lesions (Fig. 7), linear extension of contrast media into the superior labrum and the biceps anchor is seen. The criteria for differentiation between this type of lesion and a sublabral recess as a common anatomic variant (Fig. 6e) are superior or lateral extension of contrast media or, if the cleft is oriented medially, irregular margins and/or a wide separation between labrum and glenoid. In the bucket-handle tears of types 3 and 4, the fragment can be more or less dislocated inferiorly. In a type 3 lesion, the fragment is typically triangular and separated from the intact biceps insertion, whereas in a type 4 lesion the bucket-handle consists of the superior labrum and a portion of the biceps tendon. In patients with anterior shoulder instability, SLAP lesions typically represent the superior extension of an anteroinferior labroligamentous injury, with the Bankart-Perthes lesion and the SLAP type 2 lesion as the most common combination.

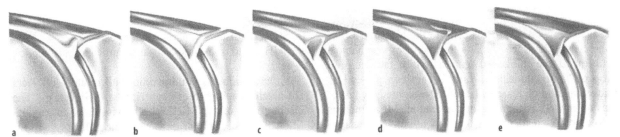

Fig. 6 a-e. SLAP lesions. **a** type 1; **b** type 2; **c** type 3; **d** type 4. **e** Sublabral recess (normal variant). (Modified from Woertler and Waldt, 2006)

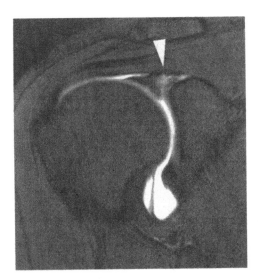

Fig. 7. SLAP type 2 lesion. Coronal fat-suppressed T1-weighted MRA shows superior extension of contrast media into the superior labrum and biceps anchor (*arrowhead*). Note the irregular margins of the tear

Biceps Tendinopathy and Tear

Tendinopathy of the long head of the biceps tendon can result from chronic overuse or tendon instability. The majority of degenerative lesions are, however, associated with impingement and rotator cuff pathology. Degenerative changes most commonly affect the horizontal portion of the biceps tendon and therefore are usually best depicted on sagittal MRI. The findings associated with tendinosis include increased caliber, irregular contour and increased signal intensity of the tendon on short TE images (Fig. 8). Although these signs have a high sensitivity, their specificity is relatively low.

Complete tears of the biceps tendon represent the end stage of the chronic degeneration that follows tendinosis and partial tearing. Spontaneous rupture therefore usually occurs with minor trauma or even during a normal movement. The "Popeye sign" is a pathognomonic clinical presentation in which there is distal retraction of the muscle belly following complete rupture of the long head of the biceps tendon. Nonetheless, the deformity is not produced by all tears, because dislocation of the distal

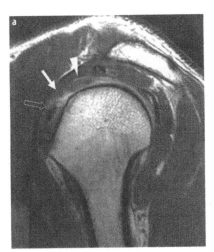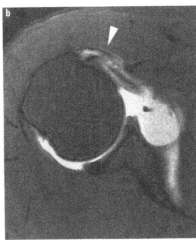

Fig. 8 a, b. Pulley lesion. **a** Sagittal T1-weighted MRA shows discontinuity of the superior glenohumeral ligament (*closed arrow*), partial tear of the superior portion of the subscapularis tendon (*open arrow*), and the increased signal intensity of a thickened biceps tendon due to tendinosis (*arrowhead*). **b** Transverse fat-suppressed T1-weighted MRA demonstrates a subscapularis tendon tear and a slight medial subluxation of the biceps tendon (*arrowhead*)

portion of the tendon can be prevented or limited by fibrous tissue that had formed adjacent to the tendon during the degenerative process prior to the tear, by fibrous adherence to the subscapularis tendon, or by mechanical fixation of the thickened tendon within the bicipital groove ("autotenodesis"). Partial tears can present as thickening and increased T1- and T2-weighted signal intensity as well as thinning of the tendon. MRI findings with complete tears range from discontinuity of the horizontal portion of the tendon to complete absence of visualization.

Rotator Interval

The rotator interval is a triangular space that is exclusively covered by capsular structures and bordered by the anterior free edge of the supraspinatus tendon superiorly, the superior free edge of the subscapularis tendon inferiorly, and the coracoid process medially. The intertubercular sulcus and transverse ligament represent the apex of this triangle, the coracoid process its base. As the long head of the biceps tendons passes through the rotator and changes its course from a horizontal to a vertical orientation, it is stabilized by two structures that form a ligamentous sling, the "reflection pulley" of the biceps tendon. These structures are the coracohumeral ligament (CHL) and the superior glenohumeral ligament (SGHL).

Biceps Tendon Instability, Pulley Lesions

Subluxation and dislocation of the biceps tendon can occur in a lateral or medial direction. Subluxation is defined as partial or transient loss of contact, dislocation as complete and permanent loss of contact between the tendon and the bicipital groove.

Lateral instability of the biceps tendon is rare and has mainly been described as following fractures of the greater tuberosity. Post-traumatic deformity of the bicipital sulcus and flattening of the anterior contour of the greater tuberosity may allow the biceps tendon to sublux or dislocate laterally.

Medial instability is far more common, results from a lesion of the reflection pulley (SGHL tear) with or without an associated subscapularis tendon tear (Fig. 8), and typically leads to tendinopathy. Three different types of medial subluxation/dislocation can be distinguished: intratendinous, intra-articular, and extracapsular. In intratendinous subluxation/dislocation, the biceps tendon cuts in between the CHL and the torn fibers of the subscapularis tendon. This lesion may progress to complete detachment of the subscapularis tendon, thus allowing the biceps tendon to dislocate intra-articularly. Extracapsular dislocation with displacement of the biceps tendon superficial to the CHL and subscapularis tendon is uncommon.

Lesions of the reflection pulley were classified by Habermeyer and coworkers as follows:

1. Isolated SGHL tear
2. SGHL and subscapularis tendon tear
3. SGHL and supraspinatus tendon tear
4. SGHL and subscapularis and supraspinatus tendon tear.

Pulley lesions in combination with rotator cuff tears are much more common than isolated SGHL tears. The discontinuity of the SGHL can be visualized on sagittal MRA. Indirect signs of damage to the pulley system include tears of the superior free edge of the subscapularis and/or anterior free edge of the subscapularis tendons, subluxation or dislocation of the biceps tendon, tendinopathy, and contrast extravasation from the rotator interval on MRA.

Suggested Reading

Ahrens PM, Boileau (2007) The long head of biceps and associated tendinopathy. J Bone Joint Surg 89-B:1001-1009

Balich SM, Sheley RC, Brown TR, Sauser DD, Quinn SF (1997) MR imaging of the rotator cuff: intraobserver agreement and analysis of interpretative errors. Radiology 204:191-194

Chandnani VP, Yeager TD, Bencardino T, Christensen K, Galgliardi JA, Heitz DR, Baird DE, Hansen MF (1993) Glenoid labral tears: prospective evaluation with MR imaging, MR arthrography, and CT arthrography. AJR Am J Roentgenol 161:1229-1235

Goutallier D, Postel JM, Bernageau J, Lavau L, Voisin MC (1994) Fatty muscle degeneration in cuff ruptures. Clin Orthop Rel Res 304:78-83

Habermeyer P, Magosch P, Pritsch M, Scheibel MT, Lichtenberg S (2004) Anterosuperior impingement of the shoulder as a result of pulley lesions: A prospective arthroscopic study. J Shoulder Elbow Surg 13:5-12

Hansen MF (1993) Glenoid labral tears: prospective evaluation with MR imaging, MR arthrography, and CT arthrography. AJR 161:1229-1235

Kassarjian A, Bencardino JT, Palmer WE (2004) MR imaging of the rotator cuff. Magn Reson Imaging Clin N Am 12:39-60

Morag Y, Jacobson JA, Shields G, Rajani R, Jamadar DA, Miller B, Hayes CW (2005) MR arthrography of rotator interval, long head of the biceps brachii, and biceps pulley of the shoulder. Radiology 235:21-30

Palmer WE, Brown JH, Rosenthal DI (1993) Rotator cuff evaluation with fat-suppressed MR arthrography. Am J Roentgenol 188:683-687

Palmer WE, Caslowitz PL (1995) Anterior shoulder instability: diagnostic criteria determined from prospective analysis of 121 MR arthrograms. Radiology 197:819-825

Patte D (1990) Classification of rotator cuff lesions. Clin Orthop Rel Res 254:81-86

Snyder SJ, Karzel RP, Del-Pizzo W, Ferkel RD, Friedmann MJ (1990) SLAP lesions of the shoulder. Arthroscopy 6:274-279

Tirman PFJ, Bost FW, Gravin GJ, Peterfy CG, Mall JC, Steinbach LS, Feller JF, Crues JV 3rd (1994) Posterosuperior glenoid impingement of the shoulder: findings at MR imaging and MR arthrography with arthroscopic correlation. Radiology 193:431-436

Tuite MJ, Cirillo RL, De Smet AA, Orwin JF (2000) Superior labrum anterior-posterior (SLAP) tears: evaluation of three MR signs on T2-weighted images. Radiology 215:841-845

Waldt S, Bruegel M, Mueller D, Holzapfel K, Imhoff AB, Rummeny E, Woertler K (2006) Rotator cuff tears: assessment with MR arthrography in 275 cases with arthroscopic correlation. Eur Radiol 17:491-498

Waldt S, Burkart A, Imhoff AB, Bruegel M, Rummeny EJ, Woertler K (2005) Anterior shoulder instability: performance

Elbow Imaging with an Emphasis on MRI

Lynne S. Steinbach[1], Marco Zanetti[2]

[1] Department of Radiology, University of California San Francisco, San Francisco, CA, USA
[2] Department of Radiology, University Hospital Balgrist, Zurich, Switzerland

Introduction

Imaging of the elbow can demonstrate a wide range of elbow abnormalities that involve osseous structures, articular surfaces, ligaments, muscles, tendons, bursae, and nerves. In the following discussion, the elbow anatomy – with variants and pitfalls as well as commonly encountered osseous and soft-tissue pathology – will be addressed. The emphasis will be on their magnetic resonance imaging (MRI) appearances.

Osseous Structures, Articular Surfaces

The articular surfaces of the humerus are formed by two components, the trochlea and the capitellum, which articulate with the ulna, and radius, respectively. The capitellum and trochlea are oriented with 30° of anterior angulation relative to the long axis of the humerus (Fig. 1) [1].

The ulnohumeral joint is the articulation between the trochlear (greater sigmoid) notch of the ulna and the humeral trochlea. The trochlear (greater sigmoid) notch is named for its articulation with the adjacent trochlea of the humerus. The radial (lesser sigmoid) notch is a small impression along the lateral margin of the coronoid process that articulates with the radial head. The anterior and posterior articular surfaces of the trochlear notch are separated by a small depression that is typically devoid of hyaline cartilage, called the trochlear ridge. The trochlear ridge is approximately 2-3 mm wide and 3-5 mm high [2]. Because the height corresponds to that of adjacent articular cartilage, the articular surface remains smooth (Fig. 2). On sagittal MRI or reconstructed sagittal computed tomography (CT) images, a central elevation of the trochlear articular surface corresponding to the trochlear ridge may be seen, simulating either a central osteophyte or an osteochondral lesion.

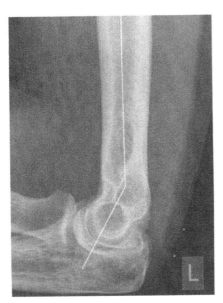

Fig. 1. The capitellum and trochlea are oriented with 30° of anterior angulation relative to the long axis of the humerus

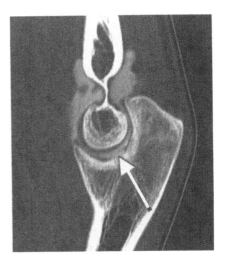

Fig. 2. A sagittal reformatted computed tomography (CT) arthrogram demonstrates the trochlear ridge (*arrow*), which separates the anterior and posterior articular surface of the trochlear notch by a small depression that is devoid of hyaline cartilage. Note that the height of the trochlear ridge corresponds to that of adjacent articular cartilage such that the articular surface remains smooth

of MR arthrography for classification of anteroinferior labroligamentous injuries. Radiology 237:578-583

Waldt S, Burkart A, Lange P, Imhoff AB, Rummeny EJ, Woertler K (2004) Diagnostic performance of MR arthrography in the assessment of superior labral anteroposterior lesions of the shoulder. AJR Am J Roentgenol 182:1271-1278

Weishaupt D, Zanetti M, Tanner A, Gerber C, Hodler J (1999) Lesions of the reflection pulley of the long biceps tendon: MR arthrographic findings. Invest Radiol 34:463-469

Woertler K, Waldt S (2006) MR imaging in sports-related glenohumeral instability. Eur Radiol 16:2622-2636

Woertler K (2007) Multimodality imaging of the postoperative shoulder. Eur Radiol 17:3038-3055

Zanetti M, Weishaupt D, Gerber C, Hodler J (1998) Tendinopathy and rupture of the tendon of the long head of the biceps brachii muscle: evaluation with MR arthography. Am J Roentgenol 170:1557-1561

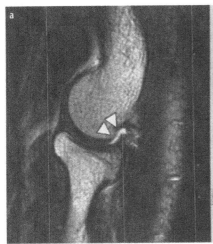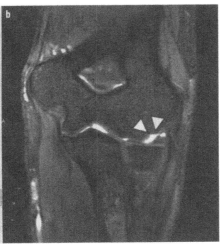

Fig. 3 a, b. Sagittal (**a**) and coronal (**b**) magnetic resonance imaging (MRI) demonstrates the normal appearance of a so-called pseudodefect of the capitellum (*arrowheads*), caused by the contour change at the posterolateral margin of the capitellum

The trochlea is a pulley-like central depression of the distal humerus. The capitellum approximates a sphere superiorly but narrows inferiorly with a distinct contour change where the anteriorly placed capitellum intersects the rough, nonarticular surface of the posterior lateral epicondyle. The imaging appearance of the abrupt contour change at the posterolateral margin of the capitellum has been termed "pseudodefect of the capitellum" [3]. It is visualized on coronal and sagittal images and should not be mistaken for an osteochondral lesion of the capitellum (Fig. 3).

Osteochondral Lesions

Osteochondral lesions of the elbow arise from several abnormal biomechanical forces, including valgus stress, repetitive hyperextension, and posterolateral rotator instability.

Valgus stress is an acute or repetitive valgus force on the elbow, with lateral impaction and shearing of the articular surfaces of the capitellum and radial head [4]. This has been termed "osteochondritis dissecans" and it is common in throwing athletes between the ages of 11 and 15 years (e.g., Little League baseball players) [5]. The same mechanism produces sprains and tears of the ulnar collateral ligament and medial epicondylitis, as described below. Osteochondritis dissecans of the elbow involves primarily the capitellum, but reports have described this process in the radial aspects of the trochlea due to valgus stress, with the latter possibly due to a combination of repetitive hyperextension and hypovascularity in this region [6]. Osteochondritis dissecans remains controversial, primarily due to debate over its etiology.

Another mechanism for osteochondral injury of the capitellum, recently described in two articles in the radiology literature, is that of posterolateral rotary instability (PLRI), which is caused by failure of a component of the radial collateral ligament complex, the lateral ulnar collateral ligament (LUCL) [7, 8]. This osteochondral lesion has been termed the "Osborne-Cotterill" lesion, named for the authors who were the first to describe "an osteochondral fracture in the posterolateral margin of the capitellum with or without a crater or shovel-like defect in the radial head" [9].

Post-traumatic osteochondral lesions such as osteochondritis dissecans and the Osborne Cotterill lesion present on MRI as irregularities of the chondral surface, disruption or irregularity of the subchondral bone plate, and or the presence of a fracture line. The cartilage may demonstrate chondral abnormalities only, in which case the lesion would not be referred to as osteochondral. The acuity of the lesion and a post-traumatic etiology are implied by the presence of marrow-edema-like changes or fracture. The role of imaging is to provide information regarding the integrity of the overlying articular cartilage, the viability of the separated fragment, and the presence of associated intra-articular bodies. Both CT and MRI, with and without arthrography, can provide this information to varying degrees. MRI, with its excellent soft-tissue contrast, allows direct visualization of the articular cartilage and of the character of the the osteochondral lesion interface with native bone (Fig. 4). The presence of joint fluid at this interface, manifested as increased signal intensity on fluid-sensitive MRI, generally indicates an unstable lesion. The introduction of contrast into the articulation in conjunction with MRI can be helpful in two ways: (1) to facilitate the identification of intra-articular bodies, and (2) to establish whether there is communication of the bone-fragment interface with the articulation by following the route of contrast, which would provide even stronger evidence for an unstable fragment [10, 11]. ArthroCT can also be used for this evaluation.

Close inspection of the location of the capitellum on coronal and sagittal MRI is important to distinguish a true osteochondral lesion from the normal surface irreg-

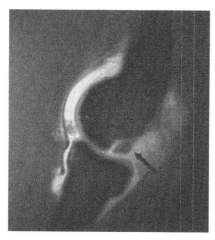

Fig. 4. A sagittal fat-suppressed T1-weighted magnetic resonance arthrogram (MRA) image demonstrates an osteochondral lesion of the posterior capitellum caused by posterolateral rotatory instability associated with lateral ulnar collateral ligament tear (*arrow*). The lesion is unstable, with contrast extending into the interface between the fragment and the parent bone

ularity produced by the above-described pseudodefect of the capitellum. The pseudodefect does not have bone-marrow reactive changes or osteochondral fracture lines. Correlation with presenting clinical history is also helpful in determining the etiology of the imaging findings.

Ligaments

Normal Ligamentous Anatomy

Three components of the medial or ulnar collateral ligaments (UCL) are traditionally described: the anterior, posterior, and transverse bundles. The largest and most important component of the UCL is the anterior bundle, a discrete focal thickening of the medial capsule arising from the inferior margin of the medial epicondyle that inserts at the sublime tubercle of the proximal ulna. The posterior bundle is a thickening of the posterior capsule that lies underneath the ulnar nerve in the cubital tunnel. The transverse bundle appears to contribute little or nothing to elbow stability [1].

The lateral or radial collateral ligaments are less discrete and variations are common. The radial collateral ligament (RCL) complex is most commonly described, consisting of four ligaments: the RCL proper, the lateral ulnar collateral ligament (LUCL), the annular ligament, and the accessory lateral collateral ligament. The RCL attaches proximally to the anteroinferior aspect of the lateral epicondyle and distally to the annular ligament and lies deep to the common extensor tendon. The LUCL attaches proximally to the anteroinferior aspect of the lateral epicondyle and distally to the supinator crest of the ulna (Fig. 6). In anatomic dissections, the humeral at-

tachment of the LUCL has been noted to be indistinguishable from that of the RCL and may be considered the posterior portion of the RCL. Hence, this ligament can be difficult to differentiate from the RCL on coronal oblique images and is reported to be poorly depicted on commonly used, routine coronal oblique sections. The LUCL usually tears near its common attachment with the RCL [12, 13].

Ligament Pathology

Valgus Instability

The principle function of the ulnar collateral ligament complex is to maintain medial joint stability to valgus stress. The anterior bundle is the most important component of the ligamentous complex, acting as the primary medial stabilizer of the elbow from 30° to 120° of flexion. The most common mechanisms of ulnar collateral ligament insufficiency are chronic attenuation, as seen in overhead or throwing athletes, and post-traumatic, usually after a fall on the outstretched arm. In the case of the latter, an acute tear of the ulnar collateral may be encountered. With throwing sports, high valgus stresses are placed on the medial aspect of the elbow. The maximum stress on the ulnar collateral ligament occurs during the late cocking and acceleration phases of throwing [14]. Repetitive insults to the ligament cause microscopic tears that progress to significant attenuation or frank tearing within its substance. Partial tears can be subtle and are well seen with magnetic resonance arthrography (MRA) (Fig. 5) [15, 16]. MRI facilitates direct visualization of the ligament complex. In chronic cases, the development of heterotopic ossification along the course of the ligament has been described [17].

Osseous stress or avulsion of the unfused medial epicondyle in children and adolescents with or without an

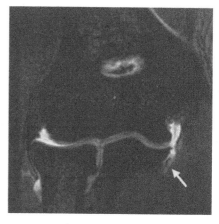

Fig. 5. A coronal fat-suppressed T1-weighted MRA image shows a partial tear of the anterior bundle of the ulnar collateral ligament, with stripping of the ligament from the sublime tubercle, called the "T sign" (*arrow*)

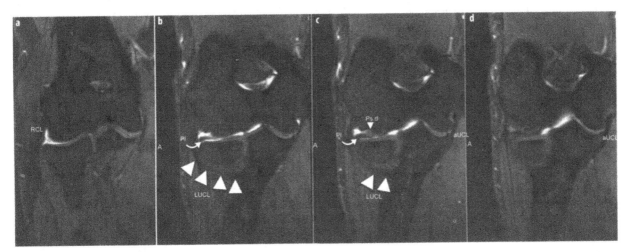

Fig. 6 a-d. Coronal MRI from the anterior to posterior aspect (**a-d**) demonstrates the proper radial collateral ligament (*RCL*) and the lateral ulnar collateral ligament (*LUCL*) (*arrowheads*). A posterolateral plica (*curved arrow*) points to the pseudodefect of the capitellum. *aUCL*, Anterior ulnar collateral ligament; *Pl*, posterolateral plica; *Psd*, pseudodefect of the capitellum

intact ulnar collateral ligament may also occur with valgus stress. Sometimes the epicondyle avulses into the joint and can simulate an osseous body. More often, it remains close to the parent bone, presenting on radiographs and cross-sectional imaging with marrow edema from stress and/or a widened gap between the medial epicondyle and the humerus, which can be subtle. Nonunion can lead to repeated valgus instability. Ultrasound [18], CT, and MRI can show these avulsions. Unlike ultrasound and CT, MRI also shows the marrow and the presence of a synchondrosis edema-like pattern, which is helpful in identifying these varying degrees of stress, even when there is no physical avulsion.

Varus Instability

Lateral elbow instability related to isolated abnormalities of the lateral collateral ligament complex arises from a stress or force applied to the medial side of the articula-tion, resulting in compression on that side, with opening of the lateral articulation and subsequent insufficiency of the radial collateral ligament. Varus stress applied to the elbow may be due to an acute injury, but rarely to repetitive stress, as encountered on the medial side. While lateral collateral ligament injuries seldom occur as the result of an isolated varus stress, other causes can commonly lead to this injury, including dislocation, subluxation, and overly aggressive surgery (release of the common extensor tendon or radial head resection).

Posterolateral Rotary Instability and Elbow Dislocation

The most common pattern of recurrent elbow instability is PLRI. It represents a spectrum of pathology consisting of three stages depending on the degree of soft-tissue disruption. In stage 1, there is posterolateral subluxation of the ulna on the humerus, which results in insufficiency or tearing of the lateral ulnar collateral ligament (Fig. 7) [19-21].

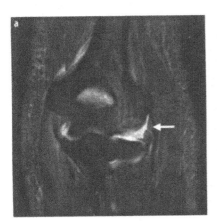 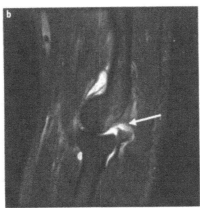

Fig. 7 a, b. Coronal (**a**) and sagittal (**b**) fat suppressed T2-weighted MRI demonstrates a tear of the proximal LUCL (*arrow*). Note the bone-marrow reactive changes in the capitellum related to the injury

In stage 2, the elbow dislocates incompletely so that the coronoid is perched under the trochlea. In this stage, the radial collateral ligament and the anterior and posterior portions of the capsule are disrupted, in addition to the lateral ulnar collateral ligament. Finally, in stage 3, the elbow dislocates fully so that the coronoid rests behind the humerus. Stage 3 is subclassified into three further categories. In stage 3A, the anterior bundle of the medial collateral ligament is intact and the elbow is stable to valgus stress after reduction. In stage 3B, the anterior bundle of the medial collateral ligament is disrupted so that the elbow is unstable with valgus stress. In stage 3C, the entire distal humerus is stripped of soft tissues, rendering the elbow grossly unstable even when a splint or cast is applied with the elbow in a semi-flexed position. This classification system is helpful, as each stage has specific clinical, radiographic, and pathologic features that are predictable and have implications for treatment [20].

Subluxation or dislocation of the elbow can be associated with fractures. Fracture dislocations most commonly involve the coronoid process and radial head, a constellation of findings referred to as the "terrible triad" of the elbow, as the injury complex is difficult to treat and prone to unsatisfactory results [20]. Fractures of the radial head do not cause clinically significant instability unless the medial collateral ligament is disrupted. Shear fracture of the coronoid process of the ulna is commonly seen following elbow dislocations. It is pathognomonic of an episode of elbow subluxation or dislocation and does not represent an avulsion, since no ligaments or tendons attach to the coronoid process. Osteochondral injuries of the articular surfaces may also be seen following elbow subluxation, as described in the section on osteochondral lesions.

Another consideration with respect to elbow dislocation is that, as the ring of soft tissues is disrupted posterolaterally to medially, the capsule is torn and insufficient. Therefore, fluid in the elbow joint can escape through the capsular tear and a joint effusion, which is an indirect sign of elbow trauma on radiographs, may not be present.

Plicae

Plicae are prominent folds of the synovial membrane. Anterior-superior and posterior-superior folds are usually equal or thinner than 2 mm [22]. There is an overlap between the thicknesses of asymptomatic and symptomatic plicae, but it is worth reporting these since a patient with thickened plica can present with elbow locking.

A posterior-lateral plica that extends off the radial collateral ligament is found in between the capitellum and the radial head [23] (Fig. 6). It has also been called lateral synovial fringe or the meniscus of the radiocapitellar joint. Although often asymptomatic, it can cause pain and snapping of the elbow and may produce cartilage damage as well as subchondral reactive marrow changes.

Muscles and Tendons

Normal Anatomy

The muscles and tendons about the elbow may be categorized into four muscle groups. The medial muscle group comprises the pronator teres and the wrist and flexor muscles. A common flexor tendon attaches at the medial epicondyle of the humerus. The lateral muscle group is made up of the wrist and finger extensor as well as the supinator and brachioradialis muscles. These tendons attach to the lateral epicondyle of the humerus [24]. The anterior compartment includes the biceps brachii and brachialis muscles. The distal biceps tendon attaches distally to the radial tuberosity (Fig. 8). It also attaches to the bicipital aponeurosis, which descends medially to insert onto the subcuta-

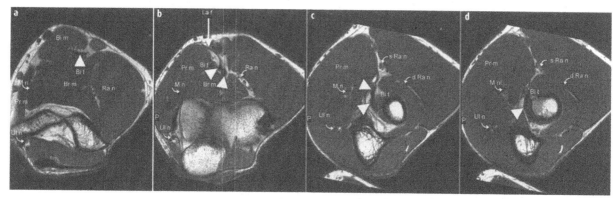

Fig. 8 a-d. Normal muscles, tendons, and nerves around the elbow. Transverse T1-weighted MRI from proximal to distal (**a-d**) demonstrates the distal biceps tendon (*Bi t, arrowheads*), which extends to the radial tuberosity. The lacertus fibrosus (*La f, arrow*) descends medially to insert onto the subcutaneous border of the upper ulna via the deep fascia of the forearm. Note that the biceps tendon may be normally bifurcated, as shown in **b** and **c** (*arrowheads*). The median nerve (*M n*) traverses the elbow deeper between the pronator teres muscle (*Pr m*) and the brachialis muscle (*Br m*). The radial nerve (*Ra n*) divides into a deep posterior interosseous nerve (*d Ra n*), motor branch, and a superficial, sensory branch (*s Ra N*). *Ul n*, Ulnar nerve; *Bi m*, biceps muscle

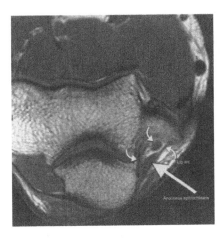

Fig. 9. Transverse T1-weighted MRI demonstrates an anconeus epitrochlearis muscle (*arrows*) that traverses the top of the cubital tunnel. *Post UCL*, Posterior band of the ulnar collateral ligament; *Ul n*, ulnar nerve; *Lig arc*, arcuate ligament

neous border of the upper ulna via the deep fascia of the forearm. It has been shown that the biceps tendon may be bifurcated in up to 25% of all individuals [25]. This anatomic variant arises from persistent division between the short head and the long head of the distal biceps brachii tendon. The posterior muscle compartment consists of the triceps and anconeus muscles. The anconeus muscle sweeps obliquely between the lateral epicondyle and olecranon. Along the posteromedial elbow, an anconeus epitrochlearis muscle – defined as an accessory muscle that traverses the top of the cubital tunnel – is found in 25% of all individuals and it may be associated with entrapment of the ulnar nerve (Fig. 9). However, the high prevalence in the asymptomatic population should be kept in mind when patients with this form of entrapment are evaluated.

Tendon and Muscle Pathology

The vast majority of pathologies encountered in the flexor and extensor groups will be isolated to the common flexor and common extensor tendons. The classification of tendon injuries about the elbow can be organized by location, acuity, and degree of injury. Tendon injury related to a single isolated event is uncommon, although exceptions do occur. More commonly, tendinous injuries in this location relate to chronic repetitive microtrauma. MRI and ultrasound are particularly well-suited to diagnose tendon pathology.

As is the case elsewhere in the body, the tendons about the elbow should be smooth linear structures of low signal intensity on MRI [26]. Abnormal morphology (attenuation or thickening) can be seen in tendinosis (also termed tendinopathy) or tear. If signal intensity becomes increased within the substance of a tendon on fluid-sensitive sequences, a tear is present. Tears can be further characterized as partial or complete. A complete tear is diagnosed by a focal area of discontinuity.

Epicondylitis and Overuse Syndromes

Chronic stress applied to the elbow is the most frequent injury in athletes, corresponding to a spectrum of pathologies with varying degrees of severity. The frequency of involvement of the common flexor and extensor tendons to the medial and lateral epicondyles, respectively, has led to the designation "epicondylitis". Anatomically, they are classified by location and are further associated with sports that incite the pathology. The injury is believed to result from extrinsic tensile overload of the tendon, which, over time, produces microscopic tears that do not heal appropriately. Although these overuse entities about the elbow are collectively referred to as "epicondylitis" for the purpose of clinical diagnosis, inflammatory osseous changes rarely occur. The imaging findings are those reflecting chronic change in the tendon, as evidenced by tendinosis alone or in conjunction with partial or complete tear. As previously mentioned, the exact pathology is determined by consideration of both morphology and the signal intensity changes on MRI. Ultrasound is also useful for evaluating epicondyliits, including as a screening tool; however, in patients with normal ultrasound, MRI can be more sensitive for discovering pathology in the symptomatic elbow [27].

Lateral epicondylitis, the most common problem in the elbow in athletes, is well-known as "tennis elbow". However, this term may be somewhat inappropriate, since 95% of the cases of lateral epicondylitis occur in people who do not play tennis [28]. Moreover, it has been estimated that 50% of people partaking in any sport in which there is overhead arm motion will develop this process [29]. It is associated with repetitive and excessive use of the wrist extensors. The pathology most commonly affects the extensor carpi radialis brevis at the common extensor tendon. A number of investigators have studied the pathology encountered in the degenerated tendon of this disease process. Histologically, necrosis, round-cell infiltration, focal calcification, and scar formation have been described [30]. There is also invasion of blood vessels, fibroblastic proliferation, and lymphatic infiltration, the combination of which is referred to as angiofibroblastic hyperplasia. As this process continues, it ultimately leads to mucoid degeneration [31, 32]. The absence of a significant inflammatory response has been emphasized repeatedly and may explain the inadequacy of the healing process.

The imaging findings of epicondylitis can include tendinosis either alone or with superimposed partial- or full-thickness tear. Intermediate to high T2 signal intensity and paratendinous soft-tissue edema-like changes are very specific for medial epicondylitis on MRI [33] (Fig. 10). Close scrutiny of the underlying ligamentous complex is necessary to exclude concomitant injury. In particular, thickening and tears of the lateral ulnar collateral ligament have been encountered with lateral epicondylitis [34]. Ultrasound has been shown to be of high sensitivity but low specificity in the detection of symptomatic lateral epicondylitis [35, 36]. In medial epicondylitis, the pathology involves the

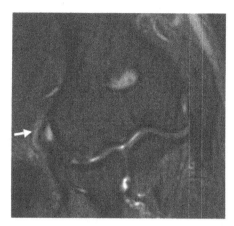

Fig. 10. Lateral epicondylitis. A partial tear of focal high signal intensity (*arrow*) is seen in the extensor carpi radialis brevis tendon on coronal fat-suppressed T2-weighted MRI

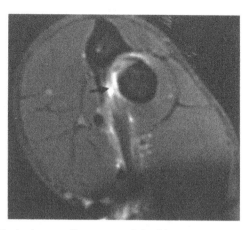

Fig. 11. An intra-tendinous tear of the biceps (*arrow*) is nicely demonstrated on this FABS axial fat-suppressed T2-weighted image of the elbow

common flexor tendon and the condition is associated primarily with golfing, pitching, and tennis. It has also been reported with javelin throwers, racquetball and squash players, swimmers, and bowlers. The pronator teres and flexor carpi radialis tendons are most frequently affected, resulting in pain and tenderness to palpation over the anterior aspect of the medial epicondyle of the humerus and origin of the common flexor tendon. The mechanism of injury includes repetitive valgus strain with pain resulting from resistance to pronation of the forearm or flexion of the wrist. The imaging findings in this process are exactly those encountered in the clinical entity of medial epicondylitis. As on the lateral side, when assessing the tendon, it is necessary to closely scrutinize the underlying collateral ligament complex to ensure integrity.

Biceps Tendon

Rupture of the tendon of the biceps brachii muscle at the elbow is rare and constitutes less than 5% of all biceps tendon injuries [37]. It usually occurs in the dominant arm of males. Injuries to the musculotendinous junction have been reported, but the most common injury is complete avulsion of the tendon from the radial tuberosity. Although the injury often occurs acutely, after a single traumatic event, the failure is thought to be due to pre-existing changes in the distal biceps tendon due to intrinsic tendon degeneration, enthesopathy at the radial tuberosity, or cubital bursal changes. The typical mechanism of injury relates to forceful hyperextension applied to a flexed and supinated forearm. Athletes involved in strength sports, such as competitive weightlifting, football and rugby, often sustain this injury. Clinically, the patient describes a history feeling a "pop" or sudden sharp pain in the antecubital fossa. The classic presentation of a complete distal biceps rupture is that of a mass in the antecubital fossa due to proximal migration of the biceps muscle belly. Accurate diagnosis is more difficult in cases of the rare partial tear of the tendon

or the more common complete tear of the tendon without retraction. The latter can occur with an intact bicipital aponeurosis, which serves to tether the ruptured tendon to the pronator flexor muscle group. A flexed abducted supinated or FABS (flexed elbow, abducted shoulder, forearm supinated) positioning of the elbow for MRI can aid in evaluation of subtle tears of the distal biceps [38].

Ultrasound and MRI diagnosis of biceps tendon pathologies becomes important in patients who do not present with the classic history or mass in the antecubital fossa and in evaluations of the integrity of the lacertus fibrosus [39, 40]. MRI diagnosis of tendon pathology, as previously mentioned, is largely dependent on morphology, signal intensity and the identification of areas of tendon discontinuity (Fig. 11). In the case of the biceps tendon, an important indirect sign of tendon pathology is the presence of cubital bursitis.

Triceps Tendon

Rupture of the triceps tendon is quite rare. The mechanism of injury has been reported to result from a direct blow to the triceps insertion, or a deceleration force applied to the extended arm with contraction of the triceps, as in a fall. Similar to the pathology encountered in the distal biceps tendon, most ruptures occur at the insertion site, although injuries to the musculotendinous junction and muscle belly have been reported. Complete ruptures are more common than partial tears. Associated findings may include olecranon bursitis, subluxation of the ulnar nerve, and fracture of the radial head. Accurate clinical diagnosis relies on the presence of local pain, swelling, ecchymosis, a palpable defect, and partial or complete loss of the ability to extend the elbow. With more than 2 cm of retraction between the origin and the insertion, a 40% loss of extension strength can result [37].

For MRI diagnosis of triceps tendon pathology, it is imperative to be aware that the appearance of the triceps tendon is largely dependent on arm position. The tendon is lax and redundant when imaged in full extension but taut in flexion. The MRI features of a tear are similar to those associated with any other tendon [26].

Bursae

There are several bursae around the elbow: the superficial olecranon bursa lies between the olecranon and subcutaneous tissues; the bicipito-radial bursa reduces the friction between biceps tendon and the tuberosity of the radius; on the medial side of the distal biceps tendon, an interosseous bursa can form (Fig. 12). En-

largement of the bicipitoradial or interosseous bursae should be recognized as structures distinct from a ganglion cyst [41]. Since the biceps does not have a tendon sheath, there is no such thing as tenosynovitis of the distal biceps.

Nerves

Three major nerves traverse the elbow joint: the ulnar, median, and radial nerves. The ulnar nerve traverses the cubital tunnel bounded by the medial humeral epicondyle, the trochlea, the posterior ulnar collateral ligament, and the arcuate ligament (Fig. 8). The nerve is accompanied in the cubital tunnel by recurrent ulnar vessels (Fig. 13). Increased signal intensity on MRI from these vessels should not be considered a neuropathy (Fig. 14). Increased signal intensity on fat-suppressed fluid-sensitive MRI is commonly (60%) seen within the ulnar nerve in asymptomatic volunteers [42].

In 80% of people, the median nerve courses between the pronator teres muscle and the brachialis muscle close to the brachial or ulnar artery. In the other 20%, the median nerve traverses the elbow deeper between the pronator teres muscle and the brachialis muscle without contacting the brachial artery or the more distal ulnar artery [42] (Fig. 9).

The radial nerve lies anteriorly between the brachialis and the brachioradialis at the level of the distal ulna and divides into a motor, deep branch, called the posterior interosseous nerve, and a superficial, sensory branch (Fig. 9). In up to 35% of individuals, the posterior interosseous nerve traverses a fibrous arch called the arcade of Frohse, where it pierces the supinator muscle [43].

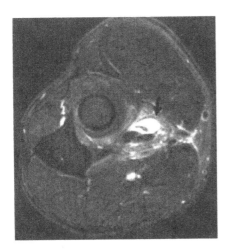

Fig. 12. An inflamed bicipitoradial bursa (*arrow*) lies lateral to the distal biceps tendon, with reactive edema-like changes around it, as seen on axial fat-suppressed T2-weighted image of the elbow obtained distal to the proximal radioulnar joint

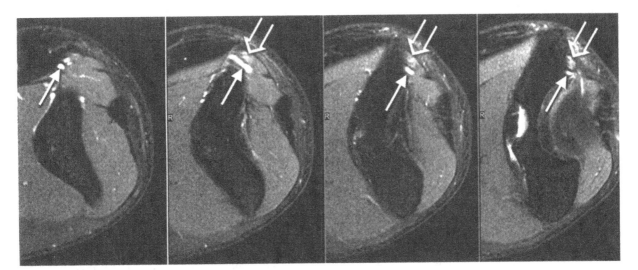

Fig. 13. Transverse intermediate-weighted fat-suppressed MRI demonstrates the ulnar nerve (*open arrow*), which is accompanied by recurrent ulnar vessels (*arrows*). This should not be interpreted as neuritis

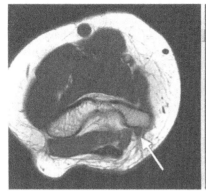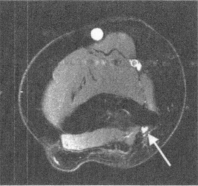

Fig. 14. Increased signal on fat-suppressed fluid-sensitive MRI is commonly (60%) seen within the ulnar nerve (*arrow*) in asymptomatic volunteers. *Left* Transverse T1-weighted and *right* transverse intermediate-weighted magnetic resonance images

Entrapment Neuropathy

The ulnar, median, and radial nerves may become compressed at the elbow, leading to symptoms of entrapment neuropathy. Abnormal nerves may have increased signal intensity on T2-weighted images, focal changes in girth, and deviation that may result from subluxation or displacement by an adjacent mass [44].

Ulnar nerve entrapment most commonly occurs in the cubital tunnel. Nerve compression may be caused by a medial trochlear osteophyte or incongruity between the trochlea and olecranon process [45]. Anatomic variations also play a role. The absence of the triangular retinaculum, the anatomic roof of the cubital tunnel, occurs in about 10% of the population; in this variant, there may be subluxation of the nerve with flexion. It is therefore necessary to include axial images of the flexed elbow in patients in whom ulnar nerve entrapment is suspected. The presence of the anomalous anconeous epitrochlearis muscle over the cubital tunnel causes static compression of the ulnar nerve (Fig. 10). In addition, there are many other causes of ulnar neuritis, including thickening of the overlying ulnar collateral ligament, medial epicondylitis, adhesions, muscle hypertrophy, direct trauma, and callus from a fracture of the medial epicondyle. The snapping medial head of the triceps muscle may also produce displacement and compression of the ulnar nerve, shown best with elbow flexion [46]. MRI can be used to identify these abnormalities and to assess the ulnar nerve itself. When compressed, the nerve may become enlarged and edematous. If conservative treatment fails, the nerve can be transposed anteriorly, deep to the flexor muscle group, or more superficially, in the subcutaneous tissue. These patients can be followed with MRI postoperatively if they become symptomatic to determine whether symptoms are secondary to scarring or infection around the area of nerve transposition.

Compression of the median nerve may be seen with osseous or muscular variants and anomalies, soft-tissue masses, and dynamic forces. In the pronator syndrome, compression occurs as the median nerve passes between the two heads of the pronator teres and under the fibrous arch of the flexor digitorum profundus.

The radial nerve can become entrapped following direct trauma, mechanical compression by a cast or overlying space-occupying mass, or a dynamic compression as a result of repeated pronation, forearm extension, and wrist flexion, as is seen in violinists and swimmers. Motor neuropathy of the hand extensors is a dominant feature when the posterior interosseous nerve is entrapped [47].

References

1. Morrey BF (1993) The elbow and its disorders. WB Saunders, Philadelphia
2. Rosenberg ZS, Beltran J, Cheung Y, Broker M (1995) MR imaging of the elbow: Normal variant and potential diagnostic pitfalls of the trochlear groove and cubital tunnel. AJR 164:415
3. Rosenberg ZS, Beltran J, Cheung YY (1994) Pseudodefect of the capitellum: Potential MR imaging pitfall. Radiology 191:821
4. Pincivero DM, Heinrichs K, Perrin DH (1994) Medial elbow stability. Clinical implications. Sports Med 18:141-148
5. Bradley JP, Petrie RS (2001) Osteochondritis dissecans of the humeral capitellum. Diagnosis and treatment. Clin Sports Med 20:565-590
6. Patel N, Weiner SD (2002) Osteochondritis dissecans involving the trochlea: report of two patients (three elbows) and review of the literature. J Pediatr Orthop 22:48-51
7. Jeon IH, Micic ID, Yamamoto N, Morrey BF (2008) Osborne-Cotterill lesion: an osseous defect of the capitellum associated with instability of the elbow. AJR Am J Roentgenol 191:727-729
8. Rosenberg ZS, Blutreich SI, Schweitzer ME et al (2008) MRI features of posterior capitellar impaction injuries. AJR Am J Roentgenol 190:435-441
9. Osborne G, Cotterill P (1966) Recurrent dislocation of the elbow. J Bone Joint Surg Br 48:340-346
10. Carrino JA, Smith DK, Schweitzer ME (1998) MR arthrography of the elbow and wrist. Semin Musculoskelet Radiol 2:397-414
11. Steinbach LS, Palmer WE, Schweitzer ME (2002) Special focus session. MR arthrography. Radiographics 22:1223-1246
12. Carrino JA, Morrison WB, Zou KH et al (2001) Lateral ulnar collateral ligament of the elbow: optimization of evaluation with two-dimensional MR imaging. Radiology 218:118-125
13. Cotten A, Jacobsen J, Brossman J et al (1997) Collateral ligaments of the elbow: conventional MR imaging and MR arthrography with coronal oblique plane and elbow flexion. Radiology 204:806-812

14. Phillips CS, Segalman KA (2002) Diagnosis and treatment of post-traumatic medial and lateral elbow ligament incompetence. Hand Clin 18:149-159

15. Schwartz ML, Al-Zahrani S, Morwessel RM, Andrews JR (1995) Ulnar collateral ligament injury in the throwing athlete: evaluation with saline-enhanced MR arthrography. Radiology 197:297

16. Steinbach LS, Schwartz M (1998) Elbow arthrography. Radiol Clin North Am 36:635-649

17. Mulligan SA, Schwartz ML, Broussard MF, Andrews JR (2000) Heterotopic calcification and tears of the ulnar collateral ligament: radiographic and MR imaging findings. AJR Am J Roentgenol 175:1099-1102

18. May DA, Disler DG, Jones EA, Pearce DA (2000) Using sonography to diagnose an unossified medial epicondyle avulsion in a child. AJR Am J Roentgenol 174:1115-1117

19. Dunning CE, Zarzour ZD, Patterson SD et al (2001) Ligamentous stabilizers against posterolateral rotatory instability of the elbow. J Bone Joint Surg Am 83-A:1823-1828

20. Potter HG, Weiland AJ, Schatz JA et al (1997) Posterolateral rotatory instability of the elbow: Usefulness of MR imaging in diagnosis. Radiology 204:185-189

21. O'Driscoll SW, Bell DF, Morrey BF (1991) Posterolateral rotatory instability of the elbow. J Bone Joint Surg 73-A:440-446

22. Awaya H, Schweitzer ME, Feng SA et al (2001) Elbow synovial fold syndrome: MR imaging findings. AJR Am J Roentgenol 177: 377-1381

23. Huang GS, Lee CH, Lee HS, Chen CY (2005) A meniscus causing painful snapping of the elbow joint: MR imaging with arthroscopic and histologic correlation. Eur Radiol 15:2411-2414

24. Ho CP (1997) MR imaging of tendon injuries in the elbow. Magn Reson Imaging Clin N Am 5:529-543

25. Dirim B, Brouha SS, Pretterklieber ML et al (2008) Terminal bifurcation of the biceps brachii muscle and tendon: anatomic considerations and clinical implications. AJR Am J Roentgenol 191:W248-255

26. Chung CB, Chew FS, Steinbach L (2004) MR imaging of tendon abnormalities of the elbow. Magn Reson Imaging Clin N Am 12:233-245, vi

27. Miller TT, Shapiro MA, Schultz E, Kalish PE (2002) Comparison of sonography and MRI for diagnosing epicondylitis. J Clin Ultrasound 30:193-202

28. Frostick SP, Mohammad M, Ritchie DA (1999) Sport injuries of the elbow. Br J Sports Med 33:301-311

29. Field LD, Savoie FH (1998) Common elbow injuries in sport. Sports Med26:193-205

30. Nirschl RP, Pettrone FA (1979) Tennis elbow. The surgical treatment of lateral epicondylitis. J Bone Joint Surg Am 61:832-839

31. Nirschl RP (1992) Elbow tendinosis/tennis elbow. Clin Sports Med 11:851-870

32. Regan W, Wold LE, Coonrad R, Morrey BF (1992) Microscopic histopathology of chronic refractory lateral epicondylitis. Am J Sports Med 20:746-749

33. Kijowski R, De Smet AA (2005) Magnetic resonance imaging findings in patients with medial epicondylitis. Skeletal Radiol 34:196-202

34. Bredella MA, Tirman PFJ, Fritz RC et al (1999) MR imaging findings of lateral ulnar collateral ligament abnormalities in patients with lateral epicondylitis. AJR Am J Roentgenol 173:1379-1382

35. Levin D, Nazarian LN, Miller TT et al (2005) Lateral epicondylitis of the elbow: US findings. Radiology 237:230-234

36. Struijs PA, Spruyt M, Assendelft WJ, van Dijk CN (2005) The predictive value of diagnostic sonography for the effectiveness of conservative treatment of tennis elbow. AJR Am J Roentgenol 185:1113-1118

37. Rettig AC (2002) Traumatic elbow injuries in the athlete. Orthop Clin North Am 33:509-522, v

38. Giuffre BM, Moss MJ (2004) Optimal positioning for MRI of the distal biceps brachii tendon: flexed abducted supinated view. AJR Am J Roentgenol 182:944-946

39. Williams BD, Schweitzer ME, Weishaupt D et al (2001) Partial tears of the distal biceps tendon: MR appearance and associated clinical findings. Skeletal Radiol 30:560-564

40. Miller TT, Adler RS (2000) Sonography of tears of the distal biceps tendon. AJR Am J Roentgenol 175:1081-1086

41. Skaf AY, Boutin RD, Weiber R et al (1999) Bicipitoradial bursitis: MR imaging findings in eight patients and anatomic data from contrast material opacification of bursae followed by routine radiography and MR imaging in cadavers. Radiology 212:111-116

42. Husarik DB, Saupe N, Pfirrmann CW et al (2009) Normal anatomy, variants and pitfalls of elbow nerve: MR findings in 60 asymptomatic volunteers. Radiology (in press)

43. Rosenberg ZS, Bencardino J, Beltran J (1997)MR features of nerve disorders at the elbow. Magn Reson Imaging Clin N Am 5:545-565

44. Bencardino JT, Rosenberg ZS (2006) Entrapment neuropathies of the shoulder and elbow in the athlete. Clin Sports Med 25:465-487, vi-vii

45. Kim YS, Yeh LR, Trudell D, Resnick D (1998) MR imaging of the major nerves about the elbow: cadaveric study examining the effect of flexion and extension of the elbow and pronation and supination of the forearm. Skeletal Radiol 27:419-426

46. Spinner RJ, Goldner RD (1998) Snapping of the medial head of the triceps and recurrent dislocation of the ulnar nerve. J Bone Joint Surg 80A:239-247

47. Yanagisawa H, Okada K, Sashi R (2001) Posterior interosseous nerve palsy caused by synovial chondromatosis of the elbow joint. Clin Radiol 56:510-514

Wrist and Hand

Louis A. Gilula

Radiology, Orthopaedic Surgery and Plastic and Reconstructive Surgery, Washington University School of Medicine, Mallinckrodt Institute of Radiology, St. Louis, MO, USA

Analysis of the Musculoskeletal System

As described by Forrester [1], the musculoskeletal system anywhere in the body can be divided into the A, B, C, D' S, starting with S. "S" stands for soft tissues, "B" is bone mineralization, "C" is cortex, cartilage, and joint-space abnormalities, and "D" is distribution of abnormalities. The application of these principles will help keep one from missing major observations. Starting with "S", the recognition of soft-tissue abnormalities will point to an area of major abnormality and should alert one to look a second or third time at the center of the area of soft-tissue swelling to see if there is an underlying abnormality. The soft tissues dorsally over the carpal bones are normally concave. When the soft tissues over the dorsum of the wrist are straight or convex, swelling is suspect. The pronator fat line lying volar to the distal radius may indicate deep swelling. Normally it should be straight or concave [2], but when it is convex outward then deep swelling should be suspect. Soft-tissue swelling along the radial and ulnar styloids may be seen with synovitis or trauma. Swelling along the radial or ulnar side of a finger joint should arouse suspicion of collateral ligament injury. Exceptions to this statement are found along the radial side of the index finger and the ulnar side of the small finger. Focal swelling circumferentially around one interphalangeal or metacarpophalangeal joint is highly suspect for capsular swelling or joint swelling. Another cause for diffuse swelling along one side of the wrist or finger can be tenosynovitis.

"A" stands for alignment. Evaluation of alignment will reveal potential deviations from normal. Angular deformities are commonly seen with arthritis. Dislocations and carpal instabilities can be recognized with abnormalities in alignment.

"B" stands for bone mineralization, of which there are several types. Acute bone demineralization can be recognized as subcortical bone loss in the metaphyseal areas and ends of bones, in areas of increased vascularity of bones. This is typified by the young person who has an injured part of the body placed in a cast, with development of rapid bone demineralization. Diffuse even demineralization is that which commonly develops over longer periods of time and may be seen in older people with diffuse osteopenia of age; it also results from prolonged disuse. Focal osteopenia, especially associated with cortical loss, raises the question of infection or a more acute inflammatory process in the area of local bone demineralization.

Representing cartilage space and cortex, "C" is a reminder to examine all of the joint spaces as well as the margins of these joints and bones for cartilage space narrowing, erosions, and other cortical abnormalities.

"D" refers to the distribution of abnormalities. This is most vividly exemplified by the distribution of erosions as classically may be seen distally in psoriasis and more proximally in rheumatoid arthritis.

Three major concepts in the wrist relate to alignment and are especially applicable to the carpal bones. In addition, the first two of these concepts are relevant throughout the body. These three concepts are "parallelism," "overlapping articular surfaces," and "three carpal arcs" [3-5]. Any anatomic structure that normally articulates with an adjacent anatomic structure should show parallelism between the articular cortices of those adjacent bones. This relates to exactly how jigsaw puzzles work. If there is a piece of a jigsaw puzzle out of place, you could see that piece losing its parallelism to adjacent pieces, thus giving rise to overlapping articular surfaces. Therefore the concept of parallelism and overlapping articular surfaces are related. Overlapping of normally articulating surfaces will result in dislocation or subluxation at the site of those overlapping surfaces. This does not apply if one bone is foreshortened or bent, as with overlapping phalanges on a posteroanterior (PA) view of a flexed finger. In that situation, one phalanx would overlap the adjacent phalanx, but in the flexed PA position one would not normally see parallel articular surfaces at that joint.

The last concept is that of three normal carpal arcs. Three carpal arcs can be drawn in any normal wrist, when the wrist and hand are in neutral position, i.e., when the third metacarpal and the radius are coaxial. Arc I is a smooth curve along the proximal convex surfaces of the scaphoid, lunate, and triquetrum. Arc II is a smooth arc drawn along the distal concave surfaces of these same three carpal bones. Arc III is a smooth arc that is drawn along the proximal convex surfaces of the capitate and hamate [3, 6]. When one of these arcs is broken at a joint or at a bone surface, then there should be something wrong with that joint, such as disruption of the ligaments, or when affecting a bone, a fracture. There are two normal exceptions to the descriptions of these arcs: In arc I, the proximal-distal dimension of the triquetrum along its radial surface may be shorter than the apposing portion of the lunate. In that situation, a broken arc I at the lunotriquetral joint is a congenital variation. Another congenital variation is the articulation of a prominent articular surface of the lunate with the hamate, i.e., a type II lunate. (In a type I lunate, there is one distal, smooth, concave surface. A type II lunate has one concave articular surface that articulates with the capitate and a second concavity, the hamate facet of the lunate that articulates with the proximal pole of the hamate). In this case, arc II may be broken at the distal surface of the lunate where there is a normal concavity at the lunate hamate joint. Similarly, in a wrist with a type II lunate, there can be a slight jog of arc III at the joint between the capitate and hamate; however, the overall outer curvatures of the capitate and hamate are still smooth. At the proximal margins of the scapholunate and lunotriquetral joints, these joints may be wider due to curvature of the respective bones. Thus, the outer curvature of these carpal bones should be examined in analyses of the carpal arcs. Also, for analysis of the scapholunate joint space width, the middle of the joint, between parallel surfaces of the scaphoid and lunate, should be evaluated for scapholunate space widening compared to a normal capitolunate joint width in that same wrist.

Analysis of the hand and wrist can be performed very promptly after an initial survey of the soft tissues by looking at the overall alignment, bone mineralization, and cortical detail as one examines the radiocarpal joints, intercarpal joints of the proximal carpal row, midcarpal joint, intercarpal joints of the distal carpal row, carpometacarpal joints, and interphalangeal joints. A thorough analysis of these surfaces and bones on all views leads to a diagnosis. It is preferable to carefully analyze the PA view of the wrist first, as this view will provide most information. The lateral and oblique views are merely used for confirmation and clarification of what is present on the PA view. An exception to this comment is the need to closely evaluate the soft tissues on the lateral and PA views. In the following sections, these principles will be applied to more specific abnormalities.

Trauma

Traumatic conditions of the wrist basically can be classified as fractures, fracture-dislocations, and soft-tissue abnormalities, including ligament instabilities. Analysis of the carpal arcs, overlapping articular surfaces, and parallelism will help determine the exact traumatic abnormality. Recognizing which bones normally parallel each

other also identifies those that have moved together as a unit away from a bone that has overlapping adjacent surfaces. A majority of the fractures and dislocations about the wrist are of the perilunate type, in which there is a dislocation with or without adjacent fractures around the lunate. The additional bones that may be fractured are named first, with the type of dislocation mentioned last. For the perilunate type of dislocations, the bone (the capitate or lunate) that centers over the radius is considered to be "in place." Therefore, if the lunate is centered over the radius, with other bones dislocated from the lunate, this would be a perilunate dislocation. If the capitate is centered over the radius and the lunate is not, this would be a lunate dislocation. A fracture of the scaphoid and capitate, with dorsal displacement of the carpus relative to the lunate and the lunate still articulating or centered over the radius, is a transscaphoid transcapitate dorsal perilunate dislocation. Another group of fracture-dislocations that occur in the wrist are the axial fracture-dislocations, in which a severe crush injury may split the wrist along an axis around a carpal bone other than the lunate, such as occurs in perihamate or peritrapezial axial dislocation, usually with fractures [7].

Ligamentous Instability

There are many types of ligament instabilities, including very subtle types; however, there are five major types of ligament instabilities that can be recognized readily based on plain radiographs. These refer to the lunate as an "intercalated segment" between the distal carpal row and the radius, similar to the middle or intercalated segment between two links in a three-link chain. On lateral view, there is normally a small amount of angulation between the capitate, lunate, and the radius. However, with increasing lunate angulation, especially as seen on lateral view, an instability pattern may be present. If the lunate tilts too far dorsally, it is called a dorsal intercalated segmental condition. If the lunate tilts too far volarly, then it is called a volar or palmar intercalated segmental condition. If the lunate is tilted too far dorsally (capitolunate angle >30° and/or a scapholunate angle >60-80°), then there is a dorsal intercalated segmental instability (DISI) pattern. Likewise, if the lunate is tilted too far volarly or palmarly (capitolunate angle >30° or a scapholunate angle <30°), this is a volar intercalated segmental instability (VISI) or palmar intercalated segmental instability (PISI) pattern. When there is a "pattern" of instability, a true instability can be further evaluated and identified with a dynamic wrist instability series, performed under fluoroscopic control [8, 9]. When there is abnormal intercarpal motion in addition to abnormal alignment, this supports the radiographic diagnosis of carpal instability. Based on a comparison with the opposite wrist, the questionable wrist can be evaluated for instability, with lateral flexion, extension, and neutral views, as well as PA and AP views, with radial, neutral, and ulnar deviation views.

Fist compression views with the patient in supine position may help widen the scapholunate joint in some patients. Ulnar carpal translation is a third type of carpal instability [8]. In an ulnar carpal translation type I, the entire carpus moves too far ulnarly, as recognized by more than one-half of the lunate positioned ulnar to the radius when the wrist and hand are in neutral position. In an ulnar carpal translation type II, the scaphoid is in normal position relative to the radial styloid, but there is scapholunate dissociation and the remainder of the carpus moves too far ulnarly, as mentioned for ulnar carpal translation type I. The fourth and fifth types of carpal instabilities relate to the carpus displacing dorsally and volarly off the radius. In a dorsal radiocarpal instability, or dorsal carpal subluxation, the carpus, as identified by the lunate, has lost its normal articulation with the radius in the lateral view and is displaced dorsally off the radius. This pattern occurs most commonly following a severe dorsally impacted distal radius fracture. In a palmar carpal subluxation, the carpal bones are normally related to the lunate and the lunate is displaced palmarly with respect to the radius. Carpal instability patterns that are detected more often by physical exam and are not usually demonstrated by radiography are not covered here.

Infection

Infection should be suspected when there is an area of cortical destruction accompanied by pronounced osteopenia. It is not uncommon to have patients present with pain and swelling. In such cases, clinically infection may be an unsuspected diagnosis when this condition is chronic, as with an indolent type of infection as tuberculosis. Soft-tissue swelling is a key point for this diagnosis as for other abnormalities of the wrist, as mentioned above. Therefore the diagnosis of infection should be considered when there is swelling, associated osteopenia, and cortical destruction or even when there is early focal joint-space loss without cortical destruction.

Neoplasia

When there is an area of abnormality, it helps to determine the gross area of involvement and then look at the center of the abnormality. If the center of abnormality is in bone, then the lesion probably originated within the bone. When the center of abnormality is in the soft tissues, a soft-tissue origin for the lesion is likely. When there is a focal area of bone loss or destruction or even a focal area of soft-tissue swelling with or without osteopenia, neoplasia is a major consideration. Whenever neoplasia is a concern on an imaging study, infection should also be considered. To analyze a lesion within a bone, the margins of the lesion should be examined to determine whether it is well-defined and if it has a thin to thick sclerotic rim. Evaluation of the endosteal surface

will reveal whether there is scalloping or concavities along the endosteal surface of the bone. Endosteal concavities representing endosteal scalloping are characteristic of cartilage tissue. Such concavities would be typical for the most common intraosseous bone lesion of hand tubular bones, an enchondroma. The matrix of the lesion should also be examined for dots of calcium, which can be seen in cartilage, or if there is a more diffuse type of bone formation, such as occurs in an osseous type of tumor, as from osteosarcoma. Analogous to elsewhere in the body, if a lesion is very well-defined and there is bone enlargement, an indolent or a less aggressive type of lesion is likely. The presence of cortical destruction supports the diagnosis of an aggressive lesion, such as malignancy or infection. To determine the extent of a lesion, magnetic resonance imaging (MRI) is the preferred imaging modality. Bone scintigraphy can be very valuable to survey for osseous lesions throughout the body, since many neoplastic conditions spread to other bones or even to the lung [10].

A soft-tissue mass lesion of the hand, especially with pressure effect on an adjacent bone, suggests giant cell tumor of tendon sheath. Ganglion is another cause for a focal swelling in the hand, but it usually occurs without underlying bone deformity. Glomus tumor is a less common, painful soft-tissue lesion that may be detected with ultrasound or MRI. Occasionally a glomus tumor causes a pressure effect on bone, especially the distal phalanx under the nail bed [10].

Arthritis

The above scheme to analyze the hand, wrist, and musculoskeletal system can be used to assess swelling, which may indicate capsular involvement and synovitis. Overall evaluation of alignment shows deviation of the fingers at the interphalangeal and metacarpophalangeal joints as well as subluxation or dislocation at the interphalangeal, metacarpophalangeal, or intercarpal or radiocarpal joints. Joint-space loss, the site of erosions, and the sites of bone production are important to recognize. By identifying the abnormalities, being certain to look carefully at the metacarpophalangeal joint capsules, especially of the index, long, and small fingers, to determine whether they are convex, indicative of capsular swelling, may indicate whether the injury is primarily a synovial arthritis, which in some cases is present in combination with osteoarthritis. Synovial arthritis is suspected when there are findings of bony destruction from erosive disease. The most common entities to consider for synovial-based arthritis are rheumatoid arthritis, then psoriasis. With osteophyte production, osteoarthritis is the most common consideration [11]. However, osteoarthritis associated with erosive disease, especially in the distal interphalangeal joints, is supportive of erosive osteoarthritis. Punched-out or well-defined lucent lesions of bone, especially about the carpometacarpal joints in well-mineralized bones, must also be considered for the robust type of rheumatoid arthritis. Among the deposition types of disease, gout is a classic example. Gout is usually associated with normal bone mineralization and punched-out lesions of bone. Gouty destruction is related to the deposition of gouty tophi, whether they are intraosseous, subperiosteal, adjacent to and outside of the periosteum, or intra-articular [11].

Metabolic Bone Disease

A classic condition of metabolic bone disease in the hands is that seen with renal osteodystrophy. Metabolic bone disease is considered when there are multiple sites of bone abnormality throughout the body, with or without diffuse osteopenia. However, some manifestations of metabolic bone disease may start or be more manifest in the hands, feet, or elsewhere in the body. One would be very suspicious of renal osteodystrophy when there is subperiosteal resorption, typically along the radial aspect of the bases of the proximal or middle phalanges, but there also may be cortical loss along the tufts of the distal phalanges. Bone resorption can also take place intra-cortically and endosteally. Again, analysis of the bones involved and associated abnormalities present can help lead to the most likely diagnosis.

Conclusions

Utilization of the above principles of the A, B, C, D's, parallelism, abnormal overlapping articular surfaces, and carpal arcs can help the clinician analyze the abnormali-ties encountered in the hand and wrist, thus allowing a most reasonable diagnosis for further evaluation of the patient.

References

1. Forrester DM, Nesson JW (1973) The ABC's of arthritis (introduction). In: Forrester DM, Nesson JW (eds) The radiology of joint disease. WB Saunders, Philadelphia, p 3
2. Curtis DJ, Downey EF Jr (1992) Soft tissue evaluation in trauma. In: Gilula LA (ed) The traumatized hand and wrist. Radiographic and anatomy correlation. WB Saunders, Philadelphia, pp 45-63
3. Gilula LA (1979) Carpal injuries: analytic approach and case exercise. AJR Am J Roentgeonol 133:503-517
4. Yin Y, Mann FA, Gilula LA, Hodge JC (1996) Roentgenographic approach to complex bone abnormalities. In: Gilula LA, Yin Y (eds) Imaging of the wrist and hand. WB Saunders, Philadelphia, pp 293-318
5. Gilula LA, Totty WG (1992) Wrist trauma: roentgenographic analysis. In: Gilula LA (ed) The traumatized hand and wrist. Radiographic and anatomy correlation. WB Saunders, Philadelphia, pp 221-239
6. Peh WCG, Gilula LA (1996) Normal disruption of carpal arcs. J Hand Surg (Am) 21:561-566
7. Garcia-Elias M, Dobyns JH, Cooney WP, Linscheid RL (1989) Traumatic axial dislocations of the carpus. J Hand Surg 14A:446-457
8. Gilula LA, Weeks PM (1978) Post-traumatic ligamentous instabilities of the wrist. Radiology 129:641-651
9. Truong NP, Mann FA, Gilula LA, Kang SW (1994) Wrist instability series: increased yield with clinical-radiologic screening criteria. Radiology192:481-484
10. Peh WCG, Gilula LA (1995) Plain film approach to tumors and tumor-like conditions of bone. Br J Hosp Med 54:549-557
11. Forrester DM, Nesson JW (1973) The radiology of joint disease. WB Saunders, Philadelphia

Imaging of the Wrist

Christian W.A. Pfirrmann

Department of Radiology, University Hospital Balgrist, Zurich, Switzerland

Introduction

Imaging of the wrist and hand is a challenging task in the field of musculoskeletal imaging. The anatomy is complex. Knowledge of normal anatomic variants, asymptomatic findings, and other diagnostic pitfalls is crucial for accurate analysis. Variants and pitfalls are commonly found as coincidental findings and may easily be misdiagnosed as relevant abnormalities. The consequences may be over-treatment. Familiarity with common disease processes and their treatment is important.

Technical Considerations and Pitfalls

Plain radiographs are the first step in imaging assessment in most cases. Many abnormalities, such as fractures, misalignment, static instabilities, inflammatory disorders, and chondrocalcinosis, may easily be diagnosed on standard radiographs. Standardized projections are important for accurate assessment. Ultrasound is excellent for the detection of soft-tissue abnormalities. especially ganglion cyst, synovitis or tenosynovitis, tendon abnormalities, and nerve abnormalities. Computed tomography (CT) is the modality of choice for the assessment of complex fractures, to differentiate fractures from bone bruise, and in the follow-up of fracture healing. Magnetic resonance (MR) arthrography is the most accurate tool for the assessment of interosseous ligament tears, lesions of the triangular fibrocartilage complex (TFCC), and, occasionally, for cartilage lesions and lesions of the extrinsic ligaments [1-3]. Standard MR, optionally with intravenous gadolinium administration, is helpful for the assessment of conditions such as the painful wrist with or without trauma, inflammatory disease, and necrosis of the scaphoid after scaphoid fracture. However, there are some important technical pitfalls to be considered.

Fractures of the distal radius are among the most common bone injuries [4]. Assessment of the distal surface of the radius is of major importance in the treatment of such fractures. The articular surface of the radius normally has a palmar tilt of 12° in women and 9° in men. Improper positioning with supination or pronation of the wrist can re-

sult in incorrect measurements of the palmar tilt. The apparent palmar tilt of the distal radius increases with forearm supination and decreases with pronation. Scaphopisocapitate (SPC) alignment is a reliable criterion to establish a reproducible neutral lateral view of the wrist (Fig. 1).

Ulnar variance is the length between the distal end of the ulna and the radius, as measured on anteroposterior radiographs. Ulnar variance refers to the distance between contiguous articular surfaces of the distal radiocarpal and ulnocarpal joints. Supination decreases the measurement of ulnar variance. Pronation increases the

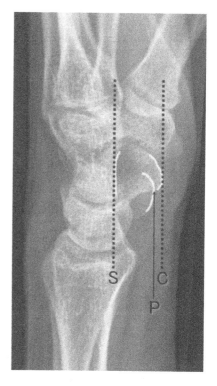

Fig. 1. The scaphopisocapitate alignment is a reliable criterion to establish a reproducible neutral lateral view of the wrist. The palmar contour of the pisiform (*P*) lies between the palmar contour of the scaphoid (*S*) and the palmar contour of the capitate (*C*)

measurement of ulnar variance by up to 2 mm. A standardized posteroanterior (PA) view of the wrist is taken with the palm flat on the table and elbow abducted to shoulder height and flexed 90°, with the forearm and wrist in neutral rotation. A standardized PA view is recognized when the extensor carpi groove is profiled at the ulnar aspect of the ulna.

Tilting of the lunate is an important element for the diagnosis of carpal instabilities. It is usually diagnosed on standardized lateral radiographs of the wrist. Dorsal tilting of the lunate is associated with an intercarpal ligament injury pattern known as dorsal intercalated segment instability. Theoretically, this diagnosis can also be made on sagittal MR images. It is usually difficult to obtain a perfectly neutral position of the wrist during MR imaging. On sagittal images the lunate apparently is more dorsally tilted than on standard lateral radiographs. Therefore, analysis of a dorsal or ventral intercalated segment instability should only be performed on standard lateral radiographs to avoid this pitfall (Fig. 2) [5].

The Triangular Fibrocartilage Complex

On MR imaging, the TFCC is a hypointense discs in all sequences. However the radial and ulnar attachments of the TFCC often show a intermediate to high signal intensity, which is a potential imaging pitfall. The ulnar attachment of the TFCC is composed of two distinct laminae: The distal lamina is orientated horizontally and extends between the articular disc and the styloid process of the ulna (Fig. 3). The proximal lamina is orientated vertically and curves from the undersurface of the articular disc to the ulnar fovea. The two laminae are separated by the ligamentum subcruentum. This fibrovascular attachment is therefore usually of intermediate signal intensity on T1- and T2-weighted images, and sometimes internal striations are seen. At the radial attachment of the TFCC, hyaline cartilage curves around the ulnar edge of the radius giving a linear area of high signal on T2 or fluid-sensitive sequences, which should not be misinterpreted as a tear. With increasing age, defects and central communication within the TFCC increase in frequency. Lesions of the TFCC are commonly classified according to the Palmer classification (Table 1) [6].

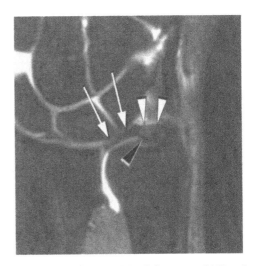

Fig. 3. Coronal intermediate-weighted, fat-saturated MR arthrography image of the wrist. The ulnar attachment of the triangular fibrocartilage complex (*white arrows*) is composed of two distinct laminae: The distal lamina is orientated horizontally (*white arrowheads*) and extends between the articular disc and the styloid process of the ulna. The proximal lamina is orientated vertically and curves from the undersurface of the articular disc to the ulnar fovea (*black arrowhead*)

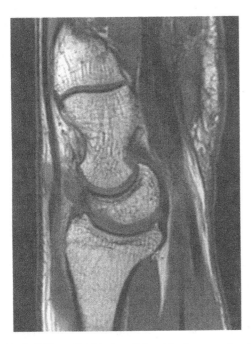

Fig. 2. Sagittal T1-weighted image of the wrist demonstrating dorsal tilting of the lunate. On sagittal images, the lunate apparently is more dorsally tilted than on standard lateral radiographs. When the patient is examined with the hand above the head, ulnar tilting is very common. Therefore, to avoid misinterpretation, analysis of a dorsal or ventral intercalated segment instability (DISI or VISI configuration) should only be performed on standard lateral radiographs

Table 1. Palmer classification of triangular fibrocartilage complex (TFCC) abnormalities. (From [6])

Class 1: Traumatic		Class 2: Degenerative	
1a	Central perforation	2a	TFCC wear
1b	Ulnar avulsion	2b	TFCC wear + lunate/ulnar chondromalacia
1c	Distal avulsion	2c	TFCC perforation + lunate/ulnar chondromalacia
1d	Radial avulsion	2d	2c + lunotriquetral ligament perforation
		2e	2d + ulnocarpal arthritis

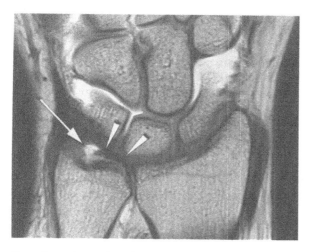

Fig. 4. Coronal T1-weighted MR arthrography image of the wrist demonstrating non-communicating and communicating defects of the TFCC near the ulnar attachment (*white arrow*). The disk (*white arrowheads*) itself is normal

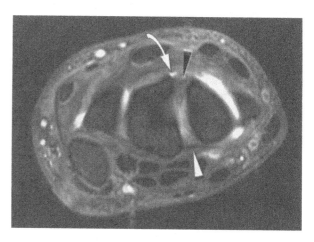

Fig. 5. Transverse (TrueFISP) MR arthrography image of the wrist demonstrating the palmar (*white arrowhead*) and dorsal (*black arrowhead*) portions of the scapholunate ligament. Note a small ganglion cyst (*curved arrow*) at the dorsal portion of the scapholunate ligament

However, defects in the TFCC often have no or little clinical significance. Zanetti and coworkers [7] have shown that radial-sided communicating TFCC defects are commonly seen bilaterally and in asymptomatic wrists. In their series of 56 patients, 64% of the communications within the TFCC were symptomatic and 46% asymptomatic; 69% of the defects were bilateral, almost all of which were located radially. Non-communicating defects were identified in 50% of symptomatic wrists and in 27% of asymptomatic wrists. Non-communicating and communicating defects of the TFCC near the ulnar attachment were more reliably associated with symptomatic wrists than radial communicating defects (Fig. 4).

Interosseous Ligament Lesions

Findings of various cadaveric and arthrographic studies have demonstrated that defects occur within the substance of the scapholunate and lunotriquetral ligaments and usually represent senescent changes in asymptomatic wrists. The scapholunate ligament and the lunotriquetral ligament are U-shaped and connect the bones of the proximal carpal row along their dorsal, palmar, and proximal margins. The ligaments have three distinct components. The palmar and dorsal portions are composed of transversely oriented, very strong collagen fibers. The largest component of the ligament is the central (also known as the proximal) segment, or pars membranacea. Histologically, it is distinctly different from the dorsal and ventral portions and is actually fibrocartilage rather than a true ligament. It is well-known that perforations in the scapholunate ligaments can be present in asymptomatic patients and are found in cadavers with no known history of wrist injury. These perforations rarely are present

before 20 years of age but occur more frequently with advancing age, reaching approximately a 50% prevalence by the eighth decade of life. In a study of Linkous and coworkers analyzing bilateral wrist arthrograms of 30 consecutive patients with a history of wrist trauma and unilateral wrist pain, bilateral tears in the central portion of the interosseous ligament were frequent [8]. However, defects in the dorsal portion of the scapholunate ligament were more common in symptomatic than in asymptomatic wrists (Fig. 5).

Capsular Ligament Lesions and Carpal Instabilities

The subject of carpal instability is complex and controversial. The patterns of carpal instability commonly are divided into dissociated and non-dissociated types. The former generally indicate more extensive ligamentous damage with injury to the interosseous (scapholunate and lunotriquetral) ligaments. Several measurements have been emphasized to define the relationship among carpal bones and to characterize the type of instability. While evaluation of carpal alignment on MR imaging can be unreliable, recent advances have focused on direct visualization of the extrinsic and capsular ligaments. Carpal coalitions are rare and have a general prevalence of 0.1%. They have a strong female predilection, and are frequently bilateral. The most common isolated carpal coalition is the lunotriquetral, followed by the capitohamate. Lunotriquetral coalitions are commonly associated with a wide scapholunate joint space. Instability tests and arthrography are often normal with respect to the scapholunate ligament in most cases. Widening of the scapholunate joint space is a normal variant that is common in patients with lunotriquetral coalition [9].

Carpal Tunnel

Carpal tunnel syndrome (CTS) is a common nerve-entrapment neuropathy affecting the median nerve within the carpal tunnel. In almost any case, clinical history, physical examination, and electromyography are sufficient for an accurate diagnosis; additional imaging, such as MR imaging, is almost never needed. Eight flexor digitorum tendons, the tendon of the flexor pollicis longus, the median nerve, and, occasionally, a persistent median artery pass through the tunnel. The last has a low incidence (2-4%). Compression of the median nerve in the carpal tunnel by a thrombosed persistent median artery has been described in several patients. Usually, a persistent median artery is asymptomatic; however, an anomalously enlarged median artery may lead to CTS. The alignment of the median nerve in the carpal tunnel, its shape, and its relationship to the flexor tendons are highly variable and dependent on wrist positioning. Because of this dynamic variability, the position of the median nerve within the carpal tunnel should not be used as a relevant diagnostic criterion. However, this characteristic may explain why certain wrist motions, flexion in particular, predispose a person to CTS. A bifid median nerve is an anatomic variation that may be associated with CTS. High division of the median nerve proximal to the carpal tunnel or bifid median nerve has been described in the surgery literature as a anomaly of the median nerve, with an incidence of 3%. It is important for the surgeon to be aware of the existence of this condition preoperatively in order to plan the carpal tunnel release [10].

Guyon's Canal Syndrome

The ulnar nerve may be compressed as it courses through Guyon's canal (ulnar tunnel). This canal is located on the ulnopalmar aspect of the wrist, superficial to the flexor retinaculum, in close proximity to the pisiform and the hamate hook [11]. It is best appreciated on axial MR images. Causes of entrapment in the region include masses, vascular injury, accessory muscles, muscle hypertrophy, fractures (hook of the hamate), and hypertrophy of the transverse carpal ligament.

Pisotriquetral Joint

The pisiform is a sesamoid bone within the flexor carpi ulnaris. Pisotriquetral joint osteoarthritis is the second most common site of osteoarthritis of the wrist and should therefore be considered in any patient with ulnar-sided wrist pain. MR arthrography in axial and sagittal planes precisely depicts the details of this joint [12].

The Type II Lunate

This is a very common variant of the wrist joint (Fig. 6). Two distinct types of lunates can be identified: type I, without a medial facet, and type II, with a medial facet that articulates with the hamate. In a series of 165 cadaveric wrists, Viegas and coworkers found a frequency of 65% of type II lunates. Significant cartilage erosion with exposed subchondral bone at the proximal pole of the hamate was evident at dissection in 44.4% of the type II lunates, while none of the type I lunates had such associated hamate pathologic conditions. The association of a hamatolunate facet with advanced cartilage damage in the proximal pole of the hamate has also been demonstrated with MR arthrography. This type II lunate, with a high incidence of associated hamate pathology, may be an unidentified cause of wrist pain on the ulnar side [13].

Ganglion Cysts

Both interosseous and soft-tissue ganglion cysts are frequent lesions about the wrist. These can be detected accurately with MR imaging using fluid-sensitive sequences and especially with ultrasound. In some instances, their origin from an intra-articular structure can be identified. The most common origin of a ganglion cyst is the interosseous ligaments. Ganglion cysts result from post-traumatic or degenerative mucoid changes of a soft-tissue structure, such as a ligament or a tendon sheath. Ganglion cysts do not communicate with the joint space primarily; rather this condition may develop secondarily.

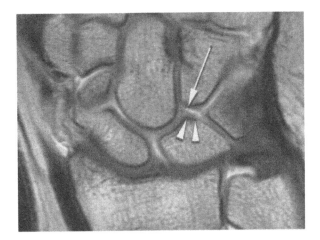

Fig. 6. Coronal T1-weighted MR arthrography image of the wrist demonstrating the association of a hamatolunate facet (type II lunate, *white arrowheads*) with advanced cartilage damage in the proximal pole of the hamate (*white arrow*)

The Carpal Boss

A bony protuberance located at the dorsum of the wrist at the base of the second or third metacarpal bone is referred to as carpal boss [14]. This bony prominence is usually caused by the presence of an os styloideum, an accessory ossification center. The os styloideum may or may not be fused with the base of the metacarpal bone. Patients typically present with complaints of pain and limitation of motion of the affected hand. The symptoms may reflect an overlying ganglion or bursitis or osteoarthritic changes at this site.

Abnormalities and Variants of Tendons and Tendons Sheath

The extensor carpi ulnaris tendon and tendon sheath are important sources of ulnar sided wrist pain. Because of their exposed location, tenosynovitis is often present. Centrally increased signal within the tendon of the extensor carpi ulnaris muscle at the level of the distal radioulnar joint is a frequent finding and may represent a normal finding. The extensor carpi ulnaris muscle is composed of two muscle bellies, one originating from the lateral epicondyle and the other from the ulnar diaphysis dorsally, with the tendon formed from spiral fibers originating from them. Histologically, the center of this tendon consists of fibrovascular tissue, explaining the high signal intensity in the center of the tendon substance. The first extensor compartment of the wrist is composed of the tendons of the abductor pollicis longus and the extensor pollicis brevis and their fascial sheath. De Quervain's disease is a localized tenosynovitis of this extensor compartment [15]. The tendon of the abductor pollicis longus is frequently composed of multiple bundles. The resulting signal changes should therefore not be misinterpreted as longitudinal tears or tendinopathy. Septations within the first extensor compartment may be an important finding for the treatment of De Quervain's disease; however, these septations may be very hard to diagnose on MR images.

Conclusions

Anatomic variants are frequent findings in imaging of the wrist and hand. They may be explained by normal physiology and/or anatomic variability, Many findings, especially changes in the TFCC and the interosseous liga-

ments, are asymptomatic; the incidence increases with age. It is not always possible to differentiate variants and artifacts from clinically relevant findings, nonetheless; it is important to know their potential etiology and clinical importance and not to over-report them as abnormalities requiring additional imaging or treatment. Thorough knowledge of normal anatomy is crucial.

References

1. Theumann NH, Pfirrmann CW, Antonio GE et al (2003) Extrinsic carpal ligaments: normal MR arthrographic appearance in cadavers. Radiology 226(1):171-179
2. Zanetti M, Saupe N, Nagy L (2007) Role of MR imaging in chronic wrist pain. Eur Radiol 17(4):927-938
3. Ruegger C, Schmid MR, Pfirrmann CW et al (2007) Peripheral tear of the triangular fibrocartilage: depiction with MR arthrography of the distal radioulnar joint. AJR Am J Roentgenol 188:187-192
4. Zanetti M, Gilula LA, Jacob HA, Hodler J (2001) Palmar tilt of the distal radius: influence of off-lateral projection initial observations. Radiology 220(3):594-600
5. Zanetti M, Hodler J, Gilula LA (1998) Assessment of dorsal or ventral intercalated segmental instability configurations of the wrist: reliability of sagittal MR images. Radiology 206(2):339-345
6. Palmer AK (1989) Triangular fibrocartilage complex lesions: a classification. J Hand Surg [Am] 14(4):594-606
7. Zanetti M, Linkous MD, Gilula LA, Hodler J (2000) Characteristics of triangular fibrocartilage defects in symptomatic and contralateral asymptomatic wrists. Radiology 216(3):840-845
8. Linkous MD, Pierce SD, Gilula LA (2000) Scapholunate ligamentous communicating defects in symptomatic and asymptomatic wrists: characteristics. Radiology 216(3):846-850
9. Metz VM, Schimmerl SM, Gilula LA, Saffar P (1993) Wide scapholunate joint space in lunotriquetral coalition: a normal variant? Radiology 188(2):557-559
10. Propeck T, Quinn TJ, Jacobson JA et al (2000) Sonography and MR imaging of bifid median nerve with anatomic and histologic correlation. AJR Am J Roentgenol 175(6):1721-1725
11. Zeiss J, Jakab E, Khimji T, Imbriglia J (1992) The ulnar tunnel at the wrist (Guyon's canal): normal MR anatomy and variants. AJR Am J Roentgenol 158(5):1081-1085
12. Theumann NH, Pfirrmann CW, Chung CB et al (2002) Pisotriquetral joint: assessment with MR imaging and MR arthrography. Radiology 222(3):763-770
13. Pfirrmann CW, Theumann NH, Chung CB et al (2002) The hamatolunate facet: characterization and association with cartilage lesions – magnetic resonance arthrography and anatomic correlation in cadaveric wrists. Skeletal Radiol 31(8):451-456
14. Conway WF, Destouet JM, Gilula LA et al (1985) The carpal boss: an overview of radiographic evaluation. Radiology 156(1): 29-31
15. Glajchen N, Schweitzer M (1996) MRI features in de Quervain's tenosynovitis of the wrist. Skeletal Radiol 25(1):63-65

MR Imaging of the Hip (Part I): Normal Labrum, Labral Tears, and Femoroacetabular Impingement

Christine B. Chung

Department of Radiology, University of California, San Diego, CA, USA

Acetabular Labrum

The acetabular labrum, similar to the labrum in the glenoid, is made up of fibrocartilaginous tissue and attaches to the margin of the acetabular rim, deepening the acetabular socket. Histologically, three separate layers are identified within the labrum: a randomly oriented fibrocartilaginous layer at the articular surface, a central lamellar layer of collagen, and a circumferentially oriented layer along the capsular surface. The composition of the labrum allows it to dissipate load stresses across the hip joint, but makes the basal layer vulnerable to shear forces. The labrum is a relatively avascular structure, resulting in a limited ability to repair itself [1]. It aids in the distribution of weight-bearing forces through the joint by maintaining a joint-fluid layer between the articular cartilage of the femur and femoral head, and by preventing lateral translation of the femur [2].

The acetabular labrum has been the subject of numerous studies that have characterized its normal magnetic resonance imaging (MRI) appearance in asymptomatic volunteer [3-5]. These studies have established that there is rather extensive variability in the appearance of the asymptomatic labrum. Although comprising large cohorts of patients, these studies certainly did not benefit from current state-of-the-art technology, including high field (≥1.5 Tesla) MRI, current coils (dedicated unilateral MRI studies), and imaging sequences. As encountered in the glenoid labrum, variation was described in the morphology, signal intensity, presence or absence as well as attachment of the labrum to the adjacent osseous acetabulum. With respect to morphology, the acetabular labrum was found to be triangular in shape in 66-94% of asymptomatic and presumably normal labra. The thickest portion of the labrum was superior and posterior, and it proved to be widest along the anterior and superior aspects of the joint. Rounded (11%) and flat (9%) labra were encountered [3]. With advancing age, labral morphology is increasingly variable, with a decreasing percentage of triangular labra. Interestingly, a difference in labral shape and size between sides was noted in 25% of volunteers in one study [5].

The most common pattern of signal intensity within the labrum is low signal intensity on all MRI sequences. This pattern of signal intensity has been reported in 44-56% of asymptomatic hips [3-7]. However, a spectrum of increased internal signal has been observed in the asymptomatic labrum, the incidence of which increased with age. Signal variations are more common in men and within the superior and anterior labrum. Variations include intermediate signal on T1-weighted and proton density-weighted images in 58% of asymptomatic labra; 37% of asymptomatic labra have intermediate signal on T2-weighted sequences [3-7]. Bright signal may be seen on T2-weighted images in up to 15% of patients. This internal signal may be globular, linear, or curvilinear and may extend to the margins of the labrum. The extension to the labral margin is one reason that differentiation of normal and abnormal labra is difficult without the benefit of intra-articular contrast material. Many factors may contribute to this internal signal. There may be extension of the osseous rim into the labral substance. Fibrocartilaginous bundles within the labral base are also contributory [1].

A consistent constellation of findings, including an absent anterior labrum accompanied by a blunted anterosuperior labrum, has been observed in 10-14% of individuals [3]. Because of the consistency of this pattern, it is believed to represent an anatomic variant rather than a pathologic finding.

The relationship between the acetabular labrum and articular cartilage is a subject of controversy (Figs. 1, 2). A separation between the articular cartilage and the labrum at the posterior aspect of the joint, the posterior labrocartilaginous cleft, has been identified as a normal variant, occurring in 22.6% of hips [8]. Whether an anterior labrocartilaginous cleft is a normal variant or a pathologic finding is unclear. A histologic study in 1981 of the fetal acetabular labrum reported the presence of defects at the anterosuperior margin of the labrum in seven of 74 specimens [9]. A similar variation was described at arthroscopy by Byrd as a "partial separation of the labrum from the lateral aspect of the bony acetabulum", noted in the anterosuperior labrum [10]. In a recent study, Studler et al. retrospectively evaluated the imaging characteristics of surgically proven sublabral recesses and labral tears in the anterior portion of the acetabulum at magnetic resonance arthrography (MRA) [11]. They found recesses to be lo-

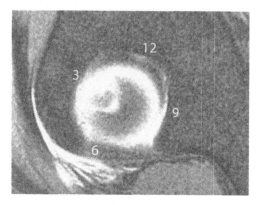

Fig. 1. Labral localization. The labrum can be localized by superimposing a clock face on the acetabulum

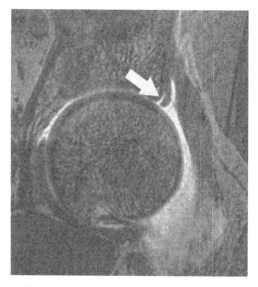

Fig. 2. Sublabral recess. A normal variation in attachment has been described between acetabulum and adjacent labrum. Coronal MRA image showing a linear space (*arrow*) between labrum and acetabulum

cated at the 8 (*n* = 7), 9 (*n* = 2), and 10 (*n* = 1) o'clock positions. The authors further noted that none of the recesses extended into the substance of the labrum or through the full thickness of the labral base. Although the shape of the majority of the recesses surgically confirmed was linear in nature, a single recess was described as "gaping."

Labral Tears

Historically, radiologists have used conventional contrast arthrography to detect labral tears. More recently, MRA has provided a useful tool for the detection of labral pathology (Fig. 3). Mintz et al. used non-contrast MRI to detect labral tears; the accuracy was similar to that of MRA. They ascribed the improved accuracy to the high-resolution technique, which afforded small pixel size and an in-plane resolution of 330-442 µm in the sagittal plane. The use of fast spin-echo technique provided differential contrast between normal and abnormal cartilage and labral tissue. Image acquisition included both wide field-of-view body coil images including both hips and dedicated images of the hip that were acquired with a surface coil [12]. Radial-sequence imaging is another technique that has been explored in conjunction with MRA and with computed tomography (CT). While the technique did not reveal additional labral pathology when used with MRA, promising sensitivity, specificity, and accuracy were obtained when used with CT [13, 14]. In preliminary reports, high field strength (3 Tesla) was shown to be a promising approach to the evaluation of labral abnormalities in the hip as well as in the detection of chondral lesions [15].

The labrum can fail either through intrinsic substance tears and/or through detachment from the adjacent acetabulum. In the literature, the term "labral tear" commonly encompasses both of these abnormalities. Detachments are more common than intrasubstance tears. Most labral pathology occurs in the anterior and anterosuperior aspect of the joint. Less commonly involved are the posterosuperior and anteroinferior portions of the

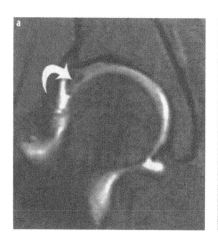

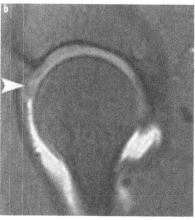

Fig. 3 a, b. Labral tear. Coronal (**a**) MRA image shows linear contrast extending into the labral substance (*curved arrow*), representing a labral tear. Corresponding sagittal (**b**) MRA image also shows the tear (*arrowhead*)

labrum. Posteroinferior pathology is unusual. Posterior lesions are typically the result of trauma or dysplasia. The tear extends beyond one quadrant in up to 32% of patients, and this extension correlates with arthroscopically unstable tears [16]. Tears at multiple separate sites may be seen in 6.9% of patients [16]. In patients with anterior and posterior tears, the sequence of events is hypothesized to be anterior damage first leading to instability and hinging of the femoral neck along the anterior rim driving the head into the posterior aspect of the joint, as seen with pincer impingement.

Labral detachments involve separation of the labrum from the acetabular rim. They are identified by contrast material interposed between the labrum and rim. Detachments may be complete or partial, with or without a displaced fragment. Labral tears are identified by the presence of intrasubstance contrast material. Tears and detachments may occur in the same labrum. Although the literature reports that up to 90% of labral pathology is in the form of a detachment, this may respresent a bias based upon our technical limitations and inability to detect more subtle pathology.

A staging system for tears based upon MRA findings was developed by Czerny et al. [17]. This staging system combines features of the perilabral recess and the presence of intrasubstance contrast. Any obliteration of the perilabral sulcus is considered abnormal. An arthroscopic classification system for labral pathology has been described. Labral tears may be longitudinal and peripheral, radial fibrillated or flap tears. In a study by Lage et al., of 267 pateints with 37 labral tears, 56.8% were radial flap, 21.6% radial fibrillated, 16.2% longitudinal peripheral, and 5.4% unstable [18]. At least one study concluded that the Czerny classification system does not correlate with the arthroscopic staging system. Further work has been introduced in this area in an attempt to develop terminology that correlates MRA appearance with the arthroscopic appearance of labral pathology [19].

Evaluation of every MRA image of the hip should include scrutiny of the articular cartilage, as labral pathology is reported to be accompanied by chondral lesions in 30% of patients. The articular cartilage of the hip is relatively thin compared to that of the knee, and defects may require a detailed inspection to be identified. Evaluation is further adversely affected by the contact between the two articular surfaces.

Femoroacetabular Impingement

Labral pathology is currently believed to most commonly result from impingement. Femoroacetabular impingement is frequently the result of anatomic alteration within the hip joint, although it is occasionally seen in patients with normal anatomy with a superphysiologic range of motion. Impingement is more typically seen in active individuals rather than in sedentary persons. Depending on the clinical and radiographic findings, two types of impingement

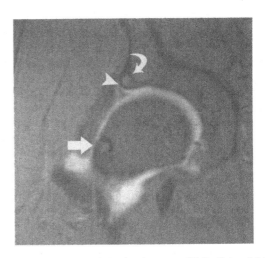

Fig. 4. Cam femoroacetabular impingement (FAI). Coronal MRA image shows the asphericity of the femoral head (*straight arrow*), cystic change at the acetabular margin (*curved arrow*), and labral tear (*arrowhead*). This constellation of findings supports the clinical diagnosis of Cam FAI in this patient

are distinguished. Pincer impingement is the acetabular cause of femoroacetabular impingement and is characterized by focal or general overcoverage of the femoral head. Cam impingement (Fig. 4) is the femoral cause of femoroacetabular impingement and is due to an aspherical portion of the femoral head-neck junction. Most patients (86%) have been reported to have a combination of the two forms of impingement, i.e., "mixed pincer and cam impingement," with only a minority (14%) reported as having the pure form of either cam or pincer impingement [20]. Intervention in these patients is directed toward restoration of normal anatomy.

Cam Impingement

The cam mechanism of impingement is the result of an abnormal femoral head-neck relationship. It is more common than pincer impingement and is typically seen in young active males. Conditions underlying cam impingement include decreased femoral anterversion, abnormal femoral head-neck offset, shallow taper between the femoral head and neck, non-spherical femoral head, a femoral neck "bump" or osseous excrescence, pistol-grip deformity, and generalized enlargement of the femoral head (coxa magna). Radiographs are extremely useful in identifying many of these anatomic alterations. Quantification of the amount of asphericity can be accomplished by the alpha angle. This is defined as the angle between the femoral neck axis and a line connecting the head center with the point of beginning asphericity of the head-neck contour. It can be measured on radiographs. An angle >50° is an indicator of an abnormally shaped femoral head-neck contour [21]. Other parameters used to quantify the amount of asphericity include the femoral offset, or the offset ratio.

In this form of impingement, osseous excrescences or enlargement of the femoral neck prevent the normal movement of the femur within the acetabulum, most commonly with flexion, internal rotation, and adduction. As a result, the abnormal head-neck junction does not "clear" the acetabulum. The anterior aspect of the neck, where most structural abnormalities occur, impinges on the anterosuperior acetabular rim. The abnormal portion of the neck acts as a wedge that is driven between the articular cartilage and labrum, leading to separation of these two structures. The primary damage on the acetabular side of the joint is to the articular cartilage. The cartilage damage begins at the margin of the joint and progresses more centrally (outside to inside delamination) as the injury progresses. As delamination continues, the articular cartilage is torn from the labrum and, initially, the labrum maintains a stable attachment to the rim. In a recent paper, Pfirrmann et al. described acetabular cartilage delamination in 52% of patients undergoing surgery for cam-type femoroacetabular impingement [22].

Pincer Impingement

The pincer mechanism of impingement is not as commonly seen as the cam mechanism. It is most typically seen in active middle-aged women. It also occurs during flexion and internal rotation. In pincer impingement, the underlying anatomic condition resides at the acetabular rim. The acetabular rim in these cases extends more laterally, with overcoverage of the femoral head, most commonly isolated to the anterosuperior aspect of this joint. This condition may be seen with excessive acetabular retroversion, protrusion acetabuli, and coxa profunda (Fig. 5). When the

femoral head rotates within the acetabulum, the neck impinges on the overextended acetabulum. The primary site of damage in this condition is the labrum. It is caught or "pinched" between the femoral neck and the acetabular rim, with the damage usually consisting of intrasubstance tearing of the labrum. Damage to the articular cartilage is secondary and, while more extensive from anterior to posterior than in cam impingement, does not extend as deeply into the joint. Contrecoup injuries are frequently observed with this type of impingement, with the contact anteriorly acting as a lever that drives the head posteriorly. These findings have been emphasized in the imaging literature [23].

References

1. Seldes RM, Tan V, Hunt J et al (2001) Anatomy, histologic features and vascularity of the adult acetabular labra. Clin Orthop Rel Res 382:232-240
2. Ferguson SJ, Bryant JT, Ganz R, Ito K (2003) An in vitro investigation of the acetabular labrum seal in hip joint mechanics. J Biomech 32:171-178
3. Lecouvet FE, Vande Berg BC, Malghem J et al (1996) MR imaging of the acetabular labrum: variations in 200 asymptomatic hips. AJR Am J Reontgenol 167(4):1025-1028
4. Cotten A, Boutry N, Demondion X et al (1998) Acetabular labrum: MRI in asymptomatic volunteers. J Comput Assist Tomogr 22(1):1-7
5. Aydingoz U, Ozturk MH (2001) MR Imaging of the acetabular labrum: a comparative study of both hips in 180 asymptomatic volunteers. Eur Radiol 11(4): 567-574
6. Czerny C, Hofmann S, Neuhold A et al (1996) Lesions of the acetabular labrum: accuracy of MR imaging and MR arthrography in detection and staging. Radiology 200(1):225-230
7. Abe I, Harada Y, Oinuma K et al (2000) Acetabular labrum: abnormal findings at MR imaging in asymptomatic hips. Radiology 216(2):576-581
8. Dinauer PA, Murphy KP, Carroll JF (2004) Sublabral sulcus at the posteroinferior acetabulum: a potential pitfall in MR arthrography diagnosis of acetabular labral tears. AJR Am J Roentgenol 183:1745-1753
9. Walker JM (1981) Histological study of the fetal development of the human acetabulum and labrum: significance in congenital hip disease. Yale J Biol Med 54:255-263
10. Byrd JW (2001) Hip arthroscopy: the supine position. Clin Sports Med 20:703-731
11. Studler U, Kalberer F, Leunig M et al (2008) MR arthrography of the hip: differentiation between an anterior sublabral recess as a normal variant and a labral tear. Radiology 249(3):947-954
12. Mintz DN, Hooper T, Connell D et al (2005) Magnetic resonance imaging of the hip: detection of labral and chondral abnormalities using noncontrast imaging. Arthroscopy 21(4):385-393
13. Yoon LS, Palmer WE, Kassarjian A (2007) Evaluation of radial-sequence imaging in detecting acetabular labral tears at hip MR arthrography. Skeletal Radiol 36:1029-1033
14. Yamamoto Y, Tonotsuka H, Ueda T, Hamada Y (2007) Usefulness of radial contrast-enhanced computed tomography for the diagnosis of acetabular labrum injury. Arthroscopy 23(12):1290-1294
15. Sundberg TP, Toomayan GA, Major NM (2006) Evaluation of the acetabular labrum at 3.0-T MR imaging compared with 1.5-T MR arthrography: preliminary experience. Radiology 238(2):706-711
16. McCarthy JC, Noble PC, Schuck MR et al (2001) The role of labral lesions to development of early degenerative hip disease. Clin Orthop Rel Res 393:25-37

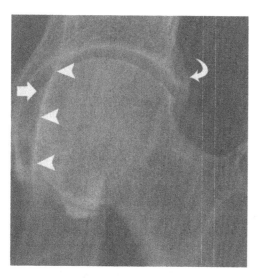

Fig. 5. Pincer femoroacetabular impingement. Plain film shows acetabular protrusion alignment of the hip with the femoral head (*arrow*) projecting medial to the ilioischial line (*arrowheads*). The labrum is ossified (*arrowhead*) in this patient, who presented with the pincer FAI

17. Czerny C, Hofmann S, Urban M et al (1999) MR arthrography of the adult acetabular-labral complex: correlation with surgery and anatomy. AJR Am J Roentgenol 173(2):345-349
18. Lage LA, Patel JV. Villar RN (1996) The acetabular labral tear: an arthroscopic classification. Arthroscopy 12: 269-272
19. Blankenbaker DG, De Smet AA, Keene JS (2007) Classification and localization of acetabular labral tears. Skeletal Radiol 36:391-397
20. Beck M, Kalhor M, Leunig M, Ganz R (2005) Hip morphology influences the pattern of damage to the acetabular cartilage: femoroacetabular impingement as a cause of early osteoarthritis of the hip. J Bone Joint Surg Br 87:1012-1018
21. Tannast M, Siebenrock KA, Anderson SA (2007) Femoroacetabular impingement: radiographic diagnosis-what the radiologist should know. AJR Am J Roentgenol 188:1540-1552
22. Pfirrmann CWA, Duc SR, Zanetti M et al (2008) MR arthrography of acetabular cartilage delamination in femoroacetabular cam impingement. Radiology 249(1):236-241
23. Pfirrmann CWA, Mengiardi B, Dora C et al (2006) Cam and pincer femoroacetabular impingement: characteristic MR arthrographic findings in 50 patients. Radiology 240(3):778-785

The Hip, Part II: Soft-Tissue Abnormalities

Cheryl Petersilge

Department of Radiology, Marymount Hospital, and Regional Radiology, Imaging Institute, Cleveland Clinic Health System, Cleveland, OH, USA

Introduction

A number of soft-tissue abnormalities need to be considered in the differential diagnosis of the painful hip and pelvis. These abnormalities primarily involve musculotendinous injuries, tendon avulsions, and bursitis. The patients involved range from active athletic individuals to the elderly. The athletes most at risk for these injuries are those engaged in sports involve kicking, sprinting, and pivoting, such as soccer and ice hockey.

Musculotendinous injuries of the hip and pelvis affect the hamstring tendons and rarely the rectus femoris tendons [1]. Other sources of pain include the iliopsoas bursitis, and in the elderly the gluteus medius and minimus tendonosis and tears. Athletic pubalgia is associated with injury to the muscles and tendons of the anterior abdominal wall and the adductor musculature of the thigh.

Athletic Pubalgia

This condition has received much attention in the musculoskeletal literature in the past few years [2, 3]. Our understanding of this condition continues to evolve both in terms of understanding the significance of imaging findings as well as correlating those findings with appropriate treatment. Previously known by many names, including sports hernia, this common cause of chronic groin pain is now known as athletic pubalgia. It is not a pre-hernia condition.

Patients with athletic pubalgia present with symptoms of chronic groin pain associated with overuse. The injuries are more frequently seen in men. Pain results from injury to one or more of the tendons along the anterior aspect of the pelvis, including the rectus abdominus, adductor longus and brevis, gracilis, and conjoined (transverses abdominus and internal oblique) tendons (Fig. 1).

Slips from the rectus abdominus and adductor longus tendons decussate along the anterior aspect of the symphysis pubis, contributing to the support of that articulation. A complex interplay among these structures contributes to the stability of the anterior pelvis. Injury to the rectus abdominus or adductor longus muscles and tendons leads to micro-instability and a sequence of events that culminates in chronic groin pain.

Radiographic changes of osteitis pubis may be one manifestation of this condition. However, these changes also may be asymptomatic. Findings include joint-space widening, superior to inferior movement, subchondral erosions, sclerosis, and cysts as well as osteophyte formation. Magnetic resonance (MR) may reveal bone marrow edema, which should be differentiated from the unilateral edema distant from the subchondral bone of the symphysis, as the latter heralds an osseous stress response/fracture. When these imaging findings are identi-

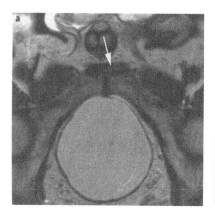
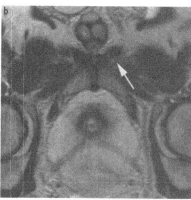

Fig. 1 a, b. T2-weighted oblique axial images perpendicular to the symphysis pubis reveal typical findings of tendonosis within the left adductor longus tendon. **a** Diffuse intermediate signal is present within the decussation of the adductor longus and rectus abdominus tendons anterior to the symphysis pubis (*arrow*). **b** More inferiorly, the intermediate signal is confined to the left adductor longus tendon (*arrow*)

fied, attention should be directed to the adductor longus and rectus abdominus muscles, looking for evidence of tendonosis, partial-thickness tendon tears, and, uncommonly, full-thickness tendon tears.

Hamstring and Rectus Femoris Injuries

The hamstring tendons consist of the tendons of the semimembranosus, semitendinosus, and long head of the biceps femoris muscles. The muscles originate from the ischial tuberosity via a conjoined tendon. The tendons cross two joints, which predisposes them to injury. The majority of hamstring injuries occur proximally in the muscle, involving the musculotendinous or myofascial junction [4, 5]. Other sites of injury include the origin from the ischial tuberosity and the distal tendons (Fig. 2). Rectus femoris tendon injuries almost always also concern the reflected or indirect head [6, 7]. The indirect head arises from the supra-acetabular ridge while the direct head arises from the anterior inferior iliac spine. Apophyseal avulsion rather than tendon disruption occurs in the skeletally immature individual.

Iliopsoas Bursitis and Tendonosis

Abnormalities of the iliopsoas bursa are quite common, with the causes ranging from direct trauma and overuse injuries in the younger active population to abnormalities resulting from arthritic conditions within the hip [8, 9]. Symptoms range from pain to a palpable mass. The abnormalities are primarily within the bursa. Associated tendon abnormalities are not common. Primary tendon abnormalities are less common although spontaneous rupture of the tendon has been reported in the older population [10].

Snapping Hip

The snapping hip syndrome has clinically been divided into several different etiologies, including external, internal, and intra-articular [11, 12]. The external form is the result of movement of the gluteus maximus tendon or iliotibial band over the greater trochanter. While this form of snapping hip is rarely imaged, imaging findings include trochanteric bursitis, iliotibial band thickening or edema, or edema within the anterior margin of the gluteus maximus muscle. Internal snapping hip is created by movement of the iliopsoas tendon across the femoral neck, lesser trochanter or iliopectineal eminence. Imaging findings include iliopsoas bursitis/tendonosis. Iliopsoas bursography may be a more definitive examination than MRI and offers a therapeutic option (steroid injection).

Greater Trochanteric Pain Syndrome

For many years, pain over the lateral aspect of the hip was diagnosed as trochanteric bursitis. With greater use of MRI in the evaluation of these patients, a spectrum of abnormalities has now been recognized, including trochanteric bursitis, tendonosis, and partial- and full-thickness tears of the gluteus medius and minimus tendons. Tendon tears occur at the insertion onto the greater trochanter. This condition is now referred to as greater trochanteric pain syndrome (GTPS), and the gluteus minimus and medius tendons are referred to as the rotator cuff of the hip [13-15]. GTPS is most commonly seen in elderly women. The tendon abnormalities always involve the gluteus medius tendon, with variable involvement of the gluteus minimus tendon (Fig. 3). Associated bursitis may involve the trochanteric (gluteus maximus) bursa, as well as the subgluteus medius and minimus bursa [16].

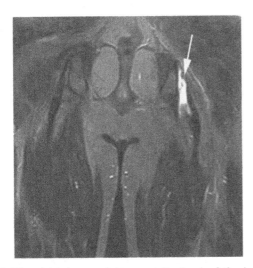

Fig. 2. T2-weighted coronal image at the level of the ischial tuberosities demonstrates a large fluid collection in the gap created by complete rupture of the hamstring tendons (*large arrow*)

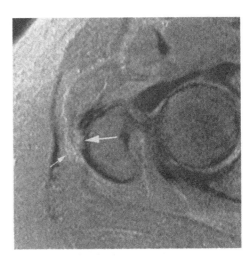

Fig. 3. Fat-saturated T1-weighted axial image after the intravenous administration of gadolinium shows a gap within the insertion of the gluteus medius tendon onto the greater trochanter (*large arrow*) and inflammatory changes within the trochanteric bursa (*small arrow*)

Thigh Splints

This injury, the result of chronic repetitive stress at the femoral insertion of the adductor longus and brevis muscles [17, 18], may also present with hip or groin pain. Imaging findings are consistent with chronic repetitive stress and include periosteal new bone formation, linear periosteal edema, and adjacent cortical or marrow edema. The abnormalities are located along the posteromedial surface of the mid-diaphysis. This anatomy may not always be included on a traditional MRI of the hip. One should consider using a wide field-of-view (FOV) on the screening short tau inversion recovery (STIR) sequence to avoid missing this injury.

References

1. Koulouris G, Connell D (2003) Evaluation of the hamstring muscle complex following acute injury. Skeletal Radiol 32:582-589
2. Omar IM, Zoga AC, Kavanagh EC et al (2008) Athletic pubalgia and "sports hernia": optimal MR imaging technique and findings. Radiographics 28:1415-1438
3. Zoga AC, Kavanagh ED, Omar IM et al (2008) Athletic pubalgia and the "sports hernia": MR imaging findings. Radiology 247:797-807
4. Koulouris G, Connell D (2003) Evaluation of the hamstring muscle complex following acute injury. Skeletal Radiol 32:582-589
5. Connell DA, Schneider-Kolsky ME et al (2004) Longitudinal study comparing sonographic and MRI assessments of acute and healing hamstring injuries. AJR Am J Roentgenol 183:975-984
6. Ouellette H, Thomas BJ, Nelson E, Torriani M (2006) MR imaging of rectus femoris origin injuries. Skeletal Radiol 35:665-672
7. Gyftopoulos S, Rosenberg ZS, Schweitzer ME, Bordalo-Rodrigues M (2008) Normal anatomy and strain of the deep musculotendinous junction of the proximal rectus femoris: MRI features. AJR Am J Roentgenol 190:182-186
8. Johnston CAM, Wiley JP, Lindsay DM, Wiseman DA (1998) Iliopsoas bursitis and tendonitis: a review. Sports Med 25:271-283
9. Wunderbaldinger P, Bremer C, Schellenberger E et al (2002) Imaging features of iliopsoas bursitis. Eur Radiol 12:409-415
10. Lecouvet FE, Demondion X, Leemrijse T et al (2005) Spontaneous rupture of the distal iliopsoas tendon: clinical and imaging findings. Eur Radiol 15:2341-2346
11. Blankenbaker DG, Tuite MJ (2006) The painful hip: new concepts. Skeletal Radiol 35:352-370
12. Vaccaro JP, Sauser DD, Beals RK (1995) Iliopsoas bursa imaging: efficacy in depicting abnormal iliopsoas tendon motion in patients with internal snapping hip syndrome. Radiology 197:853-856
13. Chung CB, Robertson JE, Cho GJ et al (1999) Gluteus medius tendon tears and avulsive injuries in elderly women: imaging findings in six patients. AJR Am J Roentgenol 173:351-353
14. Kingzett-Taylor A, Tirman P, Feller J et al (1999) Tendinosis and tears of the gluteus medius and minimus muscles as a cause of hip pain: MR imaging findings. AJR Am J Roentgenol 173:1123-1126
15. Bird PA, Oakley SP, Shnier R, Kirkham W (2001) Prospective evaluation of magnetic resonance imaging and physical examination findings in patients with greater trochanteric pain syndrome. Arthritis Rheum 44:2138-2145
16. Pfirmann CWA, Chung CB, Theumann NH et al (2001) "Greater trochanter of the hip". Attachment of the abductor mechanism and a complex of three bursae-MR imaging and MR bursography in cadavers and MR imaging in asymptomatic volunteers. Radiology 221:469-477
17. Anderson M, Kaplan P, Dussault R (2001) Adductor insertion avulsion syndrome (thigh splints). AJR Am J Roentgenol 177:673-675
18. Anderson SE, Johnston JO, O'Donell RO, Steinbach LS (2001) MR imaging of sports-related pseudotumor in children: Mid femoral diaphyseal periostitis at insertion site of adductor musculature. AJR Am J Roentgenol 176:1227-1231

Imaging of the Knee

David A. Rubin[1], Arthur A. De Smet[2]

[1] Musculoskeletal Section, Mallinckrodt Institute of Radiology, Washington University School of Medicine, St. Louis, MO, USA
[2] Radiology, University of Wisconsin School of Medicine and Public Health, Madison, WI, USA

Imaging Modalities

Conventional radiographs are the initial radiologic study in most suspected knee disorders. Radiographs demonstrate the joint spaces as well as bones, but are relatively insensitive to soft-tissue (except those composed largely of calcium or fat), destruction of medullary bone, and early loss of cartilage. A minimum radiographic examination consists of AP and lateral projections. In patients with acute trauma, performing the lateral examination cross-table allows identification of a lipohemarthrosis, an important clue to the presence of an intraarticular fracture [1]. The addition of oblique projections increases the sensitivity of the examination for nondisplaced fractures, especially those of the tibial plateau [2]. For the early detection of articular cartilage loss, a PA radiograph of both knees with the patient standing and knees mildly flexed is a useful adjunct projection. A joint space difference of 2 mm side-to-side correlates with grade III and higher chondrosis [3]. The tunnel projection is useful to demonstrate intercondylar osteophytes. In patients with anterior knee symptoms, an axial projection of the patellofemoral joint, such as a Merchant view, can evaluate the patellofemoral joint space and alignment [4].

Bone scintigraphy with an agent such as Tc^{99m}-MDP can screen the entire skeleton for metastatic disease. Scintigraphy also has a role in the detection of other radiographically occult conditions, such as nondisplaced fractures, and early stress fractures, osteomyelitis, and osteonecrosis, especially with three-phase technique. Bone scanning may add to the work-up of painful knee arthroplasties [5]. Evaluation of a potentially infected arthroplasty usually requires combining the bone scan with an additional scintigraphic examination, such as a sulfur colloid, labeled white blood cells or specific inflammatory agent scan [6].

Sonography is largely limited to an evaluation of the extraarticular soft tissues of the knee, but with careful technique at least partial visualization of the synovium and ligaments is also possible [7]. Ultrasound is useful in the evaluation of overuse conditions of the patellar tendon [8]. In addition, sonography easily demonstrates popliteal (Baker's) cysts and other fluid-containing structures [9].

Computed tomography (CT) is used most frequently to evaluate intraarticular fractures about the knee, for planning complex orthopedic procedures, and for post-operative evaluation. Maximal diagnostic information may necessitate reformatting the transversely acquired dataset into orthogonal planes and/or 3D projections [10]. To facilitate reconstructions, multidetector-row helical acquisitions with thin collimation (sub-millimeter, if possible) are preferred [11]. The combination of helical CT with arthrography results in a viable examination for the detection of internal derangements, including meniscal and articular cartilage injuries [12, 13].

Magnetic resonance (MR) imaging has emerged as the premier imaging modality for the knee. MR is the most sensitive, noninvasive test for the diagnosis of virtually all bone and soft-tissue disorders in and around the knee. Additionally, MR imaging provides information that can be used to grade pathology, guide therapy, prognosticate conditions, and evaluate treatment for a wide variety of orthopedic conditions in the knee. MR arthrography following the direct intraarticular injection of gadolinium-based contrast agents increases the value of the examination in selected knee conditions, including evaluation of the post-operative knee, detection and staging of chondral and osteochondral infractions, and discovery of intraarticular loose bodies [14-16].

High-quality knee MR imaging can be performed with high- or low-field systems with open, closed, or dedicated-extremity designs, as long as proper care is used for the technique [17, 18]. Use of a local coil is mandatory to maximize signal-to-noise ratio [19]. Images are acquired in the transverse, coronal, and sagittal planes. One study suggested adding oblique sagittal images to improve visualization of the anterior cruciate ligament [20]. Obliquity of the coronal images in selected patients can be of use in demonstrating posterolateral corner injuries [21]. A combination of different pulse sequences provides tissue contrast. Spin-echo T1-weighted images demonstrate hemorrhage as well as abnormalities of bone marrow and extraarticular structures that are bounded by fat [22, 23]. Proton-density-weighted images (long TR, short effective TE) are best for imaging fibrocartilage structures like the menisci [24]. T2 or T2*-weighted images are used for the evaluation of abnormalities of the muscles, tendons, ligaments, and articular cartilage [25, 26]. These fluid-sensitive sequences can be obtained using spin-echo, fast spin-echo, or gradient-recalled techniques. Suppressing the signal from fat increases the sensitivity for detecting marrow and soft-tissue edema [27, 28]. Three-dimensional gradient-recalled acquisitions can provide thin contiguous slices for supplemental imaging of articular cartilage [29, 30]. To consistently visualize critical structures in the knee, standard MR imaging should be done with a field-of-view no greater than 16 cm, 3- or 4-mm slice thickness, and imaging matrices of at least 256×256. Depending on the MR system and coil design, in order to achieve this spatial resolution with adequate signal-to-noise, other parameters like the number of signals averaged and the receiver bandwidth may need to be optimized [31, 32].

Specific Disorders

Bone and Articular Cartilage

Trauma

Bone pathology in the knee encompasses a spectrum of traumatic, reactive, ischemic, infectious, and neoplastic conditions. Radiography, CT, scintigraphy, and MR imaging each have a diagnostic role for these disorders.

Most fractures are visible radiographically. A lipohemarthrosis seen on a cross-table lateral examination is an important ancillary finding indicating an intraarticular fracture, which may be radiographically occult if it is nondisplaced [33]. The amount of depression and the congruence of the articular surface(s) determine the treatment and prognosis of tibial plateau fractures. The images need to depict accurately the amount of depression, as well as the presence, location, and size of any areas of articular surface step-off, gap, or die-punch depression. CT traditionally performs better than radiography for this indication, with the use of multiplanar sagittal and coronal images reconstructed from the initial transverse data [34]. At some institutions, MR has supplanted CT. The MR examination not only can show the number and position of the fracture planes, but also demonstrates associated soft-tissue lesions, such as meniscus and ligament tears, that often affect surgical planning [35-37].

Other common fractures about the knee include patellar fractures, intercondylar eminence fractures, and avulsions. Patellar fractures with a horizontal component require internal fixation when they become distracted due to retraction of the proximal fragment by the pull of the quadriceps. Fractures of the intercondylar eminence and spines of the tibia may affect the attachment points of the cruciate ligaments. Elevation of a fracture fragment can occur due to the attachment of one of the cruciate ligaments. Avulsion fractures may look innocuous, but they can signal serious ligament disruptions. For example, a fracture of the lateral tibial rim (Segond fracture) is a strong predictor of anterior cruciate ligament disruption, while an avulsions of the medial head of the fibula (arcuate fracture) indicates disruption of at least a portion of the posterolateral corner [38,39].

Bone scintigraphy, CT, or MR imaging are sensitive to radiographically occult fractures. A positive bone scan after trauma indicates a fracture, as long as no other reasons (osteoarthritis, Paget disease, etc.) are evident radiographically. However, an abnormal bone scan still does not show the number and position of the fracture lines, which impacts treatment. For this reason, and because of the low specificity of bone scintigraphy, CT and MR have largely replaced it for this indication. MR probably has an advantage over CT when there is no fracture present, because MR shows more of the soft-tissue injuries that may clinically mimic an occult fracture. On MR examination, non-fat-suppressed T1-weighted images best demonstrate fracture lines, which appear as very low-signal intensity linear or stellate lines surrounded by marrow edema, which has low signal intensity compared to marrow fat but is approximately isointense compared to muscle. On gradient-recalled, proton-density-weighted, and non-fat-suppressed T2-weighted images, fractures lines and marrow edema are often not visible. Marrow edema is most conspicuous on fat-suppressed T2-weighted or STIR images, but the amount of edema may obscure underlying fracture lines.

Injuries to the articular surfaces often produce changes in the underlying subcortical bone. In children, these injuries are usually osteochondral, while in adults they may be purely chondral or involve both the cartilage and subjacent bone. Osteochondral infractions are visible radiographically, most often those involving the lateral aspect of the medial femoral condyle. However, MR imaging is the study of choice to stage these lesions. On T2-weighted images, a thin line of fluid-intensity signal surrounding the base of the lesion combined with disruption of the articular surface indicates that the fragment is unstable. Similarly, the presence of small cysts in the base of the crater, or of an empty crater, indicates lesion instability, usually necessitating operative fixation or removal of the osteochondral fragment [40]. In these cases, the radiologist should conduct a careful search for loose bodies. Lack of any high signal at the junction between a fragment and its parent bone indicates that the lesion has healed. The most difficult cases are those in which there is a broad area of high signal that is less intense than fluid at the interface. In these instances, the high signal may represent loose connective tissue of an unstable lesion or granulation tissue in a healing lesion. MR arthrography following the direct injection of contrast is helpful in this event: contrast tracking around the base of the lesion indicates a loose, in-situ fragment [41].

In the knee, chondral injuries mimic meniscal tears clinically, but are radiographically occult. Arthroscopy, MR imaging with or without arthrography, or CT arthrography can show these injuries. Arthrographic images demonstrate contrast filling a defect in the articular cartilage. Most of the traumatic cartilage injuries are full-thickness and have sharp, vertically oriented walls (unlike degenerative cartilage lesions, which may be partial-thickness or full-thickness with sloped walls). To demonstrate small defects, non-arthrographic MR images need high-contrast resolution between joint fluid and hyaline cartilage [42]. Useful sequences include T2-weighted fast spin-echo ones, in which articular cartilage is dark and fluid is bright, or spoiled gradient-echo images, in which normal cartilage is bright and fluid is dark. A useful associated finding is a focal area of subchondral edema overlying the defect on fat-suppressed T2-weighted images. Often, the subchondral abnormality will be more conspicuous than the chondral defect [43].

Stress fractures, whether of the fatigue or insufficiency type, occur about the knee. Once healing begins, radiographs show a band of sclerosis perpendicular to the long axis of the main trabeculae, with or without focal periosteal reaction. Rarely, a cortical fracture line is visible; however, initially, stress fractures are radiographically occult. At this stage, either bone scintigraphy or MR examinations are more sensitive [44]. The imaging appearance is similar to that of traumatic fractures. Bone scans show a nonspecific, often linear focus of intense uptake, with associated increased blood flow (on three-phase scans). The MR appearance is a low signal-intensity fracture line surrounded by a larger region of marrow edema. The proximal tibia is a common location for insufficiency fractures, especially in elderly, osteoporotic patients.

MR examination is also sensitive to lesser degrees of bone trauma. Marrow edema without a fracture line in a patient with a history of chronic repetitive injury represents a "stress reaction." If the offending activity continues without giving the bone time to heal, these injuries may progress to true stress fractures and macroscopic fractures. The term "bone bruise" or "bone contusion" describes trabecular microfracture due to impaction of the bone. Impaction can be due to blunt force from an object outside the body, or more commonly, from two bones striking each other after ligament injuries, subluxations, or reductions. Bone bruises appear as reticulated, ill-defined regions in the marrow that are isointense to muscle on T1-weighted images and hyperintense on fat-suppressed T2-weighted or STIR images [45, 46]. This pattern of signal abnormality is commonly referred to as the "bone marrow edema pattern," even though granulation tissue and fibrosis dominate the histologic appearance [47]. The configuration of bone bruises is an important clue to the mechanism of injury, can account for elements of the patient's pain, and may prognosticate eventual cartilage degeneration [48-50]. However, the radiologist should avoid the temptation to label any area of marrow edema as a "bone bruise". This term is reserved for cases in which there is documented direct trauma, which may have medicolegal implications. The focal bone marrow edema pattern is nonspecific and is seen in a variety of other conditions, from ischemia, to reactive (subjacent to areas of degenerative chondrosis) changes, to neoplastic lesions, and infectious disease.

Ischemia and Infarction

Marrow infarction and osteonecrosis result from a variety of insults, including endogenous and exogenous steroids, collagen vascular diseases, alcoholism, and hemoglobinopathies. An idiopathic form also occurs in the femoral condyles [51], sometimes precipitated by a meniscal tear or meniscectomy. Articular surface infarctions appear as sclerosis of the subchondral trabeculae radiographically, eventually leading to formation of a subchondral crescent and articular surface collapse. In the diaphyses, established infarcts have a serpiginous, sclerotic margin. Evolving infarcts may not show any radiographic findings. At this stage, bone scintigraphy will be positive (albeit nonspecifically) in the reactive margin surrounding the infarcted bone. On occasion, the actual area of infarction may show decreased tracer activity. On MR images, infarctions appear as geographic areas of abnormal marrow signal, either in the medullary shaft of a long bone or in the subchondral marrow (where it is termed osteonecrosis, avascular necrosis, or AVN). The signal intensities in the subchondral fragment and reactive surrounding bone vary based on the age of the lesion and other factors. As an infarction evolves, a typical serpiginous reactive margin becomes visible, often with a pathognomonic double-line sign on T2-weighted images. This sign represents a peripheral low-signal-intensity zone of demarcation surrounded by a parallel high-signal-intensity line representing the reactive margin [52].

Replacement

Normal bone marrow around the knee is composed of a mixture of hematopoietic (red) and fatty (yellow) marrow. Processes that alter marrow composition are typically occult on all imaging modalities except for specific nuclear marrow scans (using labeled sulfur colloid, for example) and MR. Normally, areas of yellow marrow are approximately isointense to subcutaneous fat on all pulse sequences, while red marrow is approximately isointense compared to muscle. In adults, the appophyseal and epiphyseal equivalents should contain fatty marrow. The most common marrow alteration encountered around the knee is hyperplastic red marrow. This can be seen in physiologic conditions due to anemia, obesity, and cigarette smoking, as well as in athletes and persons living at high-altitudes [53, 54]. Unlike the case for pathologic marrow replacement, the signal intensity of red marrow expansion is iperintense or isointense to muscle, foci of residual yellow marrow separate islands of red marrow islands, and the process spares the epiphyses. However, in extreme cases, such as due to hemolytic anemia, the hyperplastic marrow will partially or completely replace the epiphyseal marrow [55].

Other alterations in marrow composition are less common, but relatively characteristic in their MR appearances. Radiated and aplastic marrow is typically completely fatty [56]. Fibrotic marrow is low in signal intensity on all pulse sequences, and marrow in patients with hemosiderosis shows nearly complete absence of signal [57].

Destruction

Tumors and infections destroy the trabecular and/or cortical bone. Subacute or chronic osteomyelitis produces predictable radiographic changes: cortical destruction, periosteal new bone formation, reactive medullary sclerosis, and eventually cloacae and sinus tracts. In these cases, the primary role of cross-sectional imaging is staging infection. For example, CT is useful for surgical planning to identify a sequestrum or foreign body [58]. MR imaging can also help determine treatment in chronic osteomyelitis [59], by demonstrating non-drained abscesses, and by assessing the viability of the infected bone (by the presence or absence of enhancement after intravenous contrast administration). In patients with known chronic osteomyelitis, uptake by an inflammation-sensitive nuclear agent (like gallium or labeled white blood cells) or focal high marrow signal intensity on T2-weighted MR images suggests superimposed active infection, although neither study is sufficiently specific enough to preclude biopsy, especially in cases in which the causative agent is uncertain.

Bones with acute osteomyelitis may be radiographically normal for the first two weeks of infection [60]. While CT scanning can show cortical destruction and marrow edema earlier than radiographs, MR imaging and nuclear medicine studies are typically the first line of imaging. On MR images, the marrow edema pattern is seen, but to increase the specificity of the finding, osteomyelitis should only be diagnosed when there is also cortical destruction or an adjacent soft-tissue abscess, sinus tract, or ulcer (at least in adults, in whom direct inoculation is much more common than hematogenous spread of infection) [61].

Both benign and malignant bone tumors occur commonly around the knee. Radiographs should be the initial study in these patients and are essential for predicting the biological behavior of the tumor (by analysis of the zone of transition and pattern of periostitis) as well as for identification of calcified matrix. The intraosseous extent of tumor and the presence and type of matrix are easiest to perform with CT examination. For staging beyond the bone (into the surrounding soft tissues, as skip lesions to other parts of the same bone, and to regional nodes), MR or CT are approximately equally effective [62]. In the future, PET scanning may stage some bone tumors as well. Additionally, MR imaging is at least as sensitive as bone scintigraphy for detecting metastases and at least as sensitive as radiography in patients with multiple myeloma, although MR is currently better suited to targeted regions rather than whole-body screening [63].

Degeneration

Chondrosis refers to degeneration of articular cartilage. With progressive cartilage erosion, radiographs show the typical findings of osteoarthritis, namely non-uniform joint-space narrowing and osteophyte formation. Before these findings are apparent, bone scintigraphy may show increased uptake in the subchondral bone adjacent to the arthritic cartilage. The increased tracer uptake represents accellerated bone turnover associated with cartilage dysfunction. Direct visualization of the cartilage requires a technique that can visualize the contour of the articular surface. On standard CT examination, there is inadequate contrast between articular cartilage and joint fluid to visualize surface defects, while CT arthrography using dilute contrast can show even small areas of degeneration [64]. However, MR imaging is the most commonly used imaging modality to examine degenerated cartilage.

On MR images, internal signal intensity changes do not reliably correlate with cartilage degeneration [65, 66]. Instead, the diagnosis of chondrosis is based on visualization of joint fluid (or injected contrast) within chondral defects that start at the joint surface [67]. The accuracy of MR imaging increases for deeper and wider defects. Many different sequences provide enough tissue contrast between fluid and articular cartilage. The most commonly used ones are T2-weighted fast spin-echo and fat-suppressed spoiled gradient recalled-echo sequences. T1-weighted spin-echo sequences are used in knees that have undergone arthrography with a dilute gadolinium mixture [68-70]. However, fat-suppressed T2-weighted images have the added advantage of showing reactive marrow edema in the subjacent bone (analogous to the subchondral uptake seen on bone scans), which is often associated with deep chondral defects [71, 72].

Soft Tissues

MR imaging, with or without intraarticular or intravenous contrast, is the imaging study of choice for most soft-tissue conditions in and around the knee. Ultrasound can also visualize relatively superficial structures.

Menisci

The fibrocartilagenous menisci distribute the load of the femur on the tibia and function as shock absorbers. There are two criteria for meniscal tears on MR images. The first is intrameniscal signal on a short-TE (T1-weighted, proton-density-weighted, or gradient-recalled) image that unequivocally contacts an articular surface of the meniscus. A meniscus that has an intrameniscal signal contacting the surface of the meniscus on two or more MR images is more likely to have a tear than a meniscus with only one abnormal image [73]. Intrameniscal signal that only equivocally touches the meniscal surface is no more likely torn than a meniscus containing no internal signal [74, 75]. The second criterion is abnormal meniscal shape

[24]. The normal meniscus in cross-section is triangular or bow-tie-shaped, with a sharp inner margin. Any variation from the normal shape – other than in discoid menisci or those that have undergone partial meniscectomy – represents a meniscal tear.

In addition to diagnosing meniscal tears, the radiologist should describe the features of each meniscal tear that may affect treatment. These properties include the location of the tear (medial or lateral; anterior horn, body, posterior horn, or roots; periphery or inner margin), the shape of the tear (longitudinal, horizontal, radial, or complex), the approximate length of the tear, the completeness of the tear (whether it extends partly or completely through the meniscus), and the presence or absence of associated meniscal cyst. The radiologist should also note the presence of displaced meniscal fragments, which typically occur in the intercondylar notch or outer gutters [24].

Limitations of MR imaging in diagnosing meniscal tears have been the subject of study for the past two decades with research continuing into 2008. A meta-analysis of MR studies published between 1991 and 2000 found that MR imaging is less sensitive for lateral meniscal tears than for medial meniscal tears and less specific for medial than for lateral meniscal tears [76]. A study in 2008 demonstrated that the reduced specificity of MR diagnosis of medial meniscal tears is primarily due to spontaneous healing of peripheral longitudinal tears if there is a sufficiently long interval from injury to arthroscopy [77]. The lower sensitivity for diagnosing lateral meniscal tears was confirmed in another 2008 study [78]. In that study, most of the lateral meniscal tears missed on MR imaging were not visible even in retrospect. Peripheral longitudinal tears were the most common missed tear that could be seen in retrospect [78].

A meniscal tear that heals spontaneously or following repair will often still have intrameniscal signal on short-TE images that contacts the meniscal surface. When the abnormality is also present on a T2-weighted image, when there is a displaced fragment, or when a tear occurs in a new location, the radiologist can confidently diagnose a recurrent or residual meniscal tear [79]. If none of these features is present, MR or CT examination after direct arthrography is useful. On an arthrographic examination, visualizing injected contrast within the substance of a repaired meniscus is diagnostic of a meniscal tear [80, 81]. The problem is compounded after a partial meniscectomy: in these cases both the meniscal shape and internal signal are unreliable signs of recurrent meniscal tear. Again, MR arthrography is the most useful noninvasive test for recurrent meniscal tears following partial meniscectomy [82].

Ligaments

T2-weighted images demonstrate ruptures of the cruciate, collateral, and patellofemoral ligaments. Both long-axis and cross-sectional images are important to examine. The direct sign of a ligament tear is partial or complete disruption of the ligament fibers [83]. While edema typically surrounds acutely torn ligaments, edema enveloping an intact ligament is a nonspecific finding that is also present in bursitis and other soft-tissue conditions [84]. Chronic ligament tears have a more varied appearance. Non-visualization of any ligament fibers or abnormal morphology of the scarred ligament fibers may be the only MR signs present [85]. Secondary findings of ligament tears, such as bone contusions or subluxations, are useful when present, but do not supplant the primary findings and do not reliably distinguish acute from chronic injuries [86].

Mucoid degeneration within ligaments occurs with aging in some patients. In the knee, the anterior cruciate ligament is most often affected. On MR images, the appearance is that of high-signal-intensity amorphous material between the intact ligament fibers on T2-weighted images [87]. The ligament may appear enlarged in cross-section, and often there is associated intraosseous cyst formation near the ligament attachment points. It is important to distinguish degenerated from torn ligaments because degenerated ligaments are stable and do not require surgical intervention [88].

Muscles and Tendons

The muscles around the knee are susceptible to direct and indirect injuries. Blunt trauma to a muscle results in a contusion. On T2-weighted or STIR MR images, contusions appear as high signal intensity spreading out from the point of contact in the muscle belly. Eccentric (stretching) injury results in muscle strains. On MR imaging, these are seen as regions of edema centered at the myotendinous junction, with partial or complete disruption of the tendon from the muscle in more severe cases [89]. Around the knee, muscle trauma affects the distal hamstrings, distal quadriceps, proximal gastrocnemius, soleus, popliteus, and plantaris muscles.

Chronic overuse of tendons results in degeneration or "tendonopathy", which can be painful or asymptomatic; but most importantly tendonopathy weakens tendons, placing them at risk of rupture. The patellar, quadriceps, and semimembranosus tendons are most frequently involved around the knee. In addition to MR, ultrasound can evaluate these tendons. Sonographically, a degenerated tendon appears enlarged, with loss of the normal parallel fiber architecture and often with focal hypoechoic or hyperechoic regions. A gap between the tendon fibers indicates that the process has progressed to partial or complete tear. Similarly, on MR images, focal or diffuse enlargement of a tendon with loss of its sharp margins indicates tendonopathy [90]. In those cases in which T2-weighted images show a focus of high signal intensity, surgical excision of the abnormal focus can hasten healing in refractory cases [91]. Partial or complete disruption of tendon fibers represents a tendon tear on MR imaging [92]. When macroscopic tearing is present, the radiologist should also examine the muscle belly of the affected tendon for fatty atrophy (which indicates chronicity) or edema (suggesting a more acute rupture). If the tear is complete, the retracted stump should be located on the images as well. These last two tasks may require repositioning of the MR coil.

Synovium

While radiographs can show medium and large knee effusions, other modalities better demonstrate specific synovial processes. Fluid distention of a synovial structure has water attenuation on CT images, signal isointense to fluid on MR images, and is hypoechoic or anechoic with enhanced through transmission on ultrasound images. All imaging modalities easily show popliteal or Baker's cysts, which represent distention of the posteromedial semimembranosus-gastrocnemius recess of the knee. At least 11 other named bursae occur around the knee. The most commonly diseased ones are probably the prepatellar, superficial infrapatellar, medial collateral ligament, and semimembranosus-tibial collateral ligament bursae.

Synovitis due to infection, trauma, inflammatory arthritis, or crystal disease is readily identifiable in the knee on both ultrasound and MR images. Power Doppler ultrasound or the use of ultrasound contrast agent may increase sensitivity for active synovitis [93]. On MR examination, thickening of the usually imperceptibly thin synovial membrane and enhancement of the synovium following intravenous contrast administration indicate active synovitis [94].

Synovial metaplasia and neoplasia are uncommon. In the knee, primary synovial osteochondromatosis appears as multiple cartilaginous bodies within the joint on MR images, or on radiographs or CT when the bodies are calcified [95]. The signal intensities of the bodies vary depending on their composition. Diffuse pigmented villonodular synovitis and focal nodular synovitis demonstrate proliferative synovium, which enhances following contrast administration. Hemosiderin deposition in the synovium, which appears as very low signal on all MR pulse sequences with blooming on gradient-echo images, is an important, although inconstant, clue to the diagnosis [96].

References

1. Lee JH, Weissman BN, Nikpoor N et al (1989) Lipohemarthrosis of the knee: a review of recent experiences. Radiology 173:189-191
2. Gray SD, Kaplan PA, Dussault RG et al (1997) Acute knee trauma: how many plain film views are necessary for the initial examination? Skeletal Radiol 26:298-302
3. Rosenberg TD, Paulos LE, Parker RD et al (1988) The forty-five-degree posteroanterior flexion weight-bearing radiograph of the knee. J Bone Joint Surg [Am] 70:1479-1483
4. Jones AC, Ledingham J, McAlindon T et al (1993) Radiographic assessment of patellofemoral osteoarthritis. Ann Rheum Dis 52:655-658
5. Smith SL, Wastie ML, Forster I (2001) Radionuclide bone scintigraphy in the detection of significant complications after total knee joint replacement. Clin Radiol 56:221-224
6. Pelosi E, Baiocco C, Pennone M et al (2004) 99mTc-HMPAO-leukocyte scintigraphy in patients with symptomatic total hip or knee arthroplasty: improved diagnostic accuracy by means of semiquantitative evaluation. J Nucl Med 45:438-444
7. Bouffard JA, Dhanju J (1998) Ultrasonography of the knee. Semin Musculoskelet Radiol 2:245-270
8. Khan KM, Bonar F, Desmond PM et al (1996) Patellar tendinosis (jumper's knee): findings at histopathologic examination, US, and MR imaging. Victorian Institute of Sport Tendon Study Group. Radiology 200:821-827
9. Ward EE, Jacobson JA, Fessell DP et al (2001) Sonographic detection of Baker's cysts: comparison with MR imaging. AJR Am J Roentgenol 176:373-380
10. Wicky S, Blaser PF, Blanc CH et al (2000) Comparison between standard radiography and spiral CT with 3D reconstruction in the evaluation, classification and management of tibial plateau fractures. Eur Radiol 10:1227-1232
11. Buckwalter KA, Farber JM (2004) Application of multidetector CT in skeletal trauma. Semin Musculoskelet Radiol 8:147-156
12. Mutschler C, Vande Berg BC, Lecouvet FE et al (2003) Postoperative meniscus: assessment at dual-detector row spiral CT arthrography of the knee. Radiology 228:635-641
13. Vande Berg BC, Lecouvet FE, Poilvache P et al (2002) Assessment of knee cartilage in cadavers with dual-detector spiral CT arthrography and MR imaging. Radiology 22:430-436
14. Brossmann J, Preidler KW, Daenen B et al (1996) Imaging of osseous and cartilaginous intraarticular bodies in the knee: comparison of MR imaging and MR arthrography with CT and CT arthrography in cadavers. Radiology 200:509-517
15. Sciulli RL, Boutin RD, Brown RR et al (1999) Evaluation of the postoperative meniscus of the knee: a study comparing conventional arthrography, conventional MR imaging, MR arthrography with iodinated contrast material, and MR arthrography with gadolinium-based contrast material. Skeletal Radiol 28:508-514
16. Magee T, Shapiro M, Rodriguez J, Williams D (2003) MR arthrography of postoperative knee: for which patients is it useful? Radiology 229:159-163
17. Barnett MJ (1993) MR diagnosis of internal derangements of the knee: effect of field strength on efficacy. AJR Am J Roentgenol 161:115-118
18. Franklin PD, Lemon RA, Barden HS (1997) Accuracy of imaging the menisci on an in-office, dedicated, magnetic resonance imaging extremity system. Am J Sports Med 25:382-388
19. Rubin DA, Kneeland JB (1994) MR imaging of the musculoskeletal system: technical considerations for enhancing image quality and diagnostic yield. AJR Am J Roentgenol 163:1155-1163
20. Buckwalter KA, Pennes DR (1990) Anterior cruciate ligament: oblique sagittal MR imaging. Radiology 175:276-277
21. Yu JS, Salonen DC, Hodler J et al (1996) Posterolateral aspect of the knee: improved MR imaging with a coronal oblique technique. Radiology 198:199-204
22. Vande Berg BC, Malghem J, Lecouvet FE et al (1998) 2 Classification and detection of bone marrow lesions with magnetic resonance imaging. Skeletal Radiol 7:529-545
23. Bush CH (2000) The magnetic resonance imaging of musculoskeletal hemorrhage. Skeletal Radiol 29:1-9
24. Rubin DA, Paletta GA Jr (2000) Current concepts and controversies in meniscal imaging. Magn Reson Imaging Clin N Am 8:243-270
25. Ha TPT, Li KC, Beaulieu CF et al (1998) Anterior cruciate ligament injury: fast spin-echo MR imaging with arthroscopic correlation in 217 examinations. AJR Am J Roentgenol 170:1215-1219
26. Sonin AH, Pensy RA, Mulligan ME et al (2002) Grading articular cartilage of the knee using fast spin-echo proton density-weighted MR imaging without fat suppression. AJR Am J Roentgenol 179:1159-1166

27. Kapelov SR, Teresi LM, Bradley WG et al (1993) Bone contusions of the knee: increased lesion detection with fast spine-echo MR imaging with spectroscopic fat saturation. Radiology 189:901-904

28. Weinberger E, Shaw DW, White KS et al (1995) Nontraumatic pediatric musculoskeletal MR imaging: comparison of conventional and fast-spin-echo short inversion time inversion-recovery technique. Radiology 194:721-726

29. Recht MP, Piraino DW, Paletta GA et al (1996) Accuracy of fat-suppressed three-dimensional spoiled gradient-echo FLASH MR imaging in the detection of patellofemoral articular cartilage abnormalities. Radiology 198:209-212

30. Disler DG, McCauley TR, Kelman CG et al (1996) Fat-suppressed three-dimensional spoiled gradient-echo MR imaging of hyaline cartilage defects in the knee: comparison with standard MR imaging and arthroscopy. AJR Am J Roentgenol 167:127-132

31. Woertler K, Strothmann M, Tombach B et al (2000) Detection of articular cartilage lesions: experimental evaluation of low- and high-field-strength MR imaging at 0.18 and 1.0 T. J Magn Reson Imaging 11:678-685

32. Kladny B, Gluckert K, Swoboda B et al (1995) Comparison of low-field (0.2 Tesla) and high-field (1.5 Tesla) magnetic resonance imaging of the knee joint. Arch Orthop Trauma Surg 114:281-286

33. Lee JH, Weissman BN, Nikpoor N et al (1989) Lipohemarthrosis of the knee: a review of recent experiences. Radiology 173:189-191

34. Wicky S, Blaser PF, Blanc CH et al (2000) Comparison between standard radiography and spiral CT with 3D reconstruction in the evaluation, classification and management of tibial plateau fractures. Eur Radiol 10:1227-1232

35. Kode L, Lieberman JM, Motta AO et al (1994) Evaluation of tibial plateau fractures: efficacy of MR imaging compared with CT. AJR Am J Roentgenol 163:141-147

36. Mui LW, Engelsohn E, Umans H (2007) Comparison of CT and MRI in patients with tibial plateau fracture: can CT findings predict ligament tear or meniscal injury? Skeletal Radiol 36:145-151

37. Yacoubian SV, Nevins RT, Sallis JG et al (2002) Impact of MRI on treatment plan and fracture classification of tibial plateau fractures. J Orthop Trauma 16(9):632-637

38. Campos JC, Chung CB, Lektrakul N et al (2001) Pathogenesis of the Segond fracture: anatomic and MR imaging evidence of an iliotibial tract or anterior oblique band avulsion. Radiology 219:381-386

39. Huang GS, Yu JS, Munshi M et al (2003) Avulsion fracture of the head of the fibula (the "arcuate" sign): MR imaging findings predictive of injuries to the posterolateral ligaments and posterior cruciate ligament. AJR Am J Roentgenol 180:381-387

40. De Smet AA, Ilahi OA, Graf BK (1996) Reassessment of the MR criteria for stability of osteochondritis dissecans in the knee and ankle. Skeletal Radiol 25:159-163

41. Kramer J, Stiglbauer R, Engel A et al (1992) MR contrast arthrography (MRA) in osteochondrosis dissecans. J Comput Assist Tomogr 16:254-260

42. Speer KP, Spritzer CE, Goldner JL et al (1991) Magnetic resonance imaging of traumatic knee articular cartilage injuries. Am J Sports Med 19:396-402

43. Rubin DA, Harner CD, Costello JM (2000) Treatable chondral injuries in the knee: frequency of associated focal subchondral edema. AJR Am J Roentgenol 174:1099-1106

44. Spitz DJ, Newberg AH (2002) Imaging of stress fractures in the athlete. Radiol Clin North Am 40:313-331

45. Kapelov SR, Teresi LM, Bradley WG et al (1993) Bone contusions of the knee: increased lesion detection with fast spine-echo MR imaging with spectroscopic fat saturation. Radiology 189:901-904

46. Arndt WF 3rd, Truax AL, Barnett FM et al (1996) MR diagnosis of bone contusions of the knee: comparison of coronal T2-weighted fast spin-echo with fat saturation and fast spin-echo STIR images with conventional STIR images. AJR Am J Roentgenol 166:119-124

47. Zanetti M, Bruder E, Romero J, Hodler J (2000) Bone marrow edema pattern in osteoarthritic knees: correlation between MR imaging and histologic findings. Radiology 215:835-840

48. Sanders TG, Medynski MA, Feller JF, Lawhorn KW (2000) Bone contusion patterns of the knee at MR imaging: footprint of the mechanism of injury. Radiographics 20(Spec No):S135-S151

49. Wright RW, Phaneuf MA, Limbird TJ, Spindler KP (2000) Clinical outcome of isolated subcortical trabecular fractures (bone bruise) detected on magnetic resonance imaging in knees. Am J Sports Med 28:663-667

50. Costa-Paz M, Muscolo DL, Ayerza M et al (2001) Magnetic resonance imaging follow-up study of bone bruises associated with anterior cruciate ligament ruptures. Arthroscopy 17:445-449

51. Björkengren AG, AlRowaih A, Lindstrand A et al (1990) Spontaneous osteonecrosis of the knee: value of MR imaging in determining prognosis. AJR Am J Roentgenol 154:331-336

52. Mitchell DG, Rao VM, Dalinka MK et al (1987) Femoral head avascular necrosis: correlation of MR imaging, radiographic staging, radionuclide imaging, and clinical findings. Radiology 162:709-715

53. Deutsch AL, Mink JH, Rosenfelt FP et al (1989) Incidental detection of hematopoietic hyperplasia on routine knee MR imaging. AJR Am J Roentgenol 152:333-336

54. Shellock FG, Morris E, Deutsch AL et al (1992) Hematopoietic bone marrow hyperplasia: high prevalence on MR images of the knee in asymptomatic marathon runners. AJR Am J Roentgenol 158:335-338

55. Rao VM, Mitchell DG, Rifkin MD et al (1989) Marrow infarction in sickle cell anemia: correlation with marrow type and distribution by MRI. Magn Reson Imaging 7:39-44

56. Remedios PA, Colletti PM, Raval JK et al (1988) Magnetic resonance imaging of bone after radiation. Magn Reson Imaging 6:301-304

57. Lanir A, Aghai E, Simon JS et al (1986) MR imaging in myelofibrosis. J Comput Assist Tomogr 10:634-636

58. Hernandez RJ (1985) Visualization of small sequestra by computerized tomography. Report of 6 cases. Pediatr Radiol 15:238-241

59. Mason MD, Zlatkin MB, Esterhai JL et al (1989) Chronic complicated osteomyelitis of the lower extremity: evaluation with MR imaging. Radiology 173:355-359

60. Capitano MA, Kirkpatrick JA (1970) Early roentgen observations in acute osteomyelitis. AJR Am J Roentgenol 108:488-490

61. Erdman WA, Tamburro F, Jayson HT et al (1991) Osteomyelitis: characteristics and pitfalls of diagnosis with MR imaging. Radiology 180:533-539

62. Panicek DM, Gatsonis C, Rosenthal DI et al (1997) CT and MR imaging in the local staging of primary malignant musculoskeletal neoplasms: Report of the Radiology Diagnostic Oncology Group. Radiology 202:237-246

63. Daffner RH, Lupetin AR, Dash N et al (1986) MRI in the detection of malignant infiltration of bone marrow. AJR Am J Roentgenol 146:353-358

64. Vande Berg BC, Lecouvet FE, Poilvache P et al (2002) Assessment of knee cartilage in cadavers with dual-detector spiral CT arthrography and MR imaging. Radiology 222:430-436

65. Brown TR, Quinn SF (1993) Evaluation of chondromalacia of the patellofemoral compartment with axial magnetic resonance imaging. Skeletal Radiol 22: 325-328

66. Disler DG, McCauley TR, Wirth CR et al (1995) Detection of knee hyaline cartilage defects using fat-suppressed three-dimensional spoiled gradient-echo MR imaging: comparison with standard MR imaging and correlation with arthroscopy. AJR Am J Roentgenol 165:377-382

67. Gagliardi JA, Chung EM, Chandnani VP et al (1994) Detection and staging of chondromalacia patellae: relative efficacies of conventional MR imaging, MR arthrography, and CT arthrography. AJR Am J Roentgenol 163:629-636

68. Recht MP, Kramer J, Marcelis S et al (1993) Abnormalities of articular cartilage in the knee: analysis of available MR techniques. Radiology 187:473-478

69. Sonin AH, Pensy RA, Mulligan ME et al (2002) Grading articular cartilage of the knee using fast spin-echo proton density-weighted MR imaging without fat suppression. AJR Am J Roentgenol 179:1159-1166

70. Kramer J, Recht MP, Imhof H et al (1994) Postcontrast MR arthrography in assessment of cartilage lesions. J Comput Assist Tomogr 18:218-224

71. Turner DA (2000) Subchondral bone marrow edema in degenerative chondrosis [Letter]. AJR Am J Roentgenol 175:1749-1750

72. Kijowski R, Stanton P, Fine J et al (2006) Subchondral bone marrow edema in patients with degeneration of the articular cartilage of the knee joint. Radiology 238(3):943-949

73. De Smet AA, Tuite MJ (2006) Use of the "two-slice-touch" rule for the MRI diagnosis of meniscal tears. AJR Am J Roentgenol 187:911-914

74. De Smet AA, Norris MA, Yandow DR et al (1993) MR diagnosis of meniscal tears of the knee: importance of high signal in the meniscus that extends to the surface. AJR Am J Roentgenol 161:101-107

75. Kaplan PA, Nelson NL, Garvin KL et al (1991) MR of the knee: the significance of high signal in the meniscus that does not clearly extend to the surface. AJR Am J Roentgenol 156:333-336

76. Oei EH, Nikken JJ, Verstjnen ACM et al (2003) MR imaging of the menisci and cruciate ligaments: A systematic review. Radiology 226:837-848

77. De Smet AA, Nathan DH, Graf BK et al (2008) Clinical and MRI findings associated with false-positive knee MR diagnoses of medial meniscal tears. AJR Am J Roentgenol 191:93-99

78. De Smet AA, Mukherjee R (2008) Clinical, MRI, and arthroscopic findings associated with failure to diagnose a lateral meniscal tear on knee MRI. AJR Am J Roentgenol 190:22-26

79. Lim PS, Schweitzer ME, Bhatia M et al (1999) Repeat tear of postoperative meniscus: potential MR imaging signs. Radiology 210:183-188

80. Farley TE, Howell SM, Love KF et al (1991) Meniscal tears: MR and arthrographic findings after arthroscopic repair. Radiology 180:517-522

81. Sciulli RL, Boutin RD, Brown RR et al (1999) Evaluation of the postoperative meniscus of the knee: a study comparing conventional arthrography, conventional MR imaging, MR arthrography with iodinated contrast material, and MR arthrography with gadolinium-based contrast material. Skeletal Radiol 28:508-514

82. Applegate GR, Flannigan BD, Tolin BS et al (1993) MR diagnosis of recurrent tears in the knee: value of intraarticular contrast material. AJR Am J Roentgenol 161:821-825

83. Tung GA, Davis LM, Wiggins ME et al (1993) Tears of the anterior cruciate ligament: primary and secondary signs at MR imaging. Radiology 188:661-667

84. Schweitzer ME, Tran D, Deely DM, Hume EL (1995) Medial collateral ligament injuries: evaluation of multiple signs, prevalence and location of associated bone bruises, and assessment with MR imaging. Radiology 194:825-829

85. Vahey TN, Broome DR, Kayes KJ et al (1991) Acute and chronic tears of the anterior cruciate ligament: differential features at MR imaging. Radiology181:251-253

86. Brandser EA, Riley MA, Berbaum KS et al (1996) MR imaging of anterior cruciate ligament injury: independent value of primary and secondary signs. AJR Am J Roentgenol 167:121-126

87. McIntyre J, Moelleken S, Tirman P (2001) Mucoid degeneration of the anterior cruciate ligament mistaken for ligamentous tears. Skeletal Radiol 30:312-315

88. Bergin D, Morrison WB, Carrino JA et al (2004) Anterior cruciate ligament ganglia and mucoid degeneration: coexistence and clinical correlation. AJR Am J Roentgenol 182:1283-1287

89. Nguyen B, Brandser E, Rubin DA (2000) Pains, strains, and fasciculations: lower extremity muscle disorders. Magn Reson Imaging Clin N Am 8:391-408

90. Khan KM, Bonar F, Desmond PM et al (1996) Patellar tendinosis (jumper's knee): findings at histopathologic examination, US, and MR imaging. Radiology 200:821-827

91. Shalaby M, Almekinders LC (1999) Patellar tendinitis: the significance of magnetic resonance imaging findings. Am J Sports Med 27:345-349

92. Zeiss J, Saddemi SR, Ebraheim NA (1992) MR imaging of the quadriceps tendon: normal layered configuration and its importance in cases of tendon rupture. AJR Am J Roentgenol 159:1031-1034

93. Carotti M, Salaffi F, Manganelli P et al (2002) Power Doppler sonography in the assessment of synovial tissue of the knee joint in rheumatoid arthritis: a preliminary experience. Ann Rheum Dis 61:877-882

94. Adam G, Dammer M, Bohndorf K et al (1991) Rheumatoid arthritis of the knee: value of gadopentetate dimeglumine-enhanced MR imaging. AJR Am J Roentgenol 156:125-129

95. Crotty JM, Monu JU, Pope TL Jr (1996) Synovial osteochondromatosis. Radiol Clin North Am 34:327-342

96. Lin J, Jacobson JA, Jamadar DA et al (1999) Pigmented villonodular synovitis and related lesions: the spectrum of imaging findings. AJR Am J Roentgenol 172:191-197

Ankle and Foot

George Y. El-Khoury[1], Jeremy J. Kaye[2]

[1] Division of Diagnostic Radiology – Musculoskeletal, Department of Radiology, University of Iowa, Iowa City, IA, USA
[2] Department of Radiology & Radiological Sciences, Vanderbilt University Medical Center, Nashville, TN, USA

Tendon Abnormalities

Anatomy, Function and Pathophysiology

The tendon is a densely packed connective tissue structure consisting of type I collagen fibrils embedded in a matrix of proteoglycans. Tendons are relatively hypovascular but the predominant cell is the fibroblast, or tenocyte. Tenocytes are responsible for producing and maintaining a healthy matrix. Collagen fibrils are arranged in closely packed bundles to form fascicles. Tendons that move in a straight line, such as the Achilles tendon, are surrounded by loose areolar connective tissue called the "paratenon". The paratenon is usually not visible on imaging studies unless it is surrounded by fluid on both sides. Tendons that bend sharply around corners, such as the long flexors of the foot, are subject to compressive forces and are enclosed by a tendon sheath. Tendons sheaths are lubricated by synovial fluid in order to reduce friction [1, 2].

Tendons transmit forces from muscles to bone across joints and can withstand large tensile forces. Regular exercise exerts positive, long-term effects on the structural and mechanical properties of the tendon by stimulating the synthesis of collagen fibrils. Tendons that are involved with locomotion, such as the Achilles tendon, show elastic properties. Tendons that transmit large loads under eccentric or elastic conditions are more subject to injury. Stretching a tendon to >8% of its length results in acute tear [3].

Tendons respond to stress either physiologically, by a regenerative response, or pathologically, by a degenerative response. Tissue produced during a regenerative response is structurally and functionally identical to normal tissue, whereas tissue produced during a degenerative response is of lower structural and functional quality. In the degenerative response, matrix cells are overwhelmed by the injury and unable to repair the matrix. Inadequate matrix synthesis leads to tendon degeneration, or tendinosis (tendinopathy). If the injurious activity continues, gross structural abnormalities develop in the form of partial and complete tendon tears. In the ankle and foot, the Achilles, posterior tibial, and peroneal tendons are the most commonly affected [4].

Imaging of Tendon Abnormalities

The term "paratenonitis" is used, in tendons that have a straight course, to describe inflammation of the paratenon resulting from friction [2]. On magnetic resonance imaging (MRI), there is edema of the areolar tissue around the tendon (Fig. 1). In tendons that have a tendon sheath, "tenosynovitis presents as excessive fluid within the tendon sheath [2]. With chronic tenosynovitis, as in rheumatoid arthritis, there may also be synovial proliferation. Small amounts of fluid are often seen within tendon sheaths around the ankle in asymptomatic individuals. This finding is particularly common with the flexor hallucis longus and it should be considered as a normal finding [5]. Normal ankle tendons are seen as low signal intensity structures on all MRI sequences. T2-weighted images best demonstrate abnormalities within tendons as areas of increased signal intensity [6].

Tendinosis (tendinopathy) is intratendinous degeneration that can be painful or asymptomatic. Clinically, a nodule or swelling can be palpated [1, 2]; on MRI, there is fusiform tendon thickening with or without a change in signal intensity on T2-weighted images (Fig. 2) [6].

In *partial tears*, there is underlying tendinosis and splitting of the collagen bundles. Tendon attenuation is sometimes present [1, 2]. On MRI, there is thickening of the tendon along with a linear increased signal on T2-weighted images due to splitting of the collagen bundles [6]. Affected tendons can also show fluid within the tendon sheath.

Clinically, a *complete tear* presents as a loss of function of the muscle attached to the disrupted tendon [1]. On MRI, the abnormality depends on the duration of the tear. Acute tears show tendon discontinuity, bleeding, and edema in the surrounding soft tissues. Chronic disruption manifests as retraction and thickening of the disrupted ends of the tendon. An empty tendon sheath on MRI is a definitive sign of a tendon tear.

The *Achilles tendon* is the largest tendon in the body, measuring 4-6 mm in thickness. On axial sections the tendon is curved gently, with the concavity facing anteriorly. Paratenonitis is particularly common in runners and patients typically complain of pain and crepitus. On MRI,

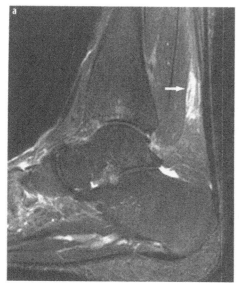

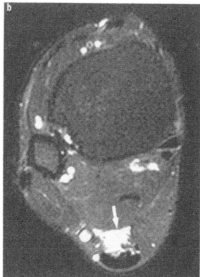

Fig. 1 a, b. Paratenonitis of the Achilles tendon in a 24 year old athlete. **a** Sagittal T2-weighted fat-suppressed image shows edema in the soft tissue anterior to the tendon (*white arrow*). **b** Axial T2-weighted fat-suppressed images shows similar findings (*white arrow*)

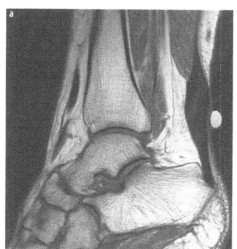

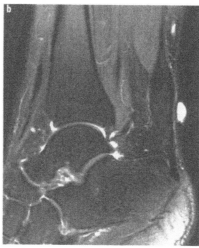

Fig. 2 a, b. Tendinosis (tendinopathy) of the Achilles tendon in a 45-year-old marathon runner. **a** T1-weighted sagittal image shows fusiform thickening of the Achilles tendon. **b** T2-weighted fat-suppressed sagittal image shows the thickened tendon but without increased signal intensity within the tendon

there is edema around the tendon but no change in size and no signal abnormalities within the tendon. Achilles tendon tendinosis is caused by cyclical loading and overuse. Long-term use of fluoroquinolone antibiotics are known to be toxic to the tenocytes and therefore predispose tendons to tendinosis and rupture. Two forms of tendinosis occur in the Achilles tendon: insertional, in which the abnormality occurs at the insertion of the tendon to the calcaneal tuberosity (Fig. 3), and non-insertional, in which the abnormality is centered 2-6 cm above the insertion of the tendon [7]. On MRI, tendinopathy shows fusiform thickening, typically without significant signal abnormalities [8]. Partial tears show tendon thickening and increased signal intensity within the substance of the tendon, especially on T2-weighted images.

Complete tear is a disabling condition and can be acute or chronic. Acute tears typically occur in sedentary middle-aged men engaged in episodic overactivity and result from forceful dorsiflexion of the foot. On MRI, acute tears show discontinuity in the tendon, edema, and hemorrhage [8, 9]. With chronic tears, a history of significant trauma is lacking. There is discontinuity of the tendon but no edema or hemorrhage.

The *posterior tibial tendon* (PTT) passes directly behind the medial malleolus and inserts primarily on the navicular tuberosity. It functions as the main inverter of subtalar joint and elevates the medial arch of the foot. A constellation of clinical signs are noted with PTT dysfunction, including ankle pain, instability, and foot deformity. As a result, the longitudinal arch of the foot col-

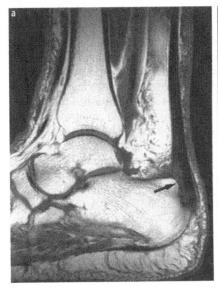
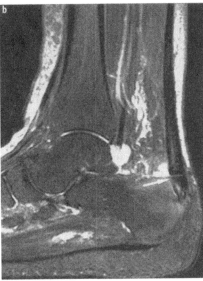

Fig. 3 a, b. Insertional tendinopathy of the Achilles tendon in a middle-age woman complaining of pain in her heel. **a** T1-weighted sagittal image showing thickening of the Achilles tendon at its insertion to the calcaneal tuberosity (*black arrow*). **b** T2-weighted fat-suppressed sagittal image shows thickening of the Achilles tendon at its insertion, small areas of increased signal intensity (*white arrow*), and fluid in the pre-Achellar bursa

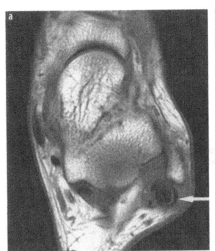
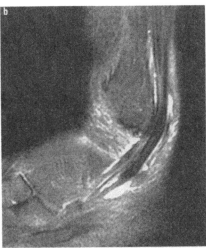

Fig. 4 a, b. Partial tears of the peroneal tendons in a 40-year-old male whose chief complaint at presentation was pain and swelling behind the lateral malleolus. **a** Axial T1-weighted image shows flattening of the peroneus brevis (*white arrow*) and thickening of the peroneus longus. **b** Sagittal T2-weighted fat-suppressed image through the lateral malleolus shows thickening and splitting of the peroneal tendons and fluid in the tendon sheath

lapses, the subtalar joint everts, the heel assumes a valgus position, and the foot abducts, producing what is known as "acquired flatfoot" [10]. Stretching or disruption of the spring, deltoid, and talocalcaneal interosseous ligaments are also implicated in acquired flatfoot. PTT dysfunction usually occurs in middle-aged obese women. PTT tendon tears typically start behind the medial malleolus as a result of shear forces. On MRI, tendinosis and partial tears show increased tendon girth, splitting, and increased signal intensity, best seen on T2-weighted images. With complete tears, the tendon sheath fills with fluid, but no tendon is identified [11, 12].

At the ankle, the *peroneal tendons* course in the fibular groove, with the peroneus brevis tendon being sandwiched between the lateral malleolus and the peroneus longus ten-

don. The peroneal tendons function as lateral stabilizers of the ankle; they also pronate and abduct the foot. On axial MRI, mild to moderate flattening or a crescentic appearance of the peroneus brevis tendon at the distal fibula is considered normal. Complete tears are uncommon; instead, tendinosis and partial tears are more frequently seen (Fig. 4) [13, 14]. Occasionally, tendon attenuation is present. The peroneus brevis in more commonly involved with tears, but often both tendons are involved. Acute peroneus longus tendon tear, at the level of the os peroneus, can occur during vigorous athletic activity. This injury is diagnosed when an acute fracture of the os peroneus is detected with distraction of the fracture fragments. Subluxation and dislocation of the peroneal tendons are commonly associated with severe calcaneal fractures. Whenever these fractures are evaluated by computed tomography (CT), attention should be paid to the position of the peroneal tendon [15]. With dislocation these tendons slip out of their normal position behind the lateral malleolus to a more anterior position along side of the malleolus.

Arthritis

All common forms of arthritis affect the ankle and foot. Most arthritides are typically diagnosed and followed on plain radiographs. *Rheumatoid arthritis* frequently involves the ankles and feet, with radiographic findings revealing periarticular soft-tissue swelling and osteopenia, marginal erosions and uniform narrowing of the joint space (Fig. 5). There is evidence in the literature that in early rheumatoid arthritis, gadolinium-enhanced MRI and ultrasound can be affective in detecting small erosions and synovial inflammation not detected by plain radiographs [16]. *Post-traumatic (secondary) osteoarthritis* of the ankle and *primary osteoarthritis* of the first metatarsophalangeal joint in the foot (hallux rigidus) are fairly common. *Calcium pyrophosphate deposition disease (CPPD)* is the most common form of crystal-induced arthropathy. Degenerative-like changes in the talonavicular joint suggest the diagnosis of CPPD. The most common site for *gout* is the foot, especially the first metatarsophalangeal joint. When tophi enlarge, they erode the para-articular bone, producing sharp, punched-out erosions with well-defined cortical margins and overhanging edges. *Reactive arthritis (Reiter's disease)* has a predilection for the peripheral joints in the lower extremities, especially the knees, ankles, and feet. The most common site of involvement in Reiter's disease is the feet, particularly the calcaneus and metatarsophalangeal joint. Enthesitis at the insertion of the Achilles tendon and origin of the plantar fascia on the calcaneus are characteristic of reactive arthritis. There is also a tendency for destructive arthritis of the small joints in the feet.

Charcot arthropathy (neuropathic arthropathy) is a destructive arthropathy most commonly seen in patients with diabetes mellitus. It is caused by diminished pain sensation and proprioception, which leave the joint without protection from repeated microtrauma. The foot and ankle are the most common sites of neuropathic arthropathy in diabetic patients. In order of frequency, the tarsometatarsal, metatarsophalangeal, and ankle joints are most frequently involved. The majority of neuropathic joints begin with a fracture or fracture dislocation (Fig. 6). Avulsion fracture

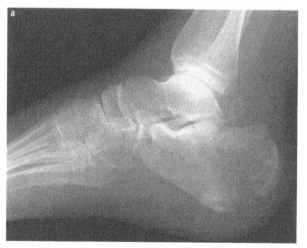

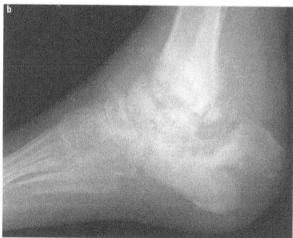

Fig. 6 a, b. A 48-year-old diabetic male who presented with swelling in the heal after a minor fall. **a** Lateral view of the foot shows an avulsion fracture with superior displacement of the calcaneal tuberosity. **b** Lateral view of the foot obtained 2 months after the initial study reveals marked bony fragmentation and disorganization of the ankle and subtalar joints. These findings are typical of Charot arthropathy

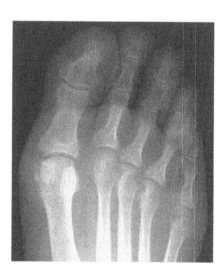

Fig. 5. A 42-year-old female diagnosed with rheumatoid arthritis 2 years earlier. AP view of the left foot shows multiple erosions in the 1st, 3rd, 4th, and 5th metatarsal heads. Small erosions are also seen in some of the phalanges

of the calcaneal tuberosity is almost pathognomonic of diabetes mellitus [17]. Fracture dislocation of Lisfranc's joint is one of the most common fractures in the Charcot foot. Neuropathic joint changes are best studied with radiography.

Radiographically, there are two types of neuropathic arthropathy: hypertrophic and atrophic. The hypertrophic type is much more common, especially in the weight-bearing joints. It shows marked disorganization, fragmentation, sclerosis, and large osteophyte formation. The atrophic type is occasionally seen, especially in the metacarpophalangeal joints. Radiographically, there is excessive bone resorption but without fragmentation, sclerosis, or large osteophytes.

Trauma

Acute trauma is fairly common in the ankle and foot, and to discuss it at all is beyond the scope of this chapter. The discussion is limited to two common albeit diagnostically challenging injuries: stress fractures and Lisfranc's (second tarsometatarsal) injuries.

Stress fractures can be classified into three types: *stress reactions, fatigue fractures, and insufficiency fractures.* A stress reaction occurs when microfractures are healing and bone is remodeling but, radiographically, a complete fracture has not yet developed. A fatigue fracture is caused by prolonged cyclical loading of healthy bone. Activities producing fatigue fractures include running, marching, and dancing. Insufficiency fractures typically occur during normal activities but in weakened bones that are deficient in mineral or elastic resistance. The second, third, and fifth metatarsals, as well as the tarsal navicular and calcaneus are the most common sites for stress fractures [18].

Radiography may be initially normal, but with time a fracture line, periosteal reaction, and callus formation develop. Only one cortex may be involved. As more callus accumulates, there is fusiform expansion of the cortex. Occasionally, more than one stress fracture is present in a foot. In the tarsal navicular, stress fractures are oriented in the sagittal plane and occur in the central third of the bone. These fractures start as incomplete fractures involving the dorsal aspect of the tarsal navicular but with time they become complete fractures extending from the dorsal to the plantar surface of the bone. In high-powered athletes, CT and MRI are effective imaging techniques if radiography is negative and there is a high suspicion of a stress fracture [19] (Fig. 7). For detecting early stress fractures, bone scanning and ultrasound may also be helpful.

Foot and ankle injuries are common in athletes, accounting for about 16% of all sports injuries. *Lisfranc's (tarsometatarsal) injuries* in athletes tend to have subtle clinical and radiographic findings and a high index of suspicion is necessary for their diagnosis [20]. When suspected, weight-bearing radiographs of the foot

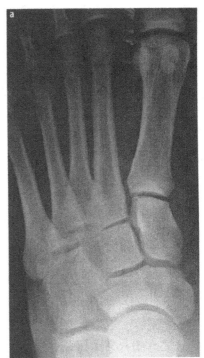

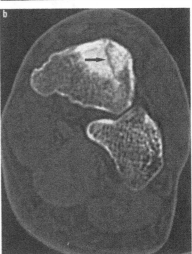

Fig. 7 a, b. Stress fracture of the tarsal navicular in an 18-year-old basketball player, who presented with pain at the medial aspect of the mid-foot of 2 weeks duration. **a** AP view of the foot showed no fracture or dislocation. **b** One month after the initial presentation, a CT scan was performed. Axial CT section through the navicular bone reveals an incomplete fracture line (*black arrow*) starting at the dorsal aspect of the navicular bone

should be obtained. Normally, the medial border of the second metatarsal aligns with the medial border of the middle cuneiform on the amteroposterior view, and the medial border of the fourth metatarsal should align with the medial border of the cuboid on the oblique view of the foot. A difference between the two feet of >2 mm in the distance between the bases of the first and second

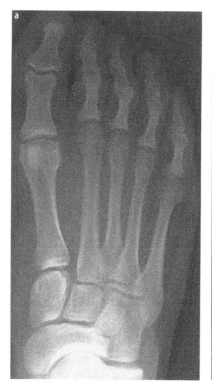
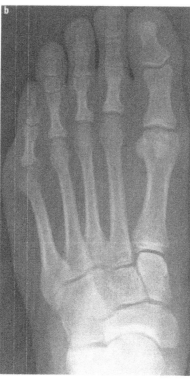

Fig. 8 a, b. Low-energy Lisfranc's injury of the left foot in a 21-year-old male athlete. **a** AP view of the left foot shows increased distance between the bases of the first and second metatarsal bones (4 mm). **b** AP view of the right foot taken for comparison shows normal relationships between the first and second metatarsals

metatarsals should raise the suspicion of a Lisfranc's injury (Fig. 8). The fleck-sign is diagnostic and consists of a small fracture fragment arising from either the lateral edge of the medial cuneiform or the medial aspect of the second metatarsal base. These fragments are the points of attachment of the Lisfranc's (tarsometatarsal) ligament, the strongest in the tarsometatarsal complex. It runs obliquely from the medial cuneiform to the plantar base of the second metatarsal [20].

Morton's Neuroma

Morton's neuroma is a non-neoplastic, perineural, fibrous proliferation involving a plantar digital nerve. It usually occurs in middle-age females. Clinical symptoms include pain and burning in the planter aspect of the forefoot. The neuroma usually occurs between the third and fourth metatarsal heads or, less frequently, between the second and third metatarsal heads. Some investigators have used MRI on normal volunteers to show that asymptomatic Morton's neuromas are fairly common. For that reason, the diagnosis of Morton's neuroma with MRI becomes relevant only when the transverse diameter of the neuroma exceeds 5 mm and its presence correlates with the clinical symptoms [21]. The lesion can be difficult to visualize on MRI, usually appearing as low signal intensity on T1- and T2-weight-

ed images. It shows moderate to marked enhancement after gadolinium administration. High-resolution ultrasonography can be very effective in diagnosing Morton's neuroma.

Plantar Fasciitis

The plantar aponeurosis consists of the medial, central, and lateral bands. The central band is also called the plantar fascia and it is the thickest and strongest component [22]. The plantar fascia originates from the medial calcaneal tuberosity. It aids in the toe-off portion of the gait and in maintaining the longitudinal arch of the foot. Plantar fasciitis is the most common cause of plantar heel pain. It can result from a number of causes, which fall into three major categories: mechanical, degenerative, and systemic [23]. Plantar fasciitis is common in obese patients and those who have flat feet. The mechanism is thought to be due to a chronic traction type injury which occurs in isolation or as a manifestation of a systemic disease, such as seronegative spondyloarthropathies, rheumatoid arthritis, gout, or systemic lupus erythematosus. In athletes, plantar fasciitis typically produces foot pain as well as fascial and perifascial inflammation. The condition is attributed to mechanical stresses – with repetitive trauma creating microtearing of the plantar fascia at its origin.

Diagnosis is usually made on clinical grounds and imaging is rarely needed. Plain radiographs are often not helpful but often obtained to rule out other conditions. MRI findings include thickening of the plantar fascia at its origin. with thickness >5 mm. There is increased signal intensity on T2-weighted images in the involved segment of the plantar fascia as well as inflammation in the adjacent soft tissues. Marrow edema in the plantar calcaneal spur can also be seen. Ultrasound has also been shown to be effective in diagnosing plantar fasciitis [24].

Tarsal Coalition

Tarsal coalition is a congenital disease in which the diagnosis is often overlooked in young patients who present with foot pain. This condition is believed to result from failure of segmentation of the primitive mesenchyme of the foot. Tarsal coalition manifests by abnormal bridging across two or more tarsal bones, but it is most commonly seen between the calcaneus and tarsal navicular or talus and calcaneus [25]. Tarsal coalition is frequently associated with spastic flatfoot, and symptoms typically appear in the teens and 20s. In most patients (90%), tarsal coalition occurs either at the middle facets of the subtalar joint or between the anterior process of the calcaneus and lateral aspect of the navicular. The prevalence of these two types is almost equal [26]. Radiographically, calcaneonavicuar coalitions can be identified consistently on an oblique view of the foot. The anterior process of the calcaneus is elongated as it extends to connect with the lateral aspect of the navicular. A secondary radiographic sign is hypoplasia of the talar head. Reossification after surgical resection of the coalition is a well-known complication. Coalitions at the middle facets of the subtalar joint can be imaged directly using the axial (Harris) view of the foot, or an oblique view of the subtalar joint of the hind foot, also known as Broden view, or by CT. Bony coalitions consist of a solid bony bridge connecting the talus and calcaneus at the sustentaculum tali. Cartilaginous and fibrous coalitions can be difficult to differentiate on imaging studies; thus, the term "fibrocartilagnous coalition" is sometimes used. Both cartilaginous and fibrous coalition show narrowing of the middle subtalar joint, with irregularity and sclerosis at the articular surfaces. Indirect radiographic signs of subtalar coalition include talar beaking [27], positive C-sign, flattening and broadening of the lateral talar process, and narrowing of the posterior talocalcaneal joint. Water-sensitive MRI sequences have been used in diagnosing tarsal coalition; they reveal bone-marrow edema at the margin of the abnormal articulation.

Tarsal Tunnel Syndrome

The tarsal tunnel is located deep to the flexor retinaculum and posterior and inferior to the medial malleolus. It contains the posterior tibial nerve, the tibialis posterior, flexor digitorum longus, and flexor hallucis longus tendons, along with the posterior tibial artery and vein [28]. Within the tarsal tunnel, the posterior tibial nerve courses distally between the flexor hallucis longus and flexor digitorum longus tendons. The posterior tibial nerve divides within the tarsal tunnel into three branches: (1) the medial calcaneal nerve, which can be the first branch of the posterior tibial nerve or can arise as a branch of the lateral plantar nerve, (2) the lateral plantar nerve, and (3) the medial plantar nerve, which is the largest branch of the posterior tibial nerve.

Tarsal tunnel syndrome is an entrapment neuropathy of the posterior tibial nerve or one of its branches. Patients typically complain of poorly localized, burning pain and paresthesias along the plantar surface of the foot and toes. The etiologies of tarsal tunnel syndrome include varicosities, trauma, fibrosis, accessory muscles, ganglion cysts, lipoma, and nerve sheath tumors. Such lesions are best visualized using MRI. Radiography is useful to rule out other abnormalities, such as fractures or osteophytes, that can occasionally cause tarsal tunnel syndrome. Ultrasound is helpful in diagnosing a mass lesion in the tarsal tunnel.

Impingement Syndromes of the Ankle

These syndromes have been recently described in the radiology literature and radiologists are becoming increasingly aware of them as a cause for chronic ankle pain. The three main impingement syndromes of the ankle are the *anterolateral, anterior* and *posterior impingement*. The diagnosis is often made on a clinical basis, and imaging beyond plain radiography is rarely required [29]. The leading causes of ankle impingement syndromes are post-traumatic injuries, usually sprains.

Anterolateral impingement syndrome is produced by entrapment of abnormal soft tissue in the anterolateral recess (or gutter) of the ankle [30]. The anterolateral recess is bounded posteromedially by the distal tibia and laterally by the lateral malleolus. Anteriorly it is bounded by the capsule of the distal tibiofibular joint, the anterior tibiofibular, anterior talofibular, and calcaneofibular ligaments. Symptoms include anterolateral pain in the ankle aggravated by supination or pronation of the foot. If advanced imaging is requested by the foot surgeon, magnetic resonance arthrography (MRA) has been shown to be reliable in demonstrating irregular or nodular contour of the soft tissues in the anterolaeral recess, although this finding in itself does not imply the presence of anterolateral impingement syndrome. Normal MRA findings, however, seem to exclude anterolateral synovial scarring [29].

Anterior impingement syndrome is characterized by anterior tibiotalar spurs that develop at the margin of the articular cartilage [29]. Imaging with plain radiography

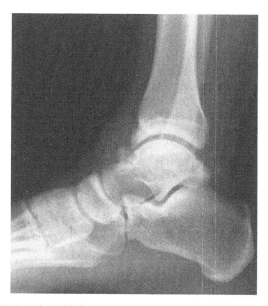

Fig. 9. Anterior ankle impingement syndrome in a 32-year-old athlete. The patient had ankle pain and limited dorsiflexion of the foot. Lateral view shows large osteophytes at the ankle joint anteriorly and possibly loose bodies within the joint

should be sufficient for showing these spurs (Fig. 9). The abnormality is common in ballet dancers and soccer players.

Posterior impingement is known by other names, such os trignom syndrome and talar compression syndrome. Common causes include the presence of an os trigonum, elongated lateral tubercle of the talus (Stieda process), and downward sloping of the posterior lip of the tibia. On MRI, bone edema in the lateral talar tubercle, os trigonum, as well as posterior ankle synovitis and tenosynovitis of the flexor hallucis longus tendon sheath suggest the diagnosis of posterior ankle impingement [30].

References

1. Teitz CC, Garrett WE Jr, Miniaci A, Mann RA (1997) Tendon problems in athletic individuals. J Bone Joint Surg 79-A(1):138-152
2. Lutter LD, Mizel MS, Pfeffer GB (1994) Tendon problems of the foot and ankle. In: Lutter LD, Mizel MS, Pfeffer GB (eds) Foot and ankle. American Academy of Orthopaedic Surgeons, Rosemont, Illinois, pp 269-282
3. O'Brien M (1992) Functional anatomy and physiology of tendons. Clin Sports Med 11(3):505-520
4. Leadbetter WB (1992) Cell-matrix response in tendon injury. Clin Sports Med 11(3):533-578
5. Schweitzer ME, van Leersum M, Ehrlich SS, Wapner K (1994) Fluid in normal and abnormal ankle joints: Amount and distribution as seen on MR images. AJR Am J Roentgenol 162:111-114
6. Campbell RSD, Grainger AJ (2001) Current concepts in imaging of tendinopathy. Clin Radiol 56:253-267
7. Myerson MS, McGarvey W (1998) Disorders of the insertion of the Achilles tendon and Achilles tendinitis. J Bone Joint Surg 80-A(12):1814-1824
8. Karjalaninen PT, Soila K, Aronen HJ et al (2000) MR imaging of overuse injuries of the Achilles tendon. AJR Am J Roentgenol 175:251-260
9. Quinn SF, Murray WT, Clark RA, Cochran CF (1987) Achilles tendon: MR imaging at 1.5 T. Radiology 164:767-770
10. Karasick D, Schweitzer ME (1993) Tear of the posterior tibial tendon causing asymmetric flatfoot: radiologic findings. AJR Am J Roentgenol 161:1237-1240
11. Khoury NJ, El-Khoury GY, Saltzman CL, Brandser EA (1996) MR imaging of posterior tibial tendon dysfunction. AJR Am J Roentgenol 167:675-682
12. Schweitzer ME, Caccese R, Karasick D et al (1993) Posterior tibial tendon tears: utility of secondary signs for MR imaging diagnosis. Radiology 188:655-659
13. Rosenberg ZS, Beltran J, Cheung YY et al (1997) MR features of longitudinal tears of the peroneus brevis tendon. AJR Am J Roentgenol 168:141-147
14. Khoury N, El-Khoury GY, Saltzman CL, Kathol MH (1996) Peroneus longus and brevis tendon tears: MR imaging evaluation. Radiology 200:833-841
15. Ohashi K, Restrepo JM, El-Khoury GY, Berbaum KS (2007) Peroneal tendon subluxation and dislocation: detection on volume-rendered images – initial experience. Radiology 242(1):252-257
16. Ostendorf B, Scherer A, Modder U, Schneider M (2004) Diagnostic value of magnetic resonance imaging of the forefeet in early rheumatoid arthritis when finding on imaging of the metacarpophalangeal joints of the hands remain normal. Arthritis Rheum 50:2094-2102
17. El-Khoury GY, Kathol MH (1980) Neuropathic fractures in patients with diabetes mellitus. Radiology 134:313-316
18. Greaney RB, Gerber FH, Laughlin RL et al (1983) Distribution and natural history of stress fractures in U.S. Marine recruits. Radiology 146:339-346
19. Kiss ZS, Khan KM, Fuller PJ (1993) Stress fractures of the tarsal navicular bone: CT findings in 55 cases. AJR Am J Roentgenol 160:111-115
20. Myerson MS, Cerrato RA (2008) Current management of tarsometatarsal injuries in the athlete. J Bone Joint Surg 90-A(11):2522-2533
21. Zanetti M, Ledermann T, Holder J (1997) Efficacy of MR imaging in patients suspected of having Morton's neuroma. AJR Am J Roentgenol 168:529-532
22. Grasel RP, Schweitzer ME, Kovalovich AM et al (1999) MR imaging of plantar fasciitis: Edema, tears, and occult marrow abnormalities correlated with outcome. AJR Am J Roentgenol 173:699-701
23. Theodorou DJ, Theodorou SJ, Kakitsubata Y et al (2000) Plantar fasciitis and fascial rupture: MR imaging findings in 26 patients supplemented with anatomic data in cadavers. RadioGraphics 20:S181-S197
24. Cardinal E, Chhem RK, Beauregard CG et al (1996) Plantar fasciitis: sonographic evaluation. Radiology 201:257-259
25. Newman JS, Newberg AH (2000) Congenital tarsal coalition: Multimodality evaluation with emphasis on CT and MR imaging. RadioGraphics 20:321-332
26. Kumar SJ, Guille JT, Lee MS, Couto JC (1992) Osseous and non-osseous coalition of the middle facet of the talocalcaneal joint. J Bone Joint Surg 74-A(4):529-535
27. Crim JR, Kjeldsberg KM (2004) Radiographic diagnosis of tarsal coalition. AJR 182:323-328
28. Erickson SJ, Quinn SF, Kneeland JB et al (1990) MR imaging of the tarsal tunnel and related spaces: Normal and abnormal findings with anatomic correlation. AJR Am J Roentgenol 155:323-328
29. Robinson P, White LM (2002) Soft-tissue and osseous impingement syndromes of the ankle: Role of imaging in diagnosis and management. RadioGraphics 22:1457-1471
30. Cerezal L, Abascal F, Canga A et al (2003) MR Imaging of ankle impingement syndromes. AJR Am J Roentgenol 181:551-559

Magnetic Resonance Imaging of Muscle

Mini N. Pathria[1], Robert D. Boutin[2]

[1] Department of Radiology, UCSD School of Medicine, San Diego, CA, USA
[2] Department of Radiology, Medical Resources Inc., Davis, CA, USA

Learning Objectives

At the end of this presentation, readers should be able to:
- Identify the normal imaging features of skeletal muscle on magnetic resonance imaging (MRI).
- Recognize that some muscle abnormalities do not produce signal alterations.
- Recognize the common patterns of muscle inflammation.
- Know the most common classification system used for muscle injury.
- Understand the evolution of hemorrhage in muscle tissues.

Normal Muscle

The MRI appearance of normal skeletal muscle is the result of the latter's admixture of muscle fibers and fat. Normal skeletal muscle shows a "striated" and "feathery" appearance, produced by the presence of high-signal fat interlaced within and between the major muscle bundles. Normal muscle is of low signal intensity on all sequences and of decreases in signal on T2-weighted images. The exterior surfaces of the muscle are smooth and typically show a mild convexity. An important anatomic region of the muscle is its myotendinous junction, where muscle fibers interdigitate with the tendon. The myotendinous junction is located at a variable distance from the site of tendon insertion.

Four common patterns of abnormal muscle are visualized with MRI: (1) muscle with abnormal morphology with normal signal; (2) mass within the muscle; (3) muscle atrophy; (4) muscle edema

Abnormal Morphology with Normal Signal

This pattern is most commonly caused by an accessory muscle, a congenital abnormality in which an anomalous extra muscle is present. The accessory muscle may be asymptomatic or present either as a palpable mass due to its effect on adjacent structures, such as nerve compression that results in denervation. Most accessory muscles are identified around the hand and foot (Fig. 1). The best-known accessory muscle is the accessory soleus, seen in the pre-Achilles fat pad. This muscle can be very large and is usually felt by the patient. Other common accessory muscles include the peroneus quartus muscle, located behind the fibula; the accessory anconeus epitrochlearis; the accessory abductor digiti minimi, in the wrist; and the anomalous lumbrical muscle, in the carpal tunnel.

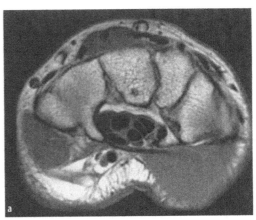

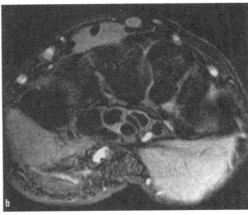

Fig. 1 a, b. Accessory muscle. This middle-aged man palpated a mass on the dorsum of his wrist. Axial T1-weighted magnetic resonance imaging (MRI) of the wrist (**a**) shows an accessory extensor digitorum manus muscle. The mass remains isointense to normal muscle on the axial T2-weighted image (**b**)

Intramuscular Mass

In this case there is a focal mass within the muscle, due to primary or secondary neoplasms or as part of a large group of non-neoplastic disorders. Metastatic disease within the muscle is relatively rare and is seen most frequently with advanced disease. The most common location for intramuscular metastasis is the paraspinal and retroperitoneal musculature (Fig. 2). Several different primary neoplasms can arise in the muscle. Common benign intramuscular neoplasms include lipoma and hemangioma. Primary intramuscular malignancies can arise from a host of tissues and include liposarcoma, malignant fibrous histiocytoma, and rhabdomyosarcoma. Non-neoplastic masses within the muscle include hematoma, abscess, myositis ossificans (see below), and inflammatory pseudotumors of muscle.

Muscle Atrophy

Muscle atrophy is the result or end stage of many muscle abnormalities, and thus is only a finding, not a diagnosis. It reflects numerous disorders that result in a loss of muscle volume and/or increased fatty infiltration of the muscle substance. Spectroscopy is more sensitive than conventional MRI for the detection of early muscle atrophy. Chronic disuse, denervation, and myopathies are the most common causes seen in clinical practice. Atrophy is generally considered irreversible.

Congenital Myopathies

Congenital myopathies result in symmetrical muscle atrophy involving multiple muscles, with a predilection in most forms for axial and truncal involvement. There are numerous forms of muscular dystrophy, with Duchenne and Becker muscular dystrophy being the most common. These typically present in childhood or adolescence as progressive proximal muscle weakness. Numerous metabolic myopathies have also been described, typically related to mitochondrial dysfunction or defects in energy metabolism. In the acute phase of muscle damage, symmetrical mild hyperintensity of the muscles can be seen. Unlike inflammatory myopathies, the subcutaneous tissues remain normal. More advanced disease typically shows pseudohypertrophy of lower-extremity muscles, particularly the calf musculature, due to excessive fatty infiltration. Ultimately, severe fatty atrophy of the muscle develops (Fig. 3).

Denervation

Muscle denervation also results in muscle atrophy, but the distribution of involvement is limited to muscles innervated by a single nerve. Acutely denervated muscle shows a paucity of findings on MRI, with signal alterations usually seen several weeks following loss of neural innervation. In subacute denervation, the denervated muscle shows high signal on T2-weighted and inversion-recovery sequences. Typically, the size of the muscle remains normal or is slightly diminished due to concomitant atrophy (Fig. 4). In chronic denervation, the muscle edema resolves, and the involved muscles undergo volume loss and fatty atrophy. The presence of fatty change implies an irreversible lesion. Clinical history and the distribution of the muscle abnormalities, which correspond to a specific nerve distribution, allow accurate diagnosis of muscle denervation.

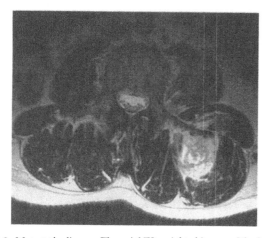

Fig. 2. Metastatic disease. The axial T2-weighted image of the lumbar spine in a patient with renal cell carcinoma shows an inhomogeneous high-signal mass in the left paraspinal musculature. Biopsy revealed that the mass represented metastatic disease

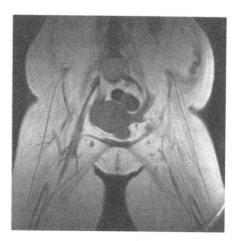

Fig. 3. Muscular dystrophy. A coronal T1-weighted image of the pelvis shows profound diffuse muscle atrophy with fatty infiltration of the muscle due to long-standing Duchenne muscular dystrophy

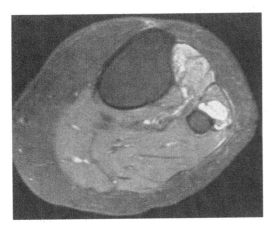

Fig. 4. Peroneal nerve denervation. An axial fat-suppressed proton-density-weighted image of the proximal calf shows a ganglion adjacent to the proximal tibiofibular joint. Due to compression of the peroneal nerve, denervation changes are apparent in the tibialis anterior muscle

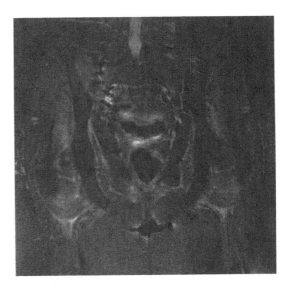

Fig. 5. Myositis. Coronal T2-weighted fat-suppressed image of the pelvis in an elderly man with myositis due to lipid-lowering statin drug therapy shows symmetric feathery muscle edema in the buttock, particularly in the quadratus femoris. There is also mild subcutaneous edema. Note the preservation of the normal muscle architecture

Muscle Edema

Muscle edema is the most common abnormality encountered in clinical practice. Diagnosis depends on assessment of the distribution of muscle abnormality, the specific distribution of signal alterations within the muscle, and evaluation of the adjacent tissues. History and biopsy are frequently necessary to establish a specific diagnosis. Common causes of muscle edema include inflammatory myositis, infection, and muscle injury.

Inflammatory Myositis

The numerous etiologies of inflammatory myositis include the classic autoimmune inflammatory myopathy autoimmune polymyositis. When associated with skin changes, the same syndrome is called dermatomyositis. Numerous other forms of autoimmune muscle inflammation are recognized. Inclusion body myositis is commonly seen in older patients and has milder clinical and MRI manifestations. The autoimmune muscle disorders produce symmetrical muscle weakness that primarily involves the proximal muscles. On MRI, widespread symmetrical muscle inflammation is the most prominent finding. The inflamed muscles are edematous but show preservation of normal muscle architecture. Associated skin and fascial edema are common.

Autoimmune myositis can also be seen in association with collagen vascular diseases, such as rheumatoid arthritis and systemic lupus erythematosus. Myositis is more often unilateral or asymmetrical in its association with collagen vascular disease than with idiopathic polymyositis. Nodular forms are also recognized. Other causes of myositis include drug reactions, particularly to lipid-lowering agents and anti-retroviral drugs; graft-versus-host disease; and paraneoplastic syndromes (Fig. 5).

Pyomyositis

This condition refers to an infiltrative deep infection of muscle, often associated with abscess formation. Nontropical pyomyositis is recognized with increasing frequency in adult patients with diabetes, AIDS, and immunosuppression. While pain is a constant symptom finding, muscle weakness is unusual. The most common causative organism is *Staphylococcus aureus*, which is responsible for 90% of cases.

Pyomyositis is typically limited to one muscle group. Involvement of the lower extremity, particularly the thigh, predominates. The muscle is typically edematous and partly necrotic. Adjacent soft-tissue inflammation may be present, but subcutaneous inflammatory changes are minimal compared to those seen in patients with cellulitis or fasciitis and are disproportionately less prominent than the muscular abnormalities. The underlying bony cortex and bone marrow are typically not involved.

On T1-weighted MRI, findings are minimal except for subcutaneous edema and mild enlargement of the affected muscles, due to the increased volume of interstitial fluid and fluid collections. The highly proteinaceous material in the center of an abscess may show intermediate signal on T1-weighted images, either diffusely or peripherally. High signal is seen within the muscle on T2-weighted images. Areas of necrosis and abscess formation are frequently seen, optimally following the administration of Gd-DTPA (Fig. 6).

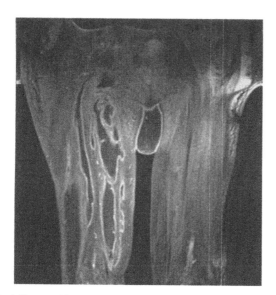

Fig. 6. Pyomyositis. This middle-aged HIV-positive male presented with a swollen painful right thigh and a fever. Gd-DTPA enhanced T1-weighted MRI shows subcutaneous and patchy muscle enhancement throughout the thigh. There are numerous loculated intramuscular abscesses with peripheral enhancement

Muscle Injury

Fascial Herniation

Herniation of muscle through an overlying fascial tear is an uncommon injury that presents as a painful mass. Muscle herniation through fascial tear is very difficult to see with MRI; instead, US is preferred for this diagnosis, because the mass can be examined during dynamic muscle contraction. On MRI, nonspecific contour irregularity of the muscle surface is often the only finding, but this may be subtle when the muscle is at rest. In some cases, the defect in the fascia itself is visible.

DOMS

Exercise can be followed by pain, muscle soreness, and muscle swelling, particularly in the poorly conditioned individual. Muscle pain developing hours or days following exercise has been termed delayed-onset muscle soreness (DOMS). Unlike the acute onset of symptoms with muscle strain, the symptoms of DOMS develop gradually, 1-2 days following exercise, peak 2-3 days following the activity, and then resolve after approximately 1 week. On T1-weighted images, mild enlargement of the muscle may be present. Increased signal is seen on T2-weighted and short tau inversion recovery (STIR) images. The muscle architecture remains preserved, as the edema parallels the muscle fascicles. Signal changes and clinical symptoms are maximal in the region of the myotendinous junction. While clinical symptoms resolve quickly, MRI signal changes of DOMS can persist for up to 80 days.

Laceration and Contusion

A muscle laceration is typically produced by direct trauma, usually a penetrating wound extending into the muscle. Less commonly, muscle can be lacerated by the sharp bone ends of a fracture. The area of the laceration can be seen on MRI as a linear defect in the muscle, filled with blood and fluid but this imaging modality is not frequently used to assess muscle laceration. Muscle injuries related to a single episode of severe trauma are subdivided into muscle strain (discussed below) and muscle contusion, depending on the mechanism of injury. A muscle strain is caused by an indirect injury, whereas a contusion is due to direct concussive trauma with a blunt, non-penetrating object. The muscle alterations of contusion are identical to those seen in high-grade strains but the location of the injury is independent of the myotendinous junction, corresponding instead with the site of impact. Contusions are more likely to be associated with extensive hemorrhage within the muscle.

Muscle Strain

Muscle strains can involve the epimysium or, more commonly, the myotendinous junction of the muscle. The myotendinous junction is vulnerable to injury because it is the structurally weakest region in the myotendinous unit, due to its limited capacity for energy absorption. Muscle strains are most common in the long fusiform muscles of the thigh or calf.

Strains are subdivided clinically into three grades. A grade 1 strain demonstrates normal muscle morphology and only mild abnormalities of muscle signal, particularly in the region of the myotendinous junction (Fig. 7).

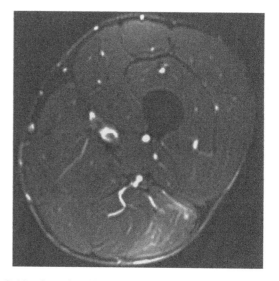

Fig. 7. Muscle strain. This man injured his hamstring during a soccer game. An axial T2-weighted image of the left thigh shows high signal localized around the myotendinous junction of the long head of the biceps femoris, consistent with a low-grade strain

In grade 2 strain, there are signal changes and mild alterations in muscle morphology. T2-weighted images show irregularity, thinning, and mild waviness of the tendon fibers. Muscle edema and hemorrhage are more prominent, often collecting in the subfascial regions around the injured muscle. More significant morphologic alterations are present in grade 3 strain, which represents a complete rupture of the myotendinous junction. Large amounts of hemorrhage may be present, obscuring the anatomy. The diagnosis is obvious if the tendon ends are retracted, producing a gap in the soft tissues at the expected position of the myotendinous junction and allowing the muscle to bunch up away from the region.

Parenchymal Hemorrhage

Hemorrhage within muscle has two different appearances depending on the pattern of bleeding. Hemorrhage dissecting within the muscle stroma, not forming a discrete collection, is known as parenchymal hemorrhage. If the blood pools in a discrete collection, the mass is referred to as a hematoma. Parenchymal hemorrhage and hematoma coexist in most cases involving extensive bleeding. Parenchymal hemorrhage does not have a brain correlate so its appearance is less well known to radiologists. Unlike hematoma, parenchymal hemorrhage has little mass effect and has a lacy, feathery appearance within the muscle, with preservation of fascial planes. Parenchymal hemorrhage is best seen on STIR or T2-weighted fat-suppressed sequences. The appearance of a subacute parenchymal bleed is very nonspecific as the blood does not undergo a prominent phase of methemoglobin formation, as is seen in hematoma.

Hematoma

Soft-tissue hemorrhage can collect as a discrete hematoma. Hematomas can be seen in the muscle, in the intermuscular fat planes, or within the subcutaneous tissues. MRI of hematomas yields highly variable depending upon their age (Fig. 8). The MRI appearance of muscle hematomas follows the same progression as in the brain but the time course may be longer and less predictable. Acute blood is of low signal intensity on both T1- and T2-weighted images due to the presence of intracellular deoxyhemoglobin. Subacute hematomas have a distinctive appearance due to formation of methemoglobin, particularly at the periphery of the hematoma. Methemoglobin produces T1 shortening, resulting in high signal within the hematoma on T1-weighted images. Fluid-fluid levels within the hematoma are common, particularly in large hematomas. In chronic hematoma, some of the iron in the methemoglobin is converted to hemosiderin and ferritin, resulting in signal loss on both T1- and T2-weighted images, producing a low-signal halo around the hematoma.

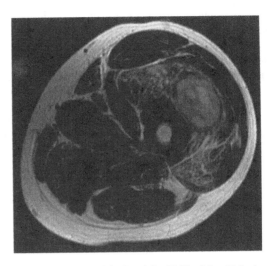

Fig. 8. Hematoma. An axial T2-weighted MR of the thigh shows a large heterogeneous mass anterior to the femur caused by a large hematoma in the vastus intermedius. There is adjacent parenchymal hemorrhage in the vastus intermedius and vastus lateralis

Myositis Ossificans

Myositis ossificans is a circumscribed mass of calcified and ossified granulation tissue that forms as a response to trauma. The early MRI appearance is that of a heterogeneous infiltrative enhancing mass that is easily mistaken for neoplasm. With maturation, a low-signal rim, due to peripheral calcification, becomes apparent. Mature myositis ossificans may show fat signal centrally due to marrow formation or there may be persistent granulation-type tissue within its central regions. Underlying periostitis is typically present with this lesion.

Compartment Syndrome

Acute compartment syndrome is a surgical emergency requiring compartment decompression. Compartment syndrome is seen most commonly in the lower extremity, typically below the knee, in patients who have suffered an injury. Any location can be involved, including the thigh, forearm, and paraspinal musculature. MRI may be performed if symptoms are confusing or unclear but is not indicated for typical compartment syndrome, which is quickly diagnosed with compartment-pressure measurement. The MRI findings are nonspecific, although the distribution of changes limited to all the muscles in a signal compartment should suggest the diagnosis. Mild swelling of the compartment and a slight increase of muscle intensity on T2-weighted images is present. Peripheral enhancement of the involved compartment may also be seen.

Chronic compartment syndrome is a poorly understood condition associated with exercise-induced swelling of muscle. In contrast to acute compartment syndrome, the muscles are less ischemic and typically do not undergo rhabdomyolysis. In long-standing chronic compartment syndrome, the muscle is often atrophic and densely fibrotic. Compartment calcification may be present, particularly in the lateral calf compartment, within the peroneal muscles. Calcific myonecrosis is an unusual condition in which either acute or chronic compartment syndrome progresses to form a chronic cystic cavity. The latter presents as a fusiform mass filled with liquefied necrotic muscle that is surrounded by a thin shell of calcification.

Rhabdomyolysis

Muscle infarction is most commonly due to massive trauma, prolonged compression resulting from immobilization, and untreated compartment syndrome. Other etiologies include vascular occlusion or vasospasm, vasculitis, and small-vessel disease in poorly controlled diabetes. T1-weighted images show minimal abnormality in the acute phase. In the involved muscles, there is mild infiltration of the intramuscular fat planes but a paucity of mass effect (Fig. 9) Rhabdomyolysis is most conspicuous on T2-weighted images, which show high signal within the abnormal muscle due to a combination of edema, necrosis, and hemorrhage. STIR and gadolinium enhancement further enhance the sensitivity of MRI.

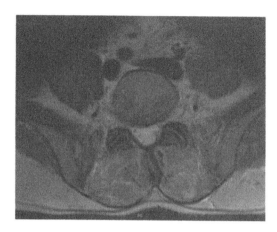

Fig. 9. Rhabdomyolysis. This man was immobilized for 3 days after taking an overdose of cocaine and other drugs. T2-weighted axial MRI shows swelling and hyperintensity of the posterior paraspinal musculature. The patient subsequently developed myoglobinuria due to extensive rhabdomyolysis

Suggested Reading

Boutin RD, Fritz RC, Steinbach LS (2002) Imaging of sports-related muscle injuries. Radiol Clin North Am 40(2):333-362

Evans GF, Haller RG, Wyrick PS et al (1998) Submaximal delayed-onset muscle soreness: Correlations between MR imaging findings and clinical measures. Radiology 208:815-820

Fleckenstein JL, Watumull D, Conner KE et al (1993) Denervated human skeletal muscle: MR imaging evaluation. Radiology 187:213-218

Glockner JF, White LM, Sundaram M, McDonald DJ (2000) Unsuspected metastases presenting as solitary soft tissue lesions: a fourteen year review. Skeletal Radiol 29:270-274

Gordon BA, Martinez S, Collins AJ (1995) Pyomyositis: characteristics at CT and MR imaging. Radiology 197:279-286

Gyftopoulos S, Rosenberg ZS, Schweitzer ME, Bordalo-Rodrigues M (2008) Normal anatomy and strains of the deep musculotendinous junction of the proximal rectus femoris: MRI features. AJR Am J Roentgenol 190:W182-W186

Holobinko JN, Damron TA, Scerpella PR, Hojnowski L (2003) Calcific myonecrosis: keys to early recognition. Skeletal Radiol 32(1):35-40

Koulouris G, Connell D (2003) Evaluation of the hamstring muscle complex following acute injury. Skeletal Radiol 32:582-589

Liu GC, Jong YJ, Chiang CH, Jaw TS (1993) Duchenne muscular dystrophy: MR grading system with functional correlation. Radiology 186:475-480

Lovitt S, Marden FA, Gundogdu B, Ostrowski ML (2004) MRI in myopathy. Neurol Clin 22(3):509-538

Mellado JM, Pérez del Palomar L, Díaz L et al (2004) Long-standing Morel-Lavallée lesions of the trochanteric region and proximal thigh: MRI features in five patients. AJR Am J Roentgenol 182:1289-1294

Moore SL, Alvin Teirstein A, Golimbu C (2005) MRI of sarcoidosis patients with musculoskeletal symptoms. AJR Am J Roentgenol 185:154-159

O'Connell MJ, Powell T, Brennan D et al (2002) Whole-body MR imaging in the diagnosis of polymyositis. AJR Am J Roentgenol 179:967-971

Özsarlak Ö, Parizel P, De Schepper A et al (2004) Whole-body MR screening of muscles in the evaluation of neuromuscular diseases. Eur Radiol 14:1489-1493

Palmer WE, Kuong SJ, Elmadbouh HM (1999) MR imaging of myotendinous strain. AJR Am J Roentgenol 173:703-709

Petersilge CA, Pathria MN, Gentili A et al (1995) Denervation hypertrophy of muscle: MR features. J Comput Assist Tomogr 19:596-600

Pfirrmann CWA, Schmid MR, Zanetti M et al (2004) Assessment of fat content in supraspinatus muscle with proton MR spectroscopy in asymptomatic volunteers and patients with supraspinatus tendon lesions. Radiology 232:709-715

Restrepo CS, Lemos DF, Gordillo H et al (2004) Imaging findings in musculoskeletal complications of AIDS. Radiographics 24:1029-1049

Sallomi D, Janzen DL, Munk PL et al (1998) Muscle denervation patterns in upper limb nerve injuries: MR imaging findings and anatomic basis. AJR Am J Roentgenol 171:779-784

Shellock FG, Fukunaga T, Mink JH, Edgerton VR (1991) Exertional muscle injury: evaluation of concentric versus eccentric actions with serial MR imaging. Radiology 179:659-664

Soler R, Rodriguez E, Aguilera C, Fernandez R (2000) Magnetic resonance imaging of pyomyositis in 43 cases. Eur J Radiol 35(1):59-64

Sookur PA, Naraghi AM, Bleakney RR et al (2008) Accessory muscles: anatomy, symptoms, and radiologic evaluation. RadioGraphics 28:481-499

Swenson SJ, Keller PL, Berquist TH et al (1985) Magnetic resonance imaging of hemorrhage. AJR Am J Roentgenol 145:921-927

Verleisdonk EJ, van Gils A, van der Werken C (2001) The diagnostic value of MRI scans for the diagnosis of chronic exertional compartment syndrome of the lower leg. Skeletal Radiol 30(6):321-325

Zeiss J, Guilliam-Haidet L (1996) MR demonstration of anomalous muscles about the volar aspect of the wrist and forearm. Clin Imag 20(3):219-221

Soft-Tissue Tumors and Tumor-Like Lesions

Suzanne E. Anderson[1], Daniel Vanel[2]

[1] Medical Imaging, The University of Notre Dame Australia, The Medical School of Sydney, Sydney, Australia
[2] Department of Radiology, Rizzoli Orthopedic Institute, University of Bologna, Bologna, Italy

Introduction

Soft tissue benign masses and potentially malignant sarcomas are unfortunately not uncommon [1-3]. Some investigators have stated that based on the morphological features and signal intensity, as demonstrated by magnetic resonance imaging (MRI) radiologists are able to precisely characterize soft-tissue lesions in some 80% of cases. However, others have noted that most imaging appearances are nonspecific and that, at most, a correct histological result based on imaging can be reached in only 25-35% of cases [2, 3].

MRI is currently the central imaging modality for investigation, used in combination with radiographs. It is generally preferred for the evaluation of all soft-tissue tumors, including diagnosis, location, and extent. Preoperatively and after adjuvant therapy for soft-tissue sarcomas, MRI is used to identify the compartment of origin and tumor extent as well as for lesion characterization, biopsy planning, and surgical resection approaches [4-7]. Percutaneous biopsy can be planned at an expert center in an interdisciplinary tumor team approach following imaging by the radiologist. This is best done in conjunction with the tumor surgeon, who will be doing the definitive surgery, and requires pre-procedural planning and knowledge in order to ensure appropriate route and site and to prevent compartment breach, which may be disastrous and threaten use-of-limb salvage surgery [5-8].

Here, the main subtypes of tumors with more specific appearances are reviewed and the approach best-employed by the radiologist in evaluating images of nonspecific soft-tissue tumors is discussed. Useful imaging features for tumor diagnosis as well as the pitfalls [8] and mimickers will be described. After a section providing general background information, this chapter is divided into three other sections, covering benign and malignant soft-tissue tumors and tumor-like lesions.

Malignant Soft-Tissue Tumors: Anatomical-Compartment and Tumor Staging

The primary aim of surgery is to provide local control of disease with adequate margins, which is best achieved through limb-salvage procedures if possible. Amputation or disarticulation is considered when the lesion is too advanced.

Imaging is involved in the three components: 1) *tumor grade*, 2) *local extent*, and 3) *presence of metastases*. The Enneking system has been adopted by the Musculoskeletal Tumor Society (MTS). Tumor grade is a measure of potential to metastasize, with low-grade sarcoma being less biologically active and high-grade sarcoma being more aggressive, although both require wide surgical resection. In general, findings highly suggestive of sarcoma include a mass >5 cm in size, or in deep tissues, or present in a child. Specific tissues act as natural barriers to tumor spread, e.g., fascial septae, articular cartilage, and bone cortex, and separate tissues into anatomic regions or spaces termed compartments. Tumor extent refers to the tumor site and its size. An intracapsular tumor is within the pseudocapsule. If the tumor extends beyond the pseudocapsule but remains within the compartment of origin, it is extracapsular *intracompartmental*. An aggressive infiltrative tumor extending beyond the compartment of origin is termed *extracompartmental* and requires more extensive radical surgery. Extracompartmental spread may also occur after a falsely placed biopsy or unplanned resection or following fracture or hemorrhage. Metastases are less nodal in this setting and more commonly occur as distant metastases to the lungs.

Soft-Tissue Tumors

A review of the patient's clinical details and, if possible, seeing the patient can greatly improve imaging diagnosis. Prior to imaging the patient should fill out a general screening questionnaire as to history of the lesion. In addition, systemic review is helpful. This can help in the management of the potential tumor based on whether it is a benign, malignant, or tumor-like lesion.

When appropriately diagnosed and treated, the patient with a soft-tissue tumor can have a good clinical outcome. However, if the tumor is locally treated with inadequate surgical margins, then the patient may be confronted with a disastrous outcome, as occurs in more than half of cases managed in this way [8]. Therefore, it is imperative that radiologists suggest the possibility of a malignant soft-tissue sarcoma at the outset.

Malignant soft-tissue tumors are best reviewed and treated at an expert center [2, 5-8]. The sensitivity and specificity of diagnostic tumor imaging has been shown to improve if experienced radiologists are involved with imaging interpretation and with the supervision of juniors in training [2]. Local staging of the tumor, with adequate demonstration of the anatomy, and further staging to determine the presence of metastases can be performed with a combination of radiographs, MRI, computed tomography (CT), and nuclear medicine studies. A more specific diagnosis can sometimes be made when radiographs are assessed in combination with MRI. These are discussed below as well as the approaches to the nonspecific soft-tissue mass.

Imaging Modalities in the Evaluation of Soft-Tissue Tumors

The choice of imaging modality will be influenced by local equipment availability and the expertise of the medical team on staff. Currently, best practice consists of using a combination of radiographs with MRI for local tumor review. The addition of CT for complex anatomical cases and wider staging, and with nuclear medicine for metastases.

Generally, radiographs are performed in two planes, reviewing the clinical mass for any underlying bony anatomy, e.g, exostosis, or congenital skeletal deformity that may be evident. They are also used to assess the presence of irregular soft-tissue calcification, which is often diagnostic or at least suggestive of a particular tumor, such as calcified phleboliths for a hemangioma, osteocartilaginous masses of synovial osteochondromatosis, or irregular calcifications suggestive of synovial sarcoma (~30% of cases) or extraskeletal osteosarcoma. In addition, the radiographic soft-tissue density can be reviewed, for example fatty tissue in a lipoma. Specific malignant features include the presence of soft-tissue calcification, bone erosion or destruction, and joint involvement.

Local staging of a tumor depends on the anatomic space (compartments) involved, which is best determined with MRI, which, as mentioned above, is considered to be the gold standard for initial tumor characterization [2], local staging, tumor extent, biopsy planning [5-7], following chemotherapy treatment and surgical planning. MRI allows for the multiplanar imaging and review of all structures, including bone, joint, and soft tissues. If the radiologist knows what the objective is prior to the examination, then he or she is more likely to be able to answer the diagnostic question posed by the patient's clinician.

Images are obtained in at least two orthogonal planes and it is prudent to have a combination of several sequences, i.e., T1- and T2-weighting as well as STIR (short tau inversion recovery) with gradient echo to identify blood products (e.g., hemosiderin). It is important to include an anatomic reference point in the MRI field, usually with an adjacent joint. A large field-of-view (FOV) can be initially used for an overview or screening of the anatomy, followed by the use of a smaller FOV for more focused imaging. Fat-suppressed T1 weighted images can demonstrate methemoglobin. STIR imaging is very useful for increasing soft-tissue conspicuity, but it should not replace T2-weighting, which has a better signal-to-noise ratio and higher resolution. Many tumors have non-specific increased signal intensity on T2-weighting, whereas only a few, such as a giant cell tumor of the tendon sheath or desmoid, are characterized by decreased signal intensity on T2-weighted images. STIR is mostly used in this setting for examining adjacent bone for any secondary tumor involvement. Although T2-weighting may be performed with or without fat suppression, it is important to realize that the T2 signal intensity of tumors depicted in the imaging literature commonly is not fat suppressed. Many tumor types have been described as having multiple fluid levels; hence this sign is nonspecific.

The administration of contrast material can be most helpful in visualizing soft-tissue tumors, to determine whether a lesion is solid or cystic (rim enhancement only), to identify areas of viable tumor to select an optimal biopsy site, and to distinguish necrotic or hemorrhagic tumor regions. Prior to contrast administration, care should be taken to look for signs of renal failure or to interview the patient regarding any risk factors related to nephrogenic fibrosis. In some centers, the contrast enhancement rate is measured and plotted against time. In general malignant tumors have greater enhancement and steeper curves than benign lesions.

Some tumor surgeons prefer having axial images with T1, T2, and STIR sequences performed at exactly the same level. This yields very reproducible images and these standard sequences are those most often referenced in the tumor imaging literature. Although the inclusion of all three sequences in the axial plane as part of the tumor imaging protocol is certainly very thorough and time-consuming, it can help with preoperative planning and provide a baseline for comparison during post-therapy MRI prior to surgery. Additional planes along the long axis of the tumor, including the adjacent joint and other pertinent anatomical landmarks, are important. Placement of a marker such as a vitamin capsule above and below the mass in question is also recommended. The visibility of these markers on the images can help to verify that the entire tumor has been imaged and that the clinical mass corresponds to the mass imaged.

MRI signal intensity may directly help with the diagnosis, as some tumors are more commonly associated with a particular appearance on T1- and T2-weighting. For example, myxomas contain gelatinous myxomatous material, often with a small region of MRI-visible fat within the wall. A mass of decreased signal intensity within a joint or associated with tendon sheaths or a mass in particular anatomical locations, such as the shoulder girdle, foot, and lower limb, on T2-weighting is highly suggestive of pigmented villonodular synovitis/giant cell tumor of the tendon sheath or desmoid. The former are often associated with advanced degenerative joint disease. Some malignant soft-tissue sarcomas have specific or suggestive MRI signal characteristics on T1- and T2-weighting that may be helpful in making the diagnosis or at least a provisional diagnosis [2, 3].

In some centers, an additional magnetic resonance angiography (MRA) sequence [9] is performed to review tumor vascularity, the normal vascular anatomy, or variants. MRA may also be useful with preoperative embolization planning in some specific cases.

CT of the local tumor depicts the anatomical site as well as the features and extent of the mass. It is used to screen for metastases in the chest, abdomen, and pelvis, with review of bone, lung, and soft-tissue settings. With multislice technique, CT angiography can be used to examine preoperative normal vascularity and tumor vascularity. In addition, CT provides excellent depiction of calcification and ossification.

High-resolution ultrasound, either alone or in combination with color Doppler imaging, allows solid structures to be distinguished from cystic ones; however this technique is operator-dependent and MRI remains the gold standard. Ultrasound is also useful for specific enquiries and for metastatic staging of the abdomen.

Nuclear-medicine bone and positron emission tomography (PET) scan are used in a soft-tissue tumor workup to determine tumor activity, and bone involvement as well as to exclude metastatic tumors. These techniques have a more significant role in the imaging of malignant lesions. PET-CT correlation allows for the review of any spurious or dubious findings.

Interventional radiology may be used to identify diagnostic features, to delineate tumor vessels and normal vascular anatomy preoperatively, and or therapeutically, such as embolization in the setting of hemorrhage.

Follow-up imaging after therapy is usually in the form of MRI and CT. These modalities clarify good treatment and response, identify residual tumor or tumor growth, and any complications, e.g., seromas, hematomas, and, less commonly, infection. Skin markers usually are placed to demarcate the surgical scar. A screen with a T2-weighted sequence is very important to visualize residual or new-growth tumor, seen as a focal high-signal mass. Tumors that were originally decreased on T2 weighting at diagnosis, for example desmoids, may require more careful review and comparison with several sequences to depict the anatomy.

Soft Tissue Tumors of Specific Appearance on MRI

Soft-tissue tumors can have specific and classical imaging appearances [2, 3]. This may relate to the clinical and surgical history, the morphological appearance of a tumor with a particular imaging mode, and the MRI signal intensities on T1- and or T2-weighting, which can reflect the chemical and tissue composition of the tumor, and its anatomic location. Examples include a stump neurinoma (after amputation), lipomatous (increased signal intensity on T1-weighting) and fibromatosis or desmoid tumor (Fig. 1), pigmented villonodular synovitis (decreased signal intensity on

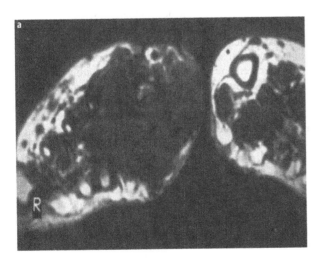
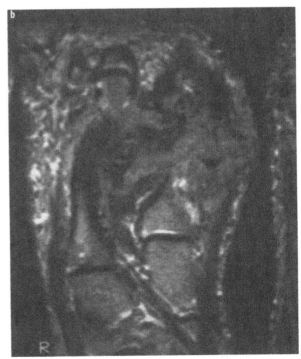

Fig. 1 a, b. T1-weighted (**a**) and T2-weighted (**b**) images through the foot show an inhomogeneous of decreased signal intensity. The mass was consistent with desmoid tumor based on MRI and histology

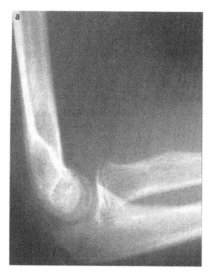 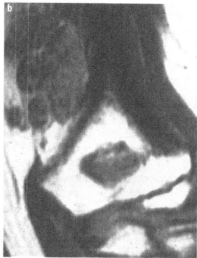 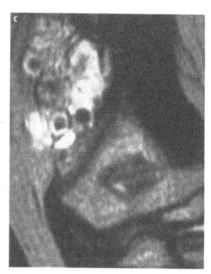

Fig. 2 a-c. Lateral radiograph shows small phlebolith anterior to humeral shaft (**a**). Coronal T1-weighted image (**b**) and corresponding T2-weighted fat suppressed image (**c**) show characteristic vascular serpinginous channels with slow flow. Together with the radiographic findings, the mass was consistent with a vascular anomaly, a hemangioma. (Courtesy of James O. Johnston)

T2-weighting), hemangiomatous (serpiginous structures; Fig. 2) and neurogenic (target sign or star sign) tumors, and elastofibroma dorsi (classic site deep to the scapular tip).

Nonspecific Tumor Findings on MRI

"Where is it before what is it?" is the rule in evaluating a tumor by MRI. If the lesion is nonspecific its exact anatomical site and extent as well as its relationship to nearby important structures, such as neurovascular bundles and joints, should be determined. In this setting at the initial stage, it is best to approach the lesion as if it were malignant. Knowledge of tumor prevalence, patient age, and tumor location are very helpful in providing an educated differential diagnosis. For this purpose, a tumor prevalence table or reference book along with compartment-anatomy diagrams should be available at the reporting site [2-7].

A general background rule is that if a soft tissue tumor is larger than 5 cm in size and is located within deep soft tissues (e.g., the thigh), and particularly if present within the pediatric age group, it should be considered as malignant until proven otherwise. Only some 5% of benign soft-tissue tumors will exceed 5 cm in diameter and only some 1% are located within deep anatomical regions [2]. Since malignant superficial tumors may have a less aggressive biology and therefore may appear benign, care should be taken and the diagnosis made by histology. Nonetheless, the histology may be also be difficult and the surgery demanding, such that good communication between team members is important.

When a definitive diagnosis is not possible, then the lesion should initially be characterized only as benign or malignant. Malignant lesions with a more autonomous growth pattern are usually large and may outstrip their blood supply, such that they are associated with hemorrhage and necrosis. This is visualized as increased T2 signal intensity which is very heterogenous in nature, as in T1-weighting. Malignancies growing within a deep space enlarge from their central origin in a centripedal fashion, pushing aside the anatomy in their path and often creating a pseudocapsule or rind. Lesions at this stage are intracapsular, remaining within the compartment of origin. The presence of a pseudocapsule can be misleading as it may not be the definitive tumor border. In fact, malignant satellite cells have been histologically found located 1 cm from this border and some even 4 cm beyond it. This may in part account for the peritumoral edema or reactive changes seen around a tumor on T2-weighting and STIR images. However, much of this region may be simply due to edema or to an inflammatory cell response [10]. Later in the tumor cycle, the perifascial planes will be breached and there is overt tumor infiltration. The tumor invades adjacent soft tissue and other structures (rarely, bone) thereby becoming extracompartmental. This aggressive feature is associated with a poorer prognosis and is influenced by cell type. It has a major impact on surgery. Other malignant characteristics include neurovascular bundle involvement, which is present in approximately 10% of patients and is more common with soft-tissue sarcomas than with bone sarcomas [11]. More commonly, the sarcoma displaces the neurovascular bundle rather than encasing it. The general rule is that when contact between the tumor and neurovascular bundle has a circumference of less than 180°, the tumor has not invaded the bundle and it may be lifted off at surgery. Abutment of the tumor to the neurovascular bundle is evidenced by a persistent T1-weighted fat plane between the two. Benign lesions are more commonly <3 cm in diameter, are increased on T1-weighting, and have smooth borders. Nonetheless, this description is a generalization and biopsy is often needed to exclude low-grade sarcoma.

Staging of a Soft-Tissue Tumor

Imaging-based staging is useful whenever a sarcoma is present within the differential diagnosis and is frequently recommended by the tumor team involved. It is prudent to stage aggressive benign lesions as well as lesions in complex anatomical locations.

Pitfalls in Tumor Imaging

The most common problem is misinterpretation of a soft-tissue lesion for benign rather than malignant, or being deceived by the presence of tumor-like processes that mimic a real tumor (pseudotumors).

The pseudocapsule of a malignant sarcoma may mimic a benign-appearing lesion. Very dense cellular homogeneous lesions with decreased signal intensity on T2-weighting, such as a fibrosarcoma, may mimic a benign lesion, such as desmoids. Pseudocystic lesions are a major pitfall, possibly appearing as a fluid-filled benign lesion such as a ganglion or myxoma. These lesions include synovial sarcomas, chondrosarcomas of soft tissue (mesenchymal or myxoid types), myxoid liposarcoma, and soft-tissue metastases, e.g. with an esophageal primary. Aspirates of fluid from these lesions notoriously lack malignant cells, giving misleading information supporting a benign diagnosis. Large hemorrhage into a malignant sarcoma may mask the tumor and may occur in malignant fibrous histiocytoma or with synovial sarcomas, making the diagnosis very difficult; however, either close up review may reveal a solid tumor component or short term follow-up may show some evidence of solid-tumor differentiation.

Treatment of Soft-Tissue Tumors

Benign tumors are identified as such based on their imaging appearances, mostly after histological confirmation, and following the exclusion of a malignancy. Resection of benign tumors is typically associated with an excellent prognosis. Rarely, some benign tumors will aggressively reoccur, such as desmoid tumor, and may require amputation if painfully and disfiguringly present in peripheral limbs.

Malignant tumors are treated according to anatomical-compartment concepts for limb salvage [8, 12, 13] after metastases and synchronous disease have been excluded.

Benign Soft-Tissue Tumors

These are defined as lesions not associated with a malignant histopathology or architectural disturbance, thus excluding a metastatic potential.

Overview of the Main Benign Soft-Tissue Tumors

The World Health Organization has compiled a list of benign soft-tissue tumors, classifying them according to histological type [1, 2] (Table 1). The incidence of these tumors is 300 per 100,000 individuals [1]. Benign soft-tissue tumors are far more common than their malignant counterparts, which have an incidence of 2 to 3 per 100,000 [1].

Table 1. Modified WHO classification: histology of benign soft-tissue tumors

Tumor group	Tumor type
Lipomatous tumors Benign	Lipoma and variations
(Myo)fibroblastic tumors Benign	Nodular fasciitis Proliferative fasciitis Proliferative myositis Myositis ossificans Ischemic fasciitis Elastofibroma Fibrotic hamartoma Fibromatosis (and subgroups) Fibroma/Fibroblastoma (and subtypes)
Intermediate	Superficial Fibromatosis Desmoid Lipofibromatosis
Fibrohistiocytic tumors Benign	Giant cell tumor of tendon sheath (GCTTS) Diffuse giant cell tumor/pigmented villonodular synovitis (PVNS)
Intermediate	Plexiform histiocytic tumor Giant cell tumor of soft tissues
Neurogenic tumors Benign	Neuroma and variants Neurofibroma and variants Benign Schwannoma (neurinoma) and variants Perineurinoma and variants
Tumors of smooth muscle Benign	(Angio)leiomyoma and variants
Pericytic tumors Benign	Glomus tumor and variants Myopericytoma
Tumors of skeletal muscle Benign	Rhabdomyoma and variants
Vascular tumors Benign	Hemangioma and variants Angiomatosis Lymphangioma
Chondroid/osseous tumors Benign	Chondroma of soft tissues
Tumors of unknown differentiation Benign	Myxoma and variants Pleomorphic hyalinizing angioectatic tumor Ectopic hamartomatosis thymoma
Intermediate	Angiomatoid fibrotic histiocytoma Ossifying fibromyxoid tumor Mixed/myoepithelial/Parachordoma

There are six main types of benign soft-tissue tumors [3]: lipoma and its variants, benign fibrotic histiocytoma, nodular fasciitis, neurogenic tumors, fibromatosis, and pigmented villonodular synovitis or giant cell tumor of the tendon sheath (summarized in Table 2). With the addition of ganglion to the list, these account for ~70% of all benign lesions [2]. This percentage is increased if vascular and lymphangiomatous lesions are also included. The age at tumor presentation is important as certain tumors are more likely to occur within particular age groups. Many of these tumors have a more characteristic appearance and will be discussed with imaging examples. Differential lists of tumor type based on MRI signal intensity are given in Tables 3 and 4.

Clinically, these present as a mass of increasing size, associated with discomfort or pain. If in the proximity of a joint there may be associated joint pain, and if near essential structures, such as a neurovascular bundle, there may be secondary features, such as nerve compression.

Table 2. The most common benign soft tissue tumors. (Adapted from [3])

Most common benign tumors	%
Lipoma and variants	16
Benign fibrotic histiocytoma	13
Nodular fascitis	11
Neurogenic tumors	10
Fibromatosis	7
PVNS/GCTTS	4

GCTTS, Giant cell tumor of tendon sheath; *PVNS*, pigmented villonodular synovitis

Table 3. Benign soft-tissue tumors commonly associated with increased signal intensity on T1-weighted MRI sequences

- Lipoma and variants
- Vascular tumors and variants (lymphangioma)
- Elastofibroma dorsi
- Subacute hemorrhage
- Myxoma (small fat component in wall)
- Tumoral calcinosis

Table 4. Benign soft-tissue tumors commonly associated with decreased signal intensity on T2 weighted MRI sequences

- Desmoid tumor/fibromatosis
- PVNS/GCTTS
- Morton's neuroma
- Hyperacute and chronic hemorrhage
- Xanthoma
- Amyloidosis
- Scar tissue
- High flow vascular malformations
- Calfication, tumoral calcinosis

GCTTS, Giant cell tumor of tendon sheath; *PVNS*, pigmented villonodular synovitis

Malignant Soft-Tissue Tumors

Overview of the Main Malignant Soft-Tissue Tumors

Characteristically, malignant soft-tissue tumors are able to invade adjacent structures and to form metastases at distant sites, resulting, if untreated, ultimately in death. While malignant soft-tissue tumors are relatively rare, they are approximately as common as multiple myeloma and twice as common as bone sarcoma [1-3]. The incidence of malignant soft tissue tumors is 2-3 per 100,000 [1, 2]. With an average mortality rate of 50%, this is relatively high, although mortality also depends on tumor stage and histology grade at time of presentation.

The World Health organization has also compiled a list of malignant soft-tissue tumors and catalogued them according to type [1, 2] (Table 5). The seven most common

Table 5. The most common malignant soft-tissue tumors. (Adapted from [3])

Tumor group	Tumor type
Lipomatous tumors Malignant	Liposarcoma and subtypes
(Myo)fibroblastic tumors Intermediate (seldom metastasize)	Solitary fibrotic tumor and hemangiopericytoma Inflammatory myofibroblastic sarcoma Low-grade myofibroblastic sarcoma Myxoinflammatory fibroblastic sarcoma Infantile fibrosarcoma
Malignant	Fibrosarcoma and subtypes
Fibrohistiocytic tumors Malignant	Malignant fibrotic histiocytoma and subgroups
Neurogenic tumors Malignant	Malignant peripheral nerve sheath tumor (MPNST) and variants
Tumors of smooth muscle Malignant	Leiomyosarcoma
Pericytic tumors Malignant	Malignant glomus tumor
Tumors of skeletal muscle Malignant	Rhabdomyosarcoma and subtypes
Vascular tumors Intermediate	Hemangioendothelioma and variants Kaposi sarcoma
Malignant	Epitheloid hemangioendothelioma Angiosarcoma of soft tissues
Chondro/osseous tumors Malignant	Mesenchymal chondrosarcoma Extraskeletal osteosarcoma
Tumors of unknown differentiation Malignant	Synovialsarcoma Epitheloid sarcoma Alveolar soft-tissue sarcoma Clear cell sarcoma Extraskeletal myxoid chondrosarcoma Extraskeletal Ewing sarcoma Primitive neuroectodermal tumor (PNET) Desmoplastic small round cell tumor Extrarenal rhabdoid tumor Malignant mesenchymoma Intimal sarcoma

Table 6. The most common malignant soft-tissue tumors. (Adapted from [3])

Most common malignant tumors	%
Malignant fibrous histiocytoma	22
Fibrosarcoma	18
Liposarcoma	17.5
Synovial sarcoma	17
Malignant peripheral nerve sheath tumor (MPNST)	5
Rhabdomyosarcoma	5
Leiomyosarcoma	4

Table 7. Malignant tumors commonly associated with increased signal intensity on T1-weighted MRI sequences

- Liposarcoma and subgroups
- Melanoma and metastases (melanin)
- Clear cell sarcoma (melanin)
- Subacute hemorrhage
- Calcification
- Myxoid material

Table 8. Malignant tumors commonly associated with decreased signal intensity on T2-weighted MRI sequences

- Fibrosarcoma
- High-grade sarcoma (compact and cellular)
- Hyperacute and chronic hemorrhage
- Scar tissue
- High-flow vascular tumors
- Calcification or products within tumor

malignant tumor types are malignant fibrous histiocytoma, fibrosarcoma, liposarcoma, synovial sarcoma, malignant peripheral nerve sheath tumor (MPNST), rhabdomyosarcoma, and leiomyosarcoma [3] (Table 6). Differential lists of MRI signal intensity are given in Tables 7 and 8.

The clinical presentation of a malignant lesion is commonly a painless slowly growing mass. Acute painful presentations are associated with tumor necrosis or hemorrhage. Some patients present at the change of seasons, as the change in clothing type is often the occasion when an anatomical asymmetry is first noticed. The commonest site is the thigh, due to the presence of a large muscle and soft-tissue bulk.

Tumor-Like Lesions

Pseudotumors are included in the differential diagnoses of benign and malignant soft-tissue tumors [14]. They are common and may be post-traumatic, sports or occupationally related, associated with aging and degenera-

tion; congenital, developmental abnormalities; normal anatomical variants; the result of overuse and joint degeneration; infection with abscess formation; or foreign-body, crystal, or inflammatory arthropathies [15-17]. Hematomas are a common finding after sports and other injuries associated with various degrees of muscle tears, as is myositis ossificans [14]. Other, less-common tumor-like lesions include those of the endocrine and metabolic group, such as tumoral calcinosis. However, with these entities, a true mass at the center of the area of abnormality is usually not seen on imaging; also, as there is serial change over time, radiographs and the clinical history can help in the differentiation of pseudotumors from benign and malignant lesions.

Conclusions

There is value in initially approaching a soft-tissue mass as a malignant lesion and in suggesting sarcoma, as this may prevent disasters. An awareness of the specific imaging features of benign and malignant tumors is very helpful. Furthermore, radiologists should develop a pragmatic and systematic approach to soft-tissue tumors of non-specific appearance. The realization that tumor-like lesions can mimic a real tumor will help in refining the differential diagnosis of soft-tissue masses. Multidisciplinary expert teams and good communication are important.

References

1. Fletcher CDM, Unni KK, Mertens F (eds) (2002) Pathology and genetics of soft tissues and bone. In: World Health Organization Classification of Tumors. IARC, Lyon
2. Kransdorf MJ, Murphey MD (1997) Imaging of soft tissues. WB Saunders, Philadelphia
3. Kransdorf MJ (1995) Benign soft tissue tumors in a large referral population: distribution of diagnosis by age, sex and location. AJR Am J Roentgenol 164:395-402
4. Campanacci M (1999) Bone and soft tissue tumors, 2ndedn. Piccin, Padua
5. Anderson MW, Temple T, Dussault RG, Kaplan PA (1999) Compartment anatomy: relevance to staging and biopsy of musculoskeletal tumors. AJR Am J Roentgenol 173:1663-1671
6. Toomayan GA, Robertson F, Major NM, Brigman BE (2006) Upper extremity compartment anatomy: clinical relevance to radiologists. Skeletal Radiol 35:195-201
7. Toomayan GA, Robertson F, Major NM (2005) Lower extremity compartmental anatomy: clinical relevance to radiologists. Skeletal Radiol 34:307-313
8. Davies AM, Mehr A, Parsonage S et al (2004) MR imaging in the assessment of residual tumour following inadequate primary excision of soft tissue sarcomas. Eur Radiol 14:506-513
9. Anderson SE, De Monaco D, Buechler U et al (2003) Imaging features of pseudoaneurysms of the hand in children and adults. AJR Am J Roentgenol 180:659-664
10. Beltran J, Simon DC, Katz W, Weis LD (1987) Increased MR signal intensity in skeletal muscle adjacent to malignant tumors: pathological correlation and clinical relevance. Radiology 162:251-255

11. Panicek DM, Go SD, Healey JH et al (1997) Soft tissue sarcoma involving bone and neurovascular structures. MR imaging prognostic factors. Radiology 205:871-875

12. Enneking WF, Spanier SS, Goodman MA (1980) The surgical staging of muscusloskeletal sarcoma. J Bone Joint Surg Am 62:1027-1030

13. Enneking WF, Spanier SS, Goodman MA (2003) A system for the surgical staging of musculoskeletal sarcoma. Clin Orthop Relat Res 415:4-18

14. Anderson SE, Johnstom JO, Steinbach LS (2008) Pseudotumors of shoulder. Eur Radiol 68:147-158

15. Anderson SE, Davies AM (2007) Pseudotumors in sports. In: Vanhoenacker FM, Maas M, Gielen (eds) Imaging in orthopedic sports injuries. Springer-Verlag, Berlin, Heidelberg New York, pp 103-118

16. Anderson SE, Johnston JO, Hertel R et al (2005) Latissimus dorsi tendonosis and tear: imaging features of a pseudotumor in five patients. AJR Am J Roentgenol 185:1145-1151

17. Tshering Vogel DW, Steinbach LS, Hertel R et al (2005) Acromioclavicular joint cysts presenting as a tumoral mass and new aspects. Skeletal Radiol 34:260-265

Bone Tumors and Tumor-Like Lesions

Mark J. Kransdorf[1,2], Mark D. Murphey[2,3]

[1] Department of Radiology, Mayo Clinic, Jacksonville, FL, USA
[2] Department of Radiologic Pathology, Armed Forces Institute of Pathology, Walter Reed Army Medical Center, Washington, DC, USA
[3] Department of Radiology and Nuclear Medicine, Uniformed Services University of the Heath Sciences, Bethesda, MD, USA

Introduction

The imaging evaluation of musculoskeletal tumors has undergone dramatic evolution with the advent of computer-assisted imaging, specifically, computed tomography (CT) and magnetic resonance imaging (MRI). Despite these sophisticated imaging modalities, the objectives of initial radiologic evaluation remain unchanged: detecting the suspected lesion, establishing a diagnosis, or, when a definitive diagnosis is not possible, formulating an appropriate differential diagnosis, and determining the radiologic staging of the lesion [1]. A detailed discussion of all bone tumors is well beyond the scope of this review; instead, we highlight the initial evaluation and staging of primary osseous neoplasms.

Initial Evaluation

The radiograph remains the initial imaging examination in evaluating bone lesions and is almost invariably the most diagnostic. The radiograph accurately predicts the biologic activity of a lesion, which is reflected in the appearance of the lesion's margin and the type and extent of accompanying periosteal reaction. In addition, the pattern of associated matrix mineralization may be a key to the underlying histology (e.g., cartilage, bone, fibro-osseous) [2-5]. Although other imaging modalities (MRI and CT) are superior to radiographs in staging a bone lesion, the radiograph remains the best modality for establishing a diagnosis, for formulating a differential, and for accurately assessing the biologic activity (separating benign from malignant lesions).

In many cases, as in patients with fibroxanthoma (nonossifying fibroma), fibrous dysplasia, osteochondroma, or enchondroma, radiographs may be virtually pathognomonic, and no further diagnostic imaging is required. In other cases, despite the lack of an unequivocal diagnosis, a benign-appearing asymptomatic lesion may require only continued radiographic follow-up in order to document long-term stability.

Advanced Imaging Techniques

Whereas MRI has emerged as the preferred advanced imaging modality for the evaluation of soft-tissue lesions, CT and MRI are often complimentary modalities for the evaluation of primary osseous tumors [6]. In a study by Tehranzadeh et al., the information obtained from CT and MRI was additive in 76% of malignant primary bone neoplasms [6]. CT scanning is superior to MRI for the detection and characterization (osteoid or chondroid) of matrix mineralization, cortical involvement and periosteal reaction [6, 7]. Although some studies suggest that CT and MRI are equivalent for the evaluation of the local extent of tumor [8], most studies note the superiority of MRI [6, 7, 9-11].

Magnetic Resonance Imaging

The excellent soft tissue contrast and multiplanar capabilities of MRI allows improved evaluation of both the intra- and extra-compartmental extent of osseous lesions, including more accurate assessment of marrow involvement and assessment of invasion of adjacent tissue planes and neurovascular structures [6, 7, 9, 11-14]. MRI has also been shown to be superior for assessing intra-articular extension as well as for identifying the presence of intra-tumoral necrosis and hemorrhage [7, 15].

While there is no single best tumor protocol, we feel MRI should be performed in at least two orthogonal planes, typically including both T1- and T2-weighted images in the axial plane, supplemented by sagittal and/or coronal images, depending on the location of the lesion. Long-axis imaging should include both a T1-weighted sequence and a water-sensitive sequence, such as short tau inversion-recovery (STIR) or fat-suppressed T2-weighted sequence. It has been our experience that standard spin-echo imaging is often most useful in establishing a specific diagnosis when possible. In addition, it is the most reproducible technique and the one most often referenced in the tumor imaging literature. This technique is the one with which we are most familiar for tumor evaluation, and it has established itself as the standard by which other imaging techniques must be judged [16]. The main disadvantage of spin-echo imaging remains the relatively long acquisition times, particularly for double-echo T2-weighted sequences [16].

Gradient-echo imaging may be a useful supplement for demonstrating hemosiderin because of this material's greater magnetic susceptibility; in general, susceptibility artifacts related to metallic material, hemorrhage, and air are accentuated on gradient-echo images [17]. STIR sequences are very useful in evaluating subtle marrow abnormalities and can be performed more quickly than T2-weighted spin-echo sequences [18], being frequently added to the conventional spin-echo sequences. Some radiologists prefer short TE/TR spin-echo and STIR sequences over typical T1- and T2-weighted spin-echo sequences. Although STIR imaging increases lesion conspicuity [18, 19], it typically has lower signal-to-noise ratios than does spin-echo imaging and is also more susceptible to degradation by motion [16, 19]. STIR imaging can be an adjunct in selective cases, but should not replace conventional spin-echo sequences. Lesions are generally well-seen on standard imaging, whereas, in our opinion, STIR and other fat-suppressed imaging techniques tend to reduce the variations in signal intensities identified on conventional spin-echo MRI that are most helpful in tissue characterization.

For suspected malignant lesions of the extremities, such as when osteosarcoma is a differential consideration, it is essential that at least one long-axis sequence be performed through the entire involved bone in order to evaluate for the presence of skip metastases. These represent a second site of disease in the same bone as the primary tumor, but they are separated by an area of normal marrow. Because the identification of skip lesions has profound clinical implications, this additional imaging sequence should be performed in appropriate cases.

Computed Tomography Scanning

As previously noted, CT scanning is superior to MRI in the detection and characterization (osteoid or chondroid) of matrix mineralization, cortical involvement, and periosteal reaction. We find it especially useful in the assessment of lesions in those areas in which the osseous anatomy is complex, such as in the spine or small bones of the hands and feet, or where the osseous detail is obscured by overlying soft tissue, such as in the pelvis. An important limitation of MRI is its relative inability to detect and characterize soft-tissue calcification [7, 20]; consequently, CT is uniquely suited to assess internal matrix obscured by marginal sclerosis associated with the lesion and not adequately evaluated by radiographs [21].

Although initial investigations maintained that CT is superior to MRI in detecting destruction of cortical bone [6, 7], more recently it has been suggested that these two modalities are comparable in this regard [22]. It has also been our experience that nonmetallic foreign bodies may be difficult to identify on MRI. In such cases, MRI shows

the changes associated with the foreign body, although the foreign body itself may have no signal and may be difficult to identify.

Contrast Enhancement

Contrast administration may be a useful adjunct in the assessment of osseous lesions; however, its use is usually dictated by the objectives of the examination. For example, it is typically required to assess the extent of soft-tissue involvement on CT scanning, while it may not be needed to assess the presence or character of matrix mineralization, periosteal reaction, or marginal sclerosis. On MRI, many lesions are well-assessed without contrast; moreover, contrast administration can also cause confusion, blurring the distinction of tumor from peritumoral edema and normal from abnormal marrow [10, 23]. Nevertheless, it may provide essential information and we find contrast imaging especially important in the assessment of lesions containing hemorrhage, myxomatous areas, or necrotic or cystic regions. Since only vascularized tissue enhances, contrast-enhanced imaging may be quite useful in directing biopsy to the solid, enhancing portions of a lesion, i.e., the portion of the lesion that harbors the diagnostic tissue, as opposed to the cystic, necrotic, or hemorrhagic, nondiagnostic components. Additionally, the pattern of enhancement may also provide clues to the diagnosis, as in the characteristic peripheral and septal enhancement pattern seen with hyaline-cartilage neoplasms.

Contrast-enhanced imaging is not without a price. The use of intravenous contrast increases the length and cost of the examination. Although contrast-enhanced MRI may provide additional information, it usually does not increase lesion conspicuity or replace the diagnostic value of T2-weighted imaging [24]. While the contrast agents used in MRI are safer than those used with CT, there is a small, but real, incidence of untoward reactions with both gadopentetate dimeglumine (Magnevist; Berlex Laboratories, Wayne, NJ) and gadoteridol (ProHance; Squibb Diagnostics, Princeton, NJ), including hypotension, laryngospasm, bronchospasm, anaphylactic shock, nephrogenic systemic fibrosis, and death, as well as a full spectrum of less serious reactions [25-27]. Consequently, contrast-enhanced imaging should be reserved for those cases in which the results influence patient management.

The response of high-grade osteosarcoma and Ewing sarcoma to chemotherapy can be monitored with dynamic enhanced MRI. This finding was established by several investigators, who proposed evaluation based on rather complicated schemes relating to factor analysis of dynamic MRI sequences and regions of interest [28, 29]. Although such systems may be useful, they have not gained wide usage. As a generality, in patients with osteosarcoma, the absence of early enhancing nodules or the presence of only one small early enhancing nodule suggests greater than 90% tumor necrosis, representing a good response to the chemotherapy; similarly, masses with early and persistent enhancement suggest a poor response to chemotherapy in both osteosarcoma and Ewing sarcoma [30]. Caution is required, however, in that in cases of Ewing sarcoma, diffusely scattered neoplastic cells may not form perceptible nodules [29, 30].

Magnetic Resonance Angiography

With the advent of computerized imaging and MR and CT angiography (MRA and CTA), the role of conventional arteriography in evaluating tumors has decreased markedly. These new techniques are capable of depicting the major vessels in a tumor bed and detecting most of the vessels seen by conventional angiographic techniques, except for those that are quite small, such as sural or geniculate arteries [32]. These small vessels are of little importance in planning limb-salvage surgery [32]. Computed imaging is more accurate in compartmental localization of lesions, as well as in determining the relationship of the lesion to the vascular structures [33]. Moreover, the angiographic findings of tumors are nonspecific; therefore, they cannot be used to reliably distinguish benign from malignant lesions. Catheter arteriography remains useful for preoperative or therapeutic embolization. Preoperative embolization of hypervascular tumors may dramatically reduce intraoperative bleeding.

Bone Scintigraphy

Bone scintigrapy with 99mTc phosphate compounds remains the modality of choice for the identification of multifocal osseous disease. While metastases may be identified with scintigraphy, their identification is less sensitive with this technique than with CT or MRI [34]. In the evaluation of primary osseous tumors, triple-phase imaging is recommended. Dynamic images demonstrate both tumor vascularity and its effects on regional vascularity.

Both benign and malignant tumors typically demonstrate increased uptake on delayed images [34]; however, the degree of uptake may have diagnostic value in specific circumstances. For example, delayed scintigraphy has been shown to be useful for differentiating chondrosarcoma from enchondroma, since chondrosarcoma typically demonstrates significant uptake on scintigraphy that is equal to or greater in intensity than in the anterior superior iliac spine (ASIS). Uptake that is less intense than in the ASIS suggests the diagnosis of enchondroma [35].

Positron emission tomography (PET) has established itself as the gold standard for metabolic imaging; while it has not replaced skeletal scintigraphy, it has several intrinsic advantages. It provides inherently superior spatial resolution and routinely includes tomographic images with multiplanar capability. Additionally, unlike skeletal scintigraphy, which primarily evaluates only the skeletal system, PET detects disease in both the osseous structures and in the surrounding soft tissues, allowing detection of pulmonary as well as nodal metastasis [36]. More-over, PET detects tumor presence directly, by reflecting the tumor's metabolic activity, rather than indirectly, as is the case in conventional scintigraphy, by demonstrating tumor involvement due to the resulting increased bone mineral turnover [36].

Staging

The staging of osseous tumors is one of the primary functions of imaging. Accurate staging is essential for appropriate planning of therapy and establishing a prognosis. Simply stated, the purpose of a staging system is to provide a standard manner in which to readily communicate the state of a malignancy. Accurate staging is essential to: (a) incorporate the most significant prognostic factors into a system that describes the progressive degrees of risk to which a patient is subject, (b) delineate progressive stages of disease that have specific implications for surgical management, and (c) provide guidelines to the use of adjunctive therapies [37]. The staging systems most commonly used are the Enneking system and the staging system of the American Joint Committee. Staging requires knowledge of the histologic grade of the lesion as well as its anatomic extent, and can only be completed following biopsy.

Enneking Staging System

The surgical staging system most commonly used in the evaluation of musculoskeletal tumors is that of Enneking [37]. It is based on the surgical grade of a tumor (G), its local extent (T), and the presence or absence of regional or distant metastases (M) [37]. The Enneking staging system was designed for the evaluation of musculoskeletal mesenchymal tumors and is not intended for use with lesions derived from marrow or the reticuloendothelial system because of their different natural histories, surgical management, and response to treatment.

Lesions are divided into two grades, low (G_1) and high (G_2), on the basis of histologic appearance. In general, low-grade lesions are well-differentiated and have a low potential for the development of metastatic disease. In contrast, high-grade lesions are generally poorly-differentiated, with a high mitotic rate and aggressive clinical course. Local extent is divided into lesions that are intracompartmental (T_1) and extracompartmental (T_2). The designation of intracompartmental indicates that the lesion remains confined to the compartment of origin. For osseous lesions, each bone is considered to be a distinct compartment. An extracompartmental lesion has extended beyond the compartment of origin. For example, an osteosarcoma is extracompartmental when extending from the bone into the adjacent soft tissue or joint. The presence (M_1) or absence (M_0) of regional or distant metastases is the third and final component of staging. On the basis of these considerations, lesions are staged as shown in Table 1.

Table 1. Enneking surgical staging of musuloskeletal sarcomas (from [38])

Stage	Grade	Site
IA	Low (G_1)	Intracompartmental (T_1)
IB	Low (G_1)	Extracompartmental (T_2)
IIA	High (G_2)	Intracompartmental (T_1)
IIB	High (G_2)	Extracompartmental (T_2)
III	Any (G)	Any (T) with metastases

Table 3. American Joint Committee on Cancer (AJCC) AJCC staging of bone sarcomas (from [38])

Stage	T	N	M	Histologic Grade (G)
IA	T_1	N_0	M_0	$G_{1,2}$ Low grade
IB	T_2	N_0	M_0	$G_{1,2}$ Low grade
IIA	T_1	N_0	M_0	$G_{3,4}$ High grade
IIB	T_2	N_0	M_0	$G_{3,4}$ High grade
III	T_3	N_0	M_0	Any G
IVA	Any T	N_0	M_{1a}	Any G
IVB	Any T	N_1	Any M	Any G
	Any T	Any N	M_{1b}	Any G

American Joint Committee on Cancer (AJCC) Staging System

The Enneking system is well-suited for the evaluation of lesions of the extremities because of its emphasis on compartmentalization. It does not, however, consider tumor size or distinguish between regional lymph node and distant metastases. In addition, the division of all lesions into either high- or low-grade may not be sufficient to be applicable to the wide range of all sarcomas. An alternative staging system is that of the American Joint Committee on Cancer (AJCC), which is based on the tumor, node, and metastasis (TNM) classification [38]. This system is more complex, with four stages and several subclassifications.

The AJCC staging system addresses the surgical grade of a tumor (G), its size and local extent (T), the presence or absence of nodal involvement (N), and the presence or absence of distal metastasis (M) [38]. Tables 2 and 3 list the classification criteria and subsequent surgical staging.

Table 2. American Joint Committee on Cancer (AJCC) AJCC staging of bone sarcomas. The AJCC Staging system uses the TMN system as described below to assess the anatomic extent of disease (from [38])

AT	Extent of primary tumor
N	Absence or presence of regional nodal involvement
M	Absence or presence of distant metastasis

Histologic grade (G)

G_1	Well-differentiated
G_2	Moderately well-differentiated
G_3	Poorly differentiated
G_4	Undifferentiated

Primary site (T)

T_1	Tumor ≤8 cm or less in greatest dimension
T_2	Tumor >8 cm in greatest dimension
T_3	Discontinuous tumors in the primary bone site

Nodal involvement (N)

N_0	No regional lymph nodal metastases
N_1	Regional lymph nodal metastases

Distant Metastasis (M)

M_0	No distant metastasis
M_{1a}	Lung metastasis present
M_{1b}	Metastasis other distant sites, including lymph nodes

Diagnosis

As previously noted, the radiograph remains the most diagnostic imaging study. While more advanced imaging provides the information needed for accurate staging, diagnosis (or differential diagnosis) begins with the radiograph and is based on the morphology of the lesion, the lesion's location, and the patient's age.

Morphology describes the presence and character of the lesion's margin and periosteal reaction, features that are a function of the interaction between the lesion and the host and are a key to biologic behavior. Morphology also includes an analysis of the matrix. If present, a mineralized matrix may be a key to the lesion's histology.

The location of a lesion is a major consideration in establishing a diagnosis and structuring a differential diagnosis. There are two components to the location of an osseous lesion: the anatomic location (which bone) and the lesion's location within the bone (epiphysis, metaphysis, metadiaphysis, or diaphysis). The latter is critical in assessment of long-bone lesions and is an essential principle of diagnosis (pictorially presented in Fig. 1). Age is also a critical consideration, with specific lesions tending to occur in specific age groups (Tables 4 and 5). For example, Langerhans cell histiocytosis localized to bone typically occurs in children and adolescents, while osseous lymphoma is most often encountered in mature adults, usually in the sixth and seventh decades. The final diagnosis, or differential, is then based on the integration of all of the above factors, also taking into consideration the prevalence of such tumors within the population.

Conclusions

Accurate diagnosis and staging of osseous tumors requires an organized and integrated approach involving the radiologist, pathologist, and surgeon. Despite the wide variety of imaging modalities available today, radiographs remain the mainstay in the evaluation of osseous

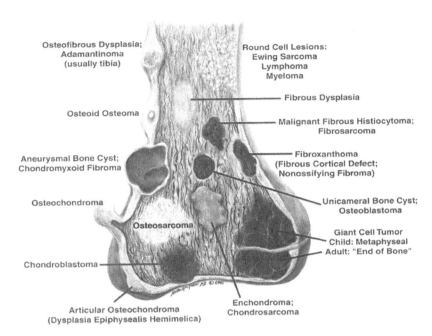

Osteofibrous Dysplasia;
Adamantinoma
(usually tibia)

Round Cell Lesions:
Ewing Sarcoma
Lymphoma
Myeloma

Fibrous Dysplasia

Osteoid Osteoma

Malignant Fibrous Histiocytoma;
Fibrosarcoma

Aneurysmal Bone Cyst;
Chondromyxoid Fibroma

Fibroxanthoma
(Fibrous Cortical Defect;
Nonossifying Fibroma)

Osteochondroma

Unicameral Bone Cyst;
Osteoblastoma

Osteosarcoma

Giant Cell Tumor
Child: Metaphyseal
Adult: "End of Bone"

Chondroblastoma

Articular Osteochondroma
(Dysplasia Epiphysealis Hemimelica)

Enchondroma;
Chondrosarcoma

Fig. 1. Preferential sites for bone tumors, based on cell type

Table 4. Age distribution of malignant osseous tumors[a]

Tumor type	Overall incidence	Incidence by decade (%)								
		1	2	3	4	5	6	7	8	9+
Osteosarcoma	29.2%	4.6	46.0	17.2	8.8	7.6	6.5	6.7	2.4	0.3
Myeloma	14.4%		0.1	1.2	5.2	15.7	29.2	29.2	15.8	3.4
Chondrosarcoma	15.8%	0.6	4.8	12.3	21.4	20.3	20.1	14.0	5.6	0.8
Lymphoma	12.3%	2.7	8.9	10.8	10.2	14.7	20.3	17.5	12.0	2.7
Ewing Sarcoma	9.5%	16.2	59.6	16.8	4.7	2.0	0.8			
Chordoma	6.3%	1.1	4.2	6.2	13.5	18.5	24.4	20.5	9.3	2.2
Fibrosarcoma	4.5%	3.1	11.4	13.3	19.2	14.5	16.7	12.9	6.3	2.4
Chondrosarcoma, dedifferentiated	2.1%		1.7	2.5	6.7	18.3	32.5	17.5	16.7	4.2
Malignant fibrous histiocytoma	1.5%	1.2	15.7	10.8	13.3	19.3	9.6	21.7	6.0	2.4
Osteosarcoma, parosteal	1.2%		17.4	39.1	27.5	10.1	5.8			
Chondrosarcoma, mesenchymal	0.6%		17.6	32.4	29.4	11.8	2.9		2.9	
Adamantinoma	0.6%	2.9	29.4	44.1	5.9	5.9	5.9		5.9	

[a] Adapted from [39], based on an analysis of 5656 malignancies, including 814 cases of myeloma diagnosed on the basis of surgical biopsy. Not included in Table 4 are 2935 cases of myeloma diagnosed on the basis of bone marrow aspirate, for a total of 8591 malignancies and an overall incidence of myeloma of 43.6%

Table 5. Age distribution of malignant osseous tumors[a]

Tumor type	Overall incidence	Incidence by decade (%)								
		1	2	3	4	5	6	7	8	9+
Osteochondroma	34.9%	11.8	47.8	18.5	10.6	5.4	3.6	1.4	0.9	
Giant cell tumor	22.8%	0.5	15.1	37.0	24.6	13.3	6.2	2.5	0.9	
Chondroma (enchondroma)	13.4%	10.7	21.8	17.0	17.0	17.3	8.1	6.6	1.2	0.3
Osteoid osteoma	13.3%	13.6	51.4	21.8	9.1	1.5	0.9	1.2	0.6	
Chondroblastoma	4.8%	2.5	58.8	14.3	10.9	4.2	8.4	0.8		
Hemangioma	4,3%	3.7	9.3	13.9	15.7	25.9	16.7	11.1	3.7	
Osteoblastoma	3.5%	6.9	41.4	32.2	10.3	3.4	3.4	1.1	1.1	
Chondromyxoid fibroma	1.8%	11.1	24.4	31.1	13.3	8.9	8.9		2.2	

[a] Adapted from [39]. based on an analysis of 2,496 benign tumors

neoplasms. Advanced imaging is, however, very useful for staging purposes and for characterization of the internal architecture of tumors and may aid significantly in limiting the differential diagnosis.

References

1. Hudson TM (1987) Radiologic-pathologic correlation of musculoskeletal lesions. Williams & Wilkins, Baltimore, pp 1-9
2. Madewell JE, Ragsdale BD, Sweet DE (1981) Analysis of solitary bone lesions. Part I. Internal margins. Radiol Clin North Am 19:715-748
3. Moser RP, Madewell JE (1987) An approach to primary bone tumors. Radiol Clin North Am 25:1049-1093
4. Ragsdale BD, Madewell JE, Sweet DE (1981) Analysis of solitary bone lesions. Part II. Periosteal reactions. Radiol Clin North Am 19:749-783
5. Sweet DE, Madewell JE, Ragsdale BD (1981) Analysis of solitary bone lesions. Part III. Matrix patterns. Radiol Clin North Am 19:785-814
6. Tehranzadeh J, Mnaymneh W, Ghavam C, Morillo G, Murphy BJ (1989) Comparison of CT and MR imaging in musculoskeletal neoplasms. J Comput Assist Tomogr 13:466-472
7. Pettersson H, Gillespy T 3rd, Hamlin DJ et al (1987) Primary musculoskeletal tumors: examination with MR imaging compared with conventional modalities. Radiology 164:237-241
8. Panicek DM, Gatsonis C, Rosenthal DI et al (1997) CT and MR imaging in the local staging of primary malignant musculoskeletal neoplasms: report of the Radiology Diagnostic Oncology Group. Radiology 202:237-246
9. Aisen AM, Martel W, Braunstein EM et al (1986) MRI and CT evaluation of primary bone and soft-tissue tumors. AJR Am J Roentgenol 146:749-756
10. Hudson TM, Hamlin DJ, Enneking WF, Pettersson H (1985) Magnetic resonance imaging of bone and soft tissue tumors: early experience in 31 patients compared with computed tomography. Skeletal Radiol 13:134-146
11. Lang P, Johnston JO, Arenal-Romero F (1988) Advances in MR imaging of pediatric musculoskeletal neoplasms. Magn Reson Imaging Clin N Am 6:579-604
12. Zimmer WD, Berquist TH, McLeod RA et al (1985) Bone tumors: magnetic resonance imaging versus computed tomography. Radiology 155:709-718
13. Vanel D, Verstraete KL, Shapeero LG (1997) Primary tumors of the musculoskeletal system. Radiol Clin North Am 35:213-237
14. Sundaram M, McLeod RA (1990) MR imaging of tumor and tumorlike lesions of bone and soft tissue. AJR Am J Roentgenol 155:817-824
15. Schima W, Amann G, Stiglbauer R et al (1994) Preoperative staging of osteosarcoma: efficacy of MR imaging in detecting joint involvement. AJR Am J Roentgenol 163:1171-1175
16. Rubin DA, Kneeland JB (1994) MR imaging of the musculoskeletal system: technical considerations for enhancing image quality and diagnostic yield. AJR Am J Roentgenol 163:1155-1163
17. Mirowitz SA (1993) Fast scanning and fat-suppression MR imaging of musculoskeletal disorders. AJR Am J Roentgenol 161:1147-1157
18. Dwyer AJ, Frank JA, Sank VJ et al (1988) Short T1 inversion-recovery pulse sequence: analysis and initial experience in cancer imaging. Radiology 168:827-836
19. Shuman WP, Baron RL, Peters MJ, Tazioli PK (1989) Comparison of STIR and spin echo MR imaging at 1.5T in 90 lesions of the chest, liver and pelvis. AJR Am J Roentgenol 152:853-859
20. Cohen MD, Weetman RM, Provisor AJ et al (1986) Efficacy of magnetic resonance imaging in 139 children with tumors. Arch Surg 121:522-529
21. Sundaram M, McLeod RA (1988) Computed tomography or magnetic resonance for evaluation of solitary tumor and tumor-like lesions of bone. Skeletal Radiol 17:393-401
22. Bloem JL, Taminiau AHM, Eulderink F et al (1988) Radiologic staging of primary bone sarcoma: MR imaging, scintigraphy, angiography, and CT correlated with pathologic examination. Radiology 169:805-810
23. Seeger LL, Widoff BE, Bassett LW et al (1991) Preoperative evaluation of osteosarcoma: value of gadopentetate dimeglumine-enhanced MR imaging. AJR Am J Roentgenol 157:347-351
24. Benedikt RA, Jelinek JS, Kransdorf MJ et al (1994) MR imaging of soft-tissue masses: role of gadopentetate dimeglumine. J Magn Reson Imaging 4:485-490
25. Jordan RM, Mintz RD (1995) Fatal reaction to gadopentetate dimeglumine. AJR Am J Roentgenol. 164:743-744
26. Tardy B, Guy C, Barral G et al (1992) Anaphylactic shock induced by intravenous gadopentetate dimeglumine. Lancet 339:494
27. Shellock FG, Hahn HP, Mink JH et al (1993) Adverse reaction to intravenous gadoteridol. Radiology 189:151-152
28. Fletcher BD, Hanna SL, Fairclough DL et al (1992) Pediatric musculoskeletal tumors: use of dynamic, contrast-enhanced MR imaging to monitor response to chemotherapy. Radiology 184:243-248
29. Shapeero LG, Henry-Amar M, Vanel D (1992) Response of osteosarcoma and Ewing sarcoma to preoperative chemotherapy: assessment with dynamic and static MR imaging and skeletal scintigraphy. Invest Radiol 27:989-991
30. Shapeero LG, Vanel D (2000) Imaging evaluation of the response of high-grade osteosarcoma and Ewing sarcoma to chemotherapy with emphasis on dynamic contrast-enhanced magnetic resonance imaging. Semin Musculoskelet Radiol 4:137-146
31. Nomikos GC, Murphey MD, Kransdorf MJ et al (2002) Primary bone tumors of the lower extremities. Radiol Clin N Amer 40:971-990
32. Swan JS, Grist TM, Sproat IA et al (1995) Musculoskeletal neoplasms: preoperative evaluation with MR angiography. Radiology 194:519-524
33. Ekelund L, Herrlin K, Rydholm A (1982) Comparison of computed tomography and angiography in the evaluation of soft tissue tumors of the extremities. Acta Radiol Diagn 23:15-28
34. Abdel-Dayem HM (1997) The role of nuclear medicine in primary bone and soft tissue tumors. Semin Nucl Med 27:355-363
35. Murphey MD, Flemming DJ, Boyea SR et al (1998) Enchondroma versus chondrosarcoma in the appendicular skeleton: differentiating features. Radiographics 18:1213-1237
36. Schulte M, Brecht-Krauss D, Werner M et al (1999) Evaluation of neoadjuvant therapy response of osteogenic sarcoma using FDG PET. J Nucl Med 40:1637-1643
37. Enneking WF, Spanier SS, Goodman MA (1980) A system for the surgical staging of musculoskeletal sarcoma. Clin Orthop 153:106-120
38. American Joint Committee on Cancer (2002) American Joint Committee on Cancer (AJCC) Staging Manual, 6th edn. www.cancerstaging.net
39. Unni KK (1996) Dahlin's bone tumors. General Aspects and data on 11,087 cases, 5th edn. Lippincott-Raven, Philadelphia, pp 1-9

Disorders of Bone Marrow

Apostolos H. Karantanas[1], David M. Panicek[2]

[1] Department of Radiology, University Hospital, Heraklion, Greece
[2] Department of Radiology, Memorial Sloan-Kettering Cancer Center, New York, NY, USA

Introduction

Distribution of Bone Marrow

Bone marrow is one of the largest organs in the body, after the osseous skeleton, skin, and body fat, and is present on nearly every magnetic resonance image obtained of the human body. Hematopoietic (red) marrow is present throughout the entire skeleton at birth, but over the ensuing two decades of life different regions of hematopoietic marrow convert to fatty (yellow) marrow. This conversion begins in the periphery of the skeleton and then symmetrically extends into the central skeleton (Fig. 1a). An additional, superimposed sequence of marrow conversion occurs in the long bones, starting in the diaphyses and progressing towards the metaphyses (particularly the distal metaphysis) (Fig. 1b). In the second decade of life, marrow in the long bones becomes predominantly fatty, except in the proximal metaphyses. In the late third decade, the marrow distribution reaches its mature state, with hematopoietic marrow occupying the axial skeleton (skull, spine, sternum, clavicles, scapulas, pelvis) as well as the proximal metaphyses of the humeri and femurs; later in life, even those regions gradually convert to fatty marrow.

At times of sustained demand for increased hematopoiesis, fatty marrow can reconvert to hematopoietic marrow. Some conditions that can initiate reconversion include heavy smoking; long-distance running; obesity; middle age in women; and chronic disorders (such as hemoglobinopathies and chronic infection) that result in anemia. Reconversion occurs in the reverse sequence from that of normal developmental conversion (i.e., from the central to the peripheral skeleton; and in long bones, from the proximal metaphyses, to the distal metaphyses, and then to the diaphyses). At MR imaging, diffuse hematopoietic marrow reconversion may be difficult to distinguish from diffuse marrow disease.

Magnetic Resonance Imaging Techniques for Evaluating Marrow

Bone marrow is composed predominantly of fat and water, the relative proportions of which affect the signal intensity of marrow at magnetic resonance imaging (MRI).

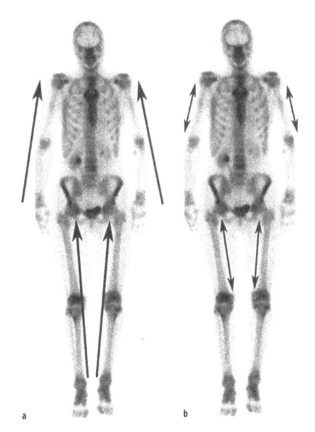

Fig. 1 a, b. Bone marrow conversion patterns. **a** The conversion of hematopoietic marrow at birth to fatty marrow occurs overall from the peripheral to the axial skeleton (*arrows*). **b** In long bones, hematopoietic marrow first converts to yellow in the diaphysis, then proceeds to the metaphysis (*double-headed arrows*). During times of increased requirement for hematopoiesis, both sequences proceed in the opposite directions to reconvert fatty marrow to hematopoietic marrow. Bone scans are used here to demonstrate the directions of marrow changes

Of note, all normal marrow contains lipid: hematopoietic marrow about 40-60%, and fatty marrow, about 95%. The signal intensity of fatty marrow is similar to that of subcutaneous fat in T1-weighted (w) spin-echo (SE) images, whereas the signal intensity of hematopoietic marrow is lower than that of subcutaneous fat but generally higher than that of muscle or intervertebral discs. Marrow lesions, whether benign or malignant, manifest similar signal intensity as muscle on T1-w SE images, which contrasts sharply with the surrounding high-signal-intensity fatty marrow. The use of a fat-suppression option is essential when obtaining fast (turbo) SE T2-w images, as both fatty marrow and tumors have similar, moderately high signal intensity on that sequence. Proton-density images are of limited use in the evaluation of marrow, as the contrast between normal marrow and most pathologic marrow processes is small.

The short-tau inversion recovery (STIR) pulse sequence, in which a specific inversion time (TI; 140-160 ms at 1.5 T) is chosen to eliminate the signal from fatty tissue, is highly sensitive in demonstrating marrow lesions. Also, STIR is less affected by magnetic-field inhomogeneities than is the fat-suppression option, resulting in more homogeneous fat suppression throughout the entire field of view.

Opposed-phase chemical-shift imaging, using a gradient-echo pulse sequence with an appropriate echo time (e.g., 2.2 ms at 1.5 T), shows loss of signal in all normal marrow due to the presence of both lipid and water in marrow-containing voxels. Tumor replaces normal marrow and does not contain lipid; therefore, tumor will not show signal loss on opposed-phase images. In fact, demonstration of fat within a bone lesion effectively excludes the presence of tumor.

Normal marrow enhances on dynamic MRI after injection of gadolinium-DTPA, but is less evident (slower) at routine T1-w SE MRI. Normal marrow enhances most in young patients and in individuals with lower marrow fat content. Strong marrow enhancement occurs in a variety of processes, such as infection, inflammation, and tumor, limiting the role of enhancement in differentiating these entities.

Diffusion-weighted imaging (DWI) provides information on the relative mobility of water molecules in a tissue. Tumor restricts the free diffusion of water molecules, and appears hyperintense at DWI.

Neoplastic Disorders

Hematologic and Solid Tumors

Malignant tumors can arise in the marrow in one of four ways: (1) from myeloid elements of marrow, resulting in leukemia, lymphoma, or multiple myeloma; (2) from mesenchymal elements of marrow, yielding a sarcoma; (3) by hematogenous dissemination (metastasis) of tumor to marrow; or (4) by direct invasion of an extraosseous tumor through the cortex into the marrow.

Leukemic infiltration of marrow generally manifests as diffusely decreased marrow signal on T1-w images, although the marrow signal may appear normal in the presence of only minimal infiltration. Myeloma cells can pro-

duce factors that suppress hematopoiesis, initially leading to an increase in surrounding marrow fat. On T1-w images, multiple myeloma typically manifests as either a variegated pattern of small hypointense lesions throughout the marrow; larger, focal marrow lesions; or diffusely low marrow signal. Like most tumors, leukemia and myeloma show high signal on T2-w images and enhance more than red marrow after administration of gadolinium-based contrast material.

The new Durie/Salmon PLUS system for initial staging of myeloma incorporates whole-body positron emission tomography (PET)/computed tomography (CT) or MRI of the spine and pelvis, rather than relying on the traditional radiographic skeletal evaluation to assess the tumor burden in the marrow. The number of marrow lesions shown at MRI correlates with both treatment outcome and overall survival. However, lesions may persist at MRI for 9-12 months after successful treatment, thus limiting the role of this modality in post-treatment follow-up. PET/CT is helpful in this situation, as active myeloma is fluorodeoxyglucose (FDG)-positive, whereas FDG uptake decreases rapidly after effective treatment.

Lymphoma deposits in marrow are usually focal or diffuse, showing signals similar to those of other tumors. In cases of multifocal lymphoma, MRI can be useful for demonstrating sites of marrow involvement and provides an alternative to relying solely on the results of routine (blind) biopsy of the posterior iliac crests to assess the marrow.

Metastases replace the normal marrow and typically manifest as intermediate signal, similar to that of muscle, on T1-w images. On fat-suppressed T2-w images, most metastases – whether lytic, blastic, or mixed – show increased signal throughout or in a peripheral rim ("halo") (Fig. 2). Some tumors, such as myxoid liposarcoma, have a propensity to metastasize to marrow without producing abnormalities on radiographs, CT, or bone scan.

The presence of marrow edema that extends far beyond the margins of a bone lesion has been shown to favor a benign etiology for the lesion. Extensive edema has been reported in association with osteoid osteoma, osteoblastoma, chondroblastoma (Fig. 3), Langerhans cell histiocytosis, and solid aneurysmal bone cyst, as well as for osteomyelitis.

Spinal Fractures: Osteoporotic vs. Metastatic

Distinguishing between benign and malignant vertebral fractures at imaging can be challenging, and clinical information may not be revealing. For example, in patients with multiple myeloma, spinal compression fractures can be due to underlying generalized osteopenia or to destructive bony changes from gross tumor deposits. Of note, a new spinal compression fracture occurring during treatment of multiple myeloma may be the result of successful tumor lysis, since, once the solid tumor mass has been destroyed, the remaining, weakened bone is no longer able to fulfill its biomechanical supporting role and thus collapses.

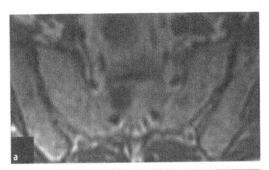
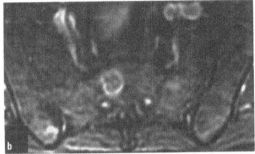
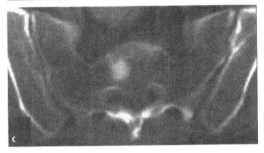

Fig. 2 a-c. Halo sign of metastasis. Lesion in sacrum has low signal on T1-weighted axial MR image (**a**) and rim ("halo") of high signal on fat-suppressed T2-weighted axial MR image (**b**). This metastasis of prostate cancer is quite blastic at computed tomography (CT) (**c**), where it might be mistaken for a bone island; however, a bone island would not show a halo sign at MRI. The blastic response of host bone trabeculae results in low signal within the lesion itself in (**b**)

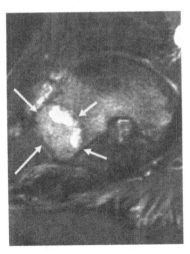

Fig. 3. Extensive marrow edema surrounding chondroblastoma. The chondroblastoma (*arrows*) in the anterior talus contains some cystic areas due to associated secondary aneurysmal bone cyst. On this sagittal fat-suppressed T2-weighted MRI images, note the extensive, poorly defined, high-signal edema present in the surrounding marrow throughout much of the talus – a helpful finding for suggesting the correct diagnosis

Various features at MRI have been reported to indicate a malignant cause for a spinal fracture, including involvement of an entire vertebral body, inhomogeneous enhancement of the vertebra, extension of signal abnormality into the pedicles, a convex contour of the collapsed vertebral body, the presence of an associated epidural mass, and a cervical or lumbosacral location of the collapsed vertebra. Features suggestive of a benign spinal fracture include the presence of a retropulsed bone fragment, preservation of fatty marrow throughout the vertebra, lack of high signal on T2-w images, only a small amount of soft tissue associated with the fracture, and the presence of a horizontal fracture plane evident on post-gadolinium images.

Reports on the utility of DWI in marrow imaging have reached contradictory conclusions. Some stated that malignant spinal compression fractures are hyperintense to normal marrow and benign (mostly osteoporotic) compression fractures are hypointense at DWI, whereas others found no substantial discriminatory findings at DWI. A recent meta-analysis concluded that the mean apparent diffusion coefficient (ADC) values obtained at DWI are significantly higher in benign spinal fractures than in malignant ones and that hypointense lesions at DWI are more likely benign. As different techniques have been used to obtain DWI, further research is needed to more fully define the role of DWI in this setting.

Therapy-Induced Marrow Changes

In some cases after successful therapy, a tumor deposit in the marrow may gradually be replaced by normal fatty marrow, whereas in others the tumor deposit may persist indefinitely as a region of abnormal signal at MRI. Reliance on the change in size of a marrow lesion alone thus may lead to an incorrect assessment of treatment response.

Conversion of a marrow lesion and its surrounding normal marrow to fatty marrow is a well-known effect of radiation therapy, manifesting as uniform, high signal intensity on T1-w images throughout the region of the radiation port.

Granulocyte-colony stimulating factor (G-CSF), a hematopoietic growth factor, is often administered to cancer patients to reduce the complications that result from myelosuppressive therapies. G-CSF stimulates the reconversion of fatty marrow to hematopoietic marrow, particularly the myeloid cell line. This stimulation produces multifocal or diffuse marrow changes at MRI that may be mistaken for the appearance of new metastases (Fig. 4). Knowing that the patient has received G-CSF is essential for proper interpretation of the marrow findings at MRI in this context.

Marrow changes are observed frequently in the long bones of patients after combined radiation therapy and chemotherapy for soft-tissue sarcoma of an extremity. Such changes are most often multiple; appear linear or curvilinear, rather than nodular or masslike; and increase or fluctuate in size on serial examinations (Fig. 5). Focal

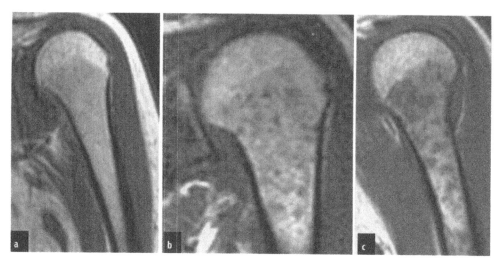

Fig. 4 a-c. Hematopoietic growth-factor (granulocyte-colony stimulating factor, G-CSF) therapy. Coronal T1-weighted MRI at baseline (**a**), 10 weeks (**b**), and 12 weeks (**c**) after the start of G-CSF therapy shows interval development of innumerable, small, low-signal foci throughout the marrow of the proximal metaphysis and diaphysis of the humerus, representing marrow reconversion. Note sparing of fatty marrow in the proximal humeral epiphysis, as would be expected except in the most extreme degrees of marrow reconversion. These findings should not be misinterpreted as metastasis

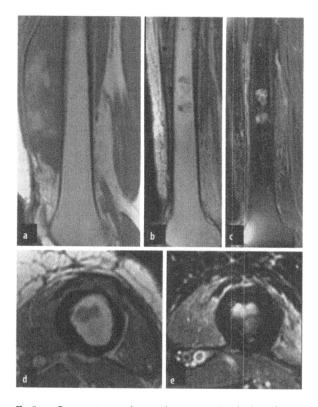

Fig. 5 a-e. Post-treatment changes in marrow, developing after radiotherapy and chemotherapy for liposarcoma. Sagittal (**a**, **b**) and axial (**d**) T1-weighted, and sagittal (**c**) and axial (**e**) fat-suppressed T2-weighted MRI before (**a**) and after (**b-e**) chemoradiation. There has been interval development of curvilinear and nodular signal changes in the marrow of the femoral shaft, within the radiation portal. These findings could easily be mistaken for marrow metastases if one relied solely on axial images

marrow lesions occur within the confines of the radiation port. Although resembling small foci of avascular necrosis at MRI in many cases, the marrow changes in one case were shown at histopathologic examination to represent gelatinous (serous) transformation of the marrow, as is seen in some patients with anorexia nervosa or AIDS. Regardless of the exact etiology, these marrow changes should not be misinterpreted as interval development of metastases.

Non-neoplastic Disorders

Bone Marrow Edema Syndrome

The clinical entity referred to as bone marrow edema (BME) syndrome is characterized by a painful joint associated with a pattern of bone marrow edema on MRI. BME shows low signal intensity on T1-w images, high signal intensity on T2-w and STIR images, and enhancement after paramagnetic contrast administration. Clinical disorders presenting with the common imaging finding of BME pattern include the transient osteoporosis or transient bone marrow edema syndrome (TBMES), regional migratory osteoporosis (RMO), and reflex sympathetic dystrophy (RSD).

Transient Osteoporosis

Transient osteoporosis most commonly involves the hip (TOH) followed by the knee, ankle, and foot. The condition affects healthy middle-aged men and, albeit rarely, women in the third trimester of pregnancy. TOH is demonstrated on MRI together with BME – usually obvious within 48 h after the onset of symptoms – associated with a joint effusion (Fig. 6). Periarticular osteopenia is often seen in radiographs obtained 3-6 weeks after symptoms arise. The syndrome is characterized by acute disabling pain and functional disability, without a history of previous trauma. The pathogenesis of the disease remains unclear, and there are no specific biochemical or serological findings in the peripheral blood. Symptoms gradually subside in parallel with the BME on follow-up clinical and MRI examinations in 4-9 months based on conservative treatment, such as restricted weight bearing, antiresorptive medications, and analgesics.

The term "TBMES" was introduced to describe the presence of a bone marrow edema pattern without radiographic evidence of osteopenia. Many clinicians believe that this syndrome is indistinguishable from TOH; rather, that it presents clinically prior to the development of osteopenia on radiographs.

Regional Migratory Osteoporosis

This condition is defined as sequential polyarticular arthralgia of the weight-bearing joints, associated with severe focal osteoporosis. RMO mainly affects middle-aged men, with a clinical presentation and course identical to that of TOH and typically without a history of trauma or injury. It has been reported that migration of symptoms occurs in 5-41% of patients with hip BME; such migration may occur within one joint or different joints and over an unpredictable time interval after the initial onset of symptoms. The commonest pattern of spread is proximal to distal in the lower limb, with the joint nearest the diseased one being the next to be involved. An association with systemic osteoporosis has been hypothesized, and thus dual-energy x-ray absorptiometry (DEXA) of the spine is suggested in this group of patients. The retrospective MRI feature of migrating BME confirms the diagnosis of RMO (Fig. 6).

The term "transient regional osteoporosis" has been proposed to describe the localized BME syndrome that includes both TOH and RMO.

Reflex Sympathetic Dystrophy

The terms RSD, algodystrophy, chronic regional pain syndrome, and Sudeck syndrome have been used in the literature to describe the same clinical entity. RSD is characterized by three distinct stages: acute, dystrophic, and atrophic. The presenting symptom is a dull, burning pain of rapid or gradual onset. On MRI, the bone marrow in the acute stage may show spotty areas of BME, usual-

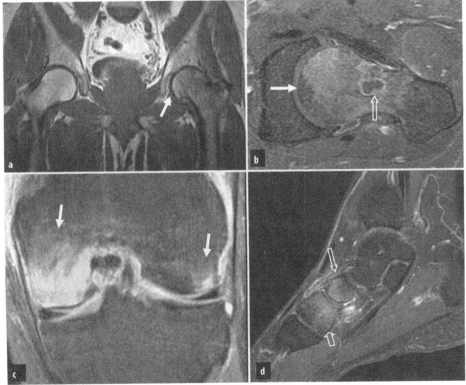

Fig. 6 a-d. Transient and migrating bone marrow edema (BME) syndrome in a 49-year-old patient presenting with a painful left hip. Coronal T1-weighted (**a**) and oblique axial fat-suppressed, contrast-enhanced T1-weighted SE MRI (**b**) shows BME that spares the subchondral area (*solid arrows*), suggesting transient osteoporosis of the hip. A herniation pit is also seen (*open arrow*). The hip symptoms resolved, but the patient presented with ipsilateral knee and foot pain 11 months after the onset of hip symptoms. The coronal fat-suppressed proton density-weighted turbo spin-echo (PD-TSE) MRI (**c**) shows bone marrow edema in the medial femoral condyle and, to a lesser extent, in the lateral condyle (*arrows*). Sagittal fat-suppressed, contrast-enhanced T1-weighted spin-echo MRI (**d**) shows enhancing edema in the midfoot (*arrows*). The findings are suggestive of transient migrating osteoporosis. Complete resolution of all symptoms occurred 9 months later

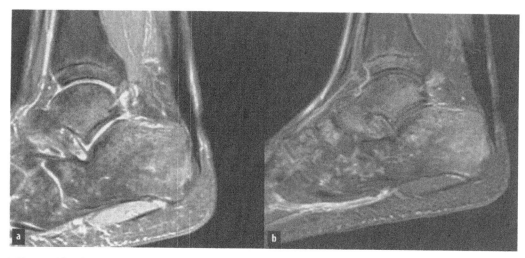

Fig. 7 a, b. A 42-year-old patient with a previously repaired tear of the Achilles tendon later presented with typical clinical signs of Sudeck's algodystrophy. Sagittal fat-suppressed PD-TSE (**a**) and contrast-enhanced T1-weighted (**b**) MRI shows diffuse, patchy, enhancing areas of bone marrow edema in the midfoot and hindfoot

ly diffuse throughout an anatomical area (Fig. 7). As yet, there are no data indicating how often and how long the BME persists in these patients. A history of trauma and the presence of secondary changes such as skin atrophy, sensimotor alterations, or contractures may be helpful in distinguishing this condition from the other types of BME syndromes. RSD has a poor prognosis, unlike the self-limited nature of TOH or RMO.

Osteonecrosis

Osteonecrosis (ON) usually involves adults in their third to fifth decades of life. Males and females are nearly equally affected in most series. In 80% of patients with os-

teonecrosis, predisposing factors, such as administration of steroids, excessive alcohol consumption, sickle-cell disease, lupus erythematosus, or renal transplantation, can be identified. Many studies have shown that patients with ON of the femoral head lack typical findings of BME in TOH in the early stages of the disease, and that BME is never found before the appearance of band patterns at MRI. Indeed, the band pattern is the initial MRI finding of early ON. Studies have shown that BME developed after the onset of hip pain and correlated significantly with the subsequent collapse of the femoral head, suggesting progression to advanced ON (Fig. 8). In addition, BME in ON highly correlates with necrotic volume and worsening of hip pain, thus representing a poor prognostic sign of the disease.

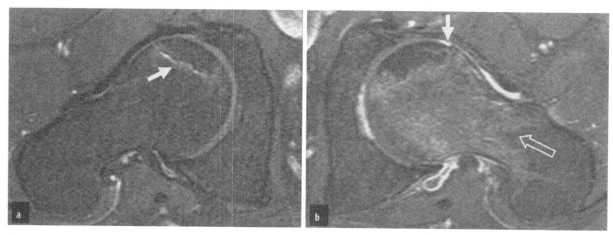

Fig. 8 a, b. A 32-year-old man with a renal transplant and a painful left hip. Oblique axial fat-suppressed, contrast-enhanced T1-weighted spin-echo MRI. **a** The osteonecrotic lesion in the right hip shows a typical band-like configuration (*solid arrow*), without associated marrow edema. **b** Diffuse marrow edema in the left femoral head and neck (*open arrow*) may be the result of the mild articular collapse (*solid arrow*)

Spontaneous Osteonecrosis of the Knee

A common cause of acute knee pain is spontaneous osteonecrosis of the knee (SONK). Initially described by Ahlback et al. in 1968 in the medial femoral condyle, it is usually a disease of the elderly, occurring after the sixth decade of life. The overall prevalence of SONK is 3.4% in patients over the age of 50 years, and it is three times more common in women than in men. Pain is typically sudden in onset and well-localized. The pain may also be present at rest and frequently causes significant functional impairment. There is no history of an acute injury. The precise etiology of this condition remains unclear; traumatic as well as vascular theories have been proposed. The prevailing theory is that the weight-bearing articular surface of the knee is subjected to altered stresses and is thus predisposed to development of a subchondral insufficiency fracture. This alteration in biomechanics can be related to an unstable meniscal tear or prior meniscal resection. Yamamoto et al. reported that lesions diagnosed as SONK were subchondral insufficiency fractures secondary to osteoporosis, and that the osteonecrotic area was the result of the fracture. In the setting of cartilage loss due to osteoarthritis

or weakened bone due to osteopenia, the repetitive impact and stress on the subchondral bone may induce microfractures, thus leading to intraosseous marrow edema. This cycle continues, with increased marrow pressure finally resulting in necrosis. The term "insufficient bone-related arthropathy of the knee" (IBrAK) has been suggested as more appropriate and accurate than SONK in describing this condition.

During the early course of the disease, radiographs are usually normal. Later, a radiolucent subchondral region may be seen. In the late stage of SONK, radiographs may show articular collapse, which may progress to secondary osteoarthritis. MRI is more sensitive than bone scan and radiographs in the diagnosis of SONK. MRI findings of SONK include BME located at the medial femoral condyle, which is the most frequent location, or at the lateral femoral condyle and either tibial plateau. The BME pattern usually extends to the intercondylar notch or tibial tuberosity. In the acute phase of the disease, a subchondral fracture line may be obscured by the extensive BME. Later, a subchondral crescent or linear focus of low signal intensity on T1-w and often T2-w sequences may be seen. Subsequently, collapse of the subchondral bone may occur, leading to secondary degenerative changes (Fig. 9).

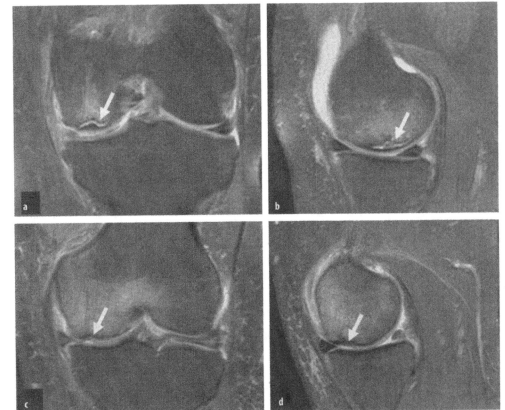

Fig. 9 a-d. Spontaneous osteonecrosis (insufficient bone-related arthropathy of the knee). Fat-suppressed coronal (**a**) and sagittal (**b**) PD-TSE MRI in an osteoporotic 70-year-old female with 4 months of pain in the left knee show extensive marrow edema in the medial femoral condyle, as well as a subchondral fracture (*arrows*). Analogous images (**c, d**) in a 77-year-old male with 7 months of pain in the left knee show minor articular collapse (*arrows*), without any obvious subchondral fracture. In both patients, the medial meniscus is degenerated

Trauma-Related BME

Trauma is the most common cause of BME. The appearance of BME at MRI after trauma (Fig. 10), regardless of its acute, subacute, or chronic nature, is similar to that due to other causes; thus, correlation with clinical history is important in assessing the significance of BME.

Bone Bruise

A bone bruise represents marrow edema and hemorrhage resulting from disrupted trabeculae following a single traumatic event. The pattern of bone bruise may suggest the mechanism of injury and, thus, the structures that might be involved. A bone bruise is commonly associated with chondral and osteochondral injuries, particularly in the growing skeleton. The term "fracture" is employed only when the overlying cortex is disrupted. Bone bruises resolve within 6-12 weeks, in parallel with clinical improvement.

Repeated trauma or friction from tendons and ligaments may also result in BME, with imaging characteristics similar to those of the bone bruise.

Stress-Related Bone Injuries

The persistent overuse of bone that is not yet habituated to new or frequently applied forces results in microscopic trabecular fractures called the *stress response.* This is the most benign event in the spectrum of stress injuries and indeed represents a physiological attempt to balance normal and maladaptive remodeling. In most such cases, MRI demonstrates BME without a fracture line. Failure of the patient to rest and allow the bone to heal results in a *fatigue fracture,* which is usually occult in early radiographs but quite obvious on MRI, which shows a low-signal-intensity fracture line and surrounding BME.

Insufficiency fractures (IF) occur when normal muscular activity is applied to a bone that is deficient in mineral and/or elastic resistance. IF may be seen in healthy women with recent gestation and prolonged lactation, as well as in elderly postmenopausal women and patients with osteopenia due to steroid administration or to metabolic or endocrine disorders. By definition, IF occur either spontaneously or after minimal trauma. Early radiographs may be normal. MRI demonstrates extensive BME surrounding a low-signal-intensity fracture line.

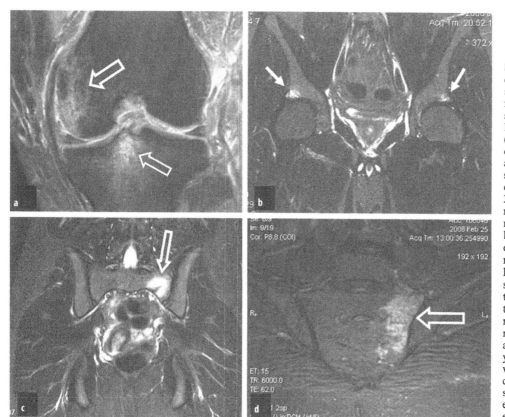

Fig. 10 a-d. Trauma-related BME. **a** Coronal fat-suppressed PD-TSE MRI in a 32-year-old male shows a bone bruise following direct trauma (*arrows*). Medial and lateral ligamentous injuries are also seen. **b** Coronal short-tau inversion recovery (STIR) MRI in a 30-year-old weekend tennis player shows a stress response in the superolateral aspect of both acetabuli (*arrows*). **c** Coronal STIR MRI in a young long-distance runner shows a low-signal-intensity stress fracture in the left sacral wing, surrounded by marrow edema (*arrow*). **d** Oblique axial STIR MRI in a 79-year-old osteoporotic woman shows an insufficiency fracture of the left sacral wing, demonstrated with bone marrow edema (*arrow*)

Radiographs obtained at 3-4 weeks after the onset of symptoms may reveal a sclerotic line that corresponds to the trabecular fracture, without any discontinuity in the cortex. Occasionally, apart from the fracture itself and the associated ipsilateral BME, BME or linear structures may be seen in other sites within the same joint, which could represent a stress response either to biomechanical stress or to a new pre-fracture state.

A pattern of BME similar to that seen with trauma may result with altered weight-bearing, such as in joints with varus or valgus deformity. Tarsal coalition may also induce a stress response manifesting as BME. The degree and duration of this kind of BME depend upon the intensity of the stimulus. A high index of suspicion for stress-related osseous injuries may help avoid unnecessary diagnostic tests and guide proper treatment.

Reactive BME

Infectious arthritis, rheumatoid arthritis, gout, and osteomyelitis should be distinguished from BME since they may present with reactive BME. A thorough history and physical examination may reveal predisposing conditions and associated systemic symptoms. Asymmetrical polyarthritis that usually involves the upper extremities, periarticular soft-tissue swelling, and marked joint effusion are some of the clinical findings that differentiate inflammatory arthritis from BME. The associated articular findings at MRI and the results of routine laboratory examinations are also helpful.

Storage and Deposition Diseases

Various storage diseases are associated with bone marrow involvement. Gaucher disease is the most prevalent lysosomal storage disorder, leading to deposition of glycocerebrosidase-loaded macrophages in the marrow. MRI is useful for elucidating the underlying cause of bone pain, with which these patients commonly present. In addition, MRI is able to quantitatively assess the degree of marrow replacement and thus to monitor the response to treatment.

Quantitative assessment of marrow siderosis in β-thalassemia major patients has been achieved with MRI, suggesting that monitoring the effectiveness of chelation treatment is also possible.

Suggested Reading

Drakonaki EE, Maris TG, Papadakis A, Karantanas AH (2007) Bone marrow changes in beta-thalassemia major: quantitative MR imaging findings and correlation with iron stores. Eur Radiol 17:2079-2087

Durie BGM (2006) The role of anatomic and functional staging in myeloma: description of Durie/Salmon plus staging system. Eur J Cancer 42:1539-1543

Hartman RP, Sundaram M, Okuno SH, Sim FH (2004) Effect of granulocyte-stimulating factors on marrow of adult patients with musculoskeletal malignancies: incidence and MRI findings. AJR Am J Roentgenol 183:645-653

Hwang S, Lefkowitz R, Landa J et al (2008) Local changes in bone marrow at MRI after treatment of extremity soft tissue sarcoma. Skeletal Radiol 38(1):11-19

Hwang S, Panicek DM (2007) Magnetic resonance imaging of bone marrow in oncology, Part 1. Skeletal Radiol 36:913-920

Hwang S, Panicek DM (2007) Magnetic resonance imaging of bone marrow in oncology, Part 2. Skeletal Radiol 36:1017-1027

Iida S, Harada Y, Shimizu K et al (2000) Correlation between bone marrow edema and collapse of the femoral head in steroid-induced osteonecrosis. AJR Am J Roentgenol 174:735-743

Ito H, Matsuno T, Minami A (2006) Relationship between bone marrow edema and development of symptoms in patients with osteonecrosis of the femoral head. AJR Am J Roentgenol 186:1761-1770

James SL, Hughes RJ, Ali KE, Saifuddin A (2006) MRI of bone marrow oedema associated with focal bone lesions. Clin Radiol 61:1003-1009

James SL, Panicek DM, Davies AM(2008) Bone marrow oedema associated with benign and malignant bone tumours. Eur J Radiol 67:11-21

Karantanas AH (2007) Acute bone marrow edema of the hip: role of MR imaging. Eur Radiol 17:2225-2236

Karantanas AH, Drakonaki E, Karachalios T et al (2008) Acute non-traumatic marrow edema syndrome in the knee: MRI findings at presentation, correlation with spinal DEXA and outcome. Eur J Radiol 67:22-33

Karantanas AH, Nikolakopoulos I, Korompilias AV et al (2008) Regional migratory osteoporosis in the knee: MRI findings in 22 patients and review of the literature. Eur J Radiol 67:34-41

Karchevsky M, Babb JS, Schweitzer ME (2008) Can diffusion-weighted imaging be used to differentiate benign from pathologic fractures? A meta-analysis. Skeletal Radiol 37:791-795

Kijowski R, Stanton O, Fine J, De Smet A (2006) Subchondral bone marrow edema in patients with degeneration of the articular cartilage of the knee joint. Radiology 238:943-949

Korompilias AV, Karantanas AH, Lykissas MG, Beris AE (2008) Transient osteoporosis. J Am Acad Orthop Surg 16:480-489

Maas M, van Kuijk C, Stoker J et al (2003) Quantification of bone involvement in Gaucher disease: MR imaging bone marrow burden score as an alternative to Dixon quantitative chemical shift MR imaging – initial experience. Radiology 229:554-561

Malizos KN, Karantanas AH, Varitimidis SE et al (2007) Osteonecrosis of the femoral head: etiology, imaging and treatment. Eur J Radiol 63:16-28

Malizos KN, Zibis AH, Dailiana Z et al (2004) MR imaging findings in transient osteoporosis of the hip. Eur J Radiol 50:238-244

Mirowitz SA, Apicella P, Reinus WR, Hammerman AM (1994) MR imaging of bone marrow lesions: relative conspicuousness on T1-weighted, fat-suppressed T2-weighted, and STIR images. AJR Am J Roentgenol 162:215-221

Montazel J-L, Divine M, Lepage E et al (2003) Normal spinal bone marrow in adults: dynamic gadolinium-enhanced MR imaging. Radiology 229:703-709

Mouloupoulos LA, Dimopoulos MA (1997) Magnetic resonance imaging of the bone marrow in hematologic malignancies. Blood 90:2127-2147

Mulligan ME, Badros AZ (2007) PET/CT and MR imaging in myeloma. Skeletal Radiol 36:5-16

Palmer WE, Levine SM, Dupuy DE (1997) Knee and shoulder fractures: association of fracture detection and marrow edema on MR images with mechanism of injury. Radiology 204:395-399

Rahmouni A, Montazel J-L, Divine M et al (2003) Bone marrow with diffuse tumor infiltration in patients with lymphoproliferative diseases: dynamic gadolinium-enhanced MR imaging. Radiology 229:710-717

Ruzal-Shapiro C, Berdon WE, Cohen MD, Abramson SJ (1991) MR imaging of diffuse bone marrow replacement in pediatric patients with cancer. Radiology 181:587-589

Schweitzer ME, Levine C, Mitchell DG et al (1993) Bull's-eyes and halos: useful MR discriminators of osseous metastases. Radiology 188:249-252

Schweitzer ME, White L (1996) Does altered biomechanics cause marrow edema? Radiology 198:851-853

Sheah K, Ouellette HA, Torriani M et al (2008) Metastatic myxoid liposarcomas: imaging and histopathologic findings. Skeletal Radiol 37:251-258

Simpfendorfer CS, Ilaslan H, Davies AM et al (2008) Does the presence of focal normal marrow fat signal within a tumor on MRI exclude malignancy? An analysis of 184 histologically proven tumors of the pelvic and appendicular skeleton. Skeletal Radiol 37:797-804

Vanel D, Bittoun J, Tardivon A (1998) MRI of bone metastases. Eur Radiol 8:1345-1351

Yamamoto T, Bullough PG (2000) Spontaneous osteonecrosis of the knee: the result of subchondral insufficiency fracture. J Bone Joint Surg Am 82A:858-866

Peripheral Arthritis

Charles S. Resnik[1], Anne Cotten[2]

[1] Department of Diagnostic Radiology, University of Maryland School of Medicine, Baltimore, MD, USA
[2] Service de Radiologie et Imagerie Musculosquelettique, Hôpital R. Salengro, Lille, France

Introduction

The correct diagnosis of peripheral arthritis is based on numerous factors, including clinical features (age and sex of the patient, duration of symptoms, clinical appearance of involved joint or joints), presence or absence of associated diseases (e.g., skin disease, uveitis, urethritis), laboratory values (e.g., markers for inflammation, serum rheumatoid factor. serum uric acid level), and various imaging features. Radiographs represent the mainstay for diagnosis and follow-up of joint damage, although magnetic resonance imaging (MRI) and sonography can be useful evaluation tools, especially in the early stages of disease. Many imaging features have to be systematically assessed to establish a correct diagnosis:

1. The distribution of joint involvement (monoarticular or polyarticular, symmetrical or asymmetrical, proximal or distal, associated axial involvement, associated enthesis involvement)
2. Soft-tissue swelling (periarticular, fusiform, nodular)
3. Joint-space narrowing (uniform, non-uniform, none)
4. Bone erosion (marginal, central, periarticular, well-defined, none)
5. Bone production (osteophytes, enthesophytes, periosteal new bone)
6. Calcification (periarticular, chondrocalcinosis)
7. Subchondral cysts
8. Periarticular osteoporosis

The sites and distribution of common arthritides of the hand and foot are shown in Fig. 1.

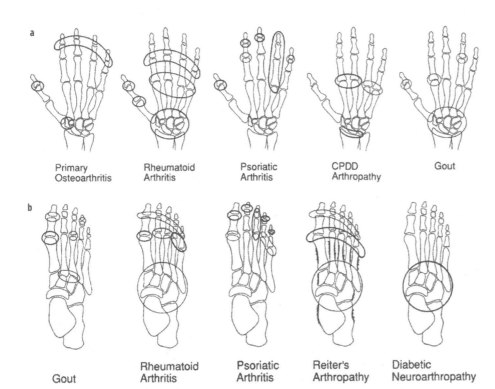

a

Primary Osteoarthritis   Rheumatoid Arthritis   Psoriatic Arthritis   CPDD Arthropathy   Gout

b

Gout   Rheumatoid Arthritis   Psoriatic Arthritis   Reiter's Arthropathy   Diabetic Neuroarthropathy

Fig. 1 a, b. Sites and distribution of common arthritides of the hand (**a**) and foot (**b**). The more common sites are encircled with *heavy lines* and the less common sites with *lighter lines*. Note the periosteal reaction (new bone formation) classically identified in Reiter's arthropathy (reactive arthritis). Note also the potential for "sausage digit" distribution in psoriatic arthritis. When joints are encircled in isolation, the distribution is random and may be isolated to any joint. (Courtesy of L.F. Rogers)

Rheumatoid Arthritis

Rheumatoid arthritis is characterized by proliferative, hypervascularized synovitis, resulting in bone erosion, cartilage damage, joint destruction, and long-term disability. Diagnosis is based on clinical, laboratory, and radiographic findings. The disease typically begins in the peripheral joints, usually the metacarpophalangeal (MCP) and proximal interphalangeal (PIP) joints, the wrists, and the metatarsophalangeal (MTP) joints, with a more or less symmetrical distribution. As the disease progresses, it affects more proximal joints.

Radiography

The initial manifestations are soft-tissue swelling and periarticular osteoporosis. These features represent indirect evidence of synovial inflammation, and their assessment is quite subjective. More specific are marginal erosions of bone that occur at the so-called bare areas between the peripheral edge of the articular cartilage and the insertion of the joint capsule. In the early stages of the disease, these may occur at the radial aspect of the second and third metacarpal heads, at the ulnar styloid process, and at the metatarsal heads, especially at the lateral aspect of the fifth metatarsal head. This is followed by diffuse narrowing of PIP, MCP, MTP, and wrist joints. Unfortunately, these features represent late consequences of synovitis. Characteristically, the distal interphalangeal (DIP) joints are spared. There is no osseous proliferation and no involvement of entheses.

Magnetic Resonance Imaging and Sonography

The development of new, powerful, but expensive, therapeutic agents for rheumatoid arthritis, such as the anti-tumor necrosis factor (TNF) agents, has created new demands on radiologists to identify patients with aggressive rheumatoid arthritis at an early stage. MRI and sonography can be useful tools in evaluating these patients. Sonography is a quick and inexpensive way to detect synovitis and tenosynovitis, whereas MRI is a more global approach to evaluating the small synovial joints of the appendicular skeleton and is more sensitive than radiography in detecting synovitis, bone-marrow edema, and bone erosions.

Seronegative Spondyloarthropathies

The seronegative spondyloarthropathies are represented by psoriatic arthritis, Reiter's syndrome (reactive arthritis), ankylosing spondylitis, colitic arthritis, and undifferentiated spondyloarthropathies. Affected persons usually are negative for serum rheumatoid factor, but a significant percentage has the HLA-B27 antigen. These diseases frequently cause symptoms in the axial skeleton, but the appendicular skeleton may also be affected, in isolation or in combination. Radiographically, these diseases differ from rheumatoid arthritis by the absence or mild nature of periarticular osteoporosis, the involvement of entheses with erosions and with new bone formation, and the asymmetrical involvement of the peripheral skeleton.

Psoriatic Arthritis

The extent of arthritis does not correlate with the degree of psoriatic skin disease, and in some cases, the skin manifestations may follow the arthritis by several years or may never develop. Psoriatic arthritis tends to involve the small joints of the hands and feet. The process is characteristically asymmetrical. Involvement of the DIP joints of the hands and toes, usually in association with psoriatic changes of the nails, or involvement of one entire digit (MCP + PIP + DIP, "sausage digit") is very suggestive of psoriatic arthritis. This arthritis is not necessarily associated with periarticular osteoporosis, and erosions are often small. In contrast, extensive osseous proliferation at the insertion of ligaments and tendons to bone (entheses) is common, as is periostitis.

At an early stage, sonography and MRI may show synovitis, tenosynovitis, and bursitis that are similar to those seen in rheumatoid arthritis. In addition, MRI may demonstrate extensive signal abnormality in the bone marrow and soft tissues far beyond the joint capsule, related to enthesitis. In patients with inflammatory polyarthralgia of the hands, these features may be useful for differentiating rheumatoid arthritis from psoriatic arthritis.

Sacroiliitis is common and resembles that seen in ankylosing spondylitis, except that it is more often asymmetrical. Spinal involvement is less common, and the paravertebral ossification that occurs in psoriatic spondylitis is typically broad, coarse, and asymmetrical in contrast to the symmetrical syndesmophytes of ankylosing spondylitis.

Reiter's Syndrome (Reactive Arthritis)

Reactive arthritis is characterized by urethritis, conjunctivitis, and mucocutaneous lesions in the oropharynx, tongue, glans penis, and skin, as well as arthritis. In general, the radiographic manifestations are similar to those of psoriatic arthritis, except that the axial skeleton is not as commonly involved and changes in the upper extremity are exceptional. The most prominent involvement is in the lower extremities, particularly the feet.

Ankylosing Spondylitis

Involvement in ankylosing spondylitis starts and is most typical in the axial skeleton (spine and sacroiliac joints), but the appendicular skeleton may also be involved, especially the feet. Radiography may demonstrate arthritis and enthesitis with erosive changes and osseous proliferation. At an early stage of the disease, sonography and MRI may be useful in showing inflammatory changes of the entheses.

Colitic Arthritis

Arthritis occurs in approximately 10% of patients with chronic inflammatory bowel disease, more commonly in ulcerative colitis than in Crohn's disease. The most common manifestation is sacroiliitis, which is similar to but not as extensive as that in ankylosing spondylitis, with bilateral symmetrical involvement. Patients are rarely symptomatic, and the radiographic findings of sacroiliitis are often noted incidentally on abdominal radiographs obtained as part of a small bowel or colon examination. Peripheral arthritis is uncommon.

Degenerative Joint Disease (Osteoarthritis)

Osteoarthritis is characterized by degeneration and shredding of articular cartilage. It mainly affects the interphalangeal joints of the fingers (sparing the MCP joints) and the weight-bearing joints (hips and knees). Degenerative joint disease occurs in two major forms: a primary form, which is a generalized disease affecting all of the aforementioned joints, and a secondary form, limited to joints affected by previous localized trauma or other joint disease. The radiographic and pathologic changes are similar in the two forms.

The general radiographic features of osteoarthritis are non-uniform joint-space narrowing, subchondral sclerosis of bone, marginal osteophytes, and subchondral cysts. Narrowing of the joint space in osteoarthritis is almost invariably uneven and more pronounced in that portion of the joint where weight-bearing stresses are greatest. In general, the greater the degree of narrowing, the more severe the associated findings of subchondral sclerosis and osteophytosis. Calcified or ossified fragments (loose bodies) may be identified within the joint and are particularly common in the knee.

The clinical and radiographic features are usually straightforward, and MRI is not used for primary diagnosis. Indeed, it should be recognized that some MRI features may be misleading, including extensive edema of subchondral bone marrow, signal changes of subchondral bone located on only one side of a joint, enhancement of subchondral cysts after intravenous gadolinium administration, and heterogeneous signal intensity of joint fluid.

Erosive Osteoarthritis

Erosive osteoarthritis is an inflammatory form of osteoarthritis that occurs primarily in postmenopausal women. It is usually limited to the interphalangeal joints of the hand. Clinically, the joints are acutely inflamed. Erosions of the central portion of articular surfaces are prominent and are superimposed on the standard radi-

ographic features of osteoarthritis. They are often more pronounced at the PIP joints. Involved joints may eventually undergo osseous ankylosis, which does not occur in non-inflammatory osteoarthritis. Inflammatory changes of these joints may also be demonstrated by MRI.

Metabolic Joint Disease

Gout

Gouty arthritis is characterized by recurring acute attacks of arthritis involving one or more joints, with an increase in the serum level of uric acid and the resulting deposition of sodium urate. The first MTP joint is the joint most often affected. Involvement of the tarsometatarsal and carpometacarpal joints frequently occurs. Over time, chronic tophaceous gout develops with a typical asymmetrical joint involvement. The tophaceous deposits occur in periarticular soft tissues and sometimes in synovium and subchondral bone. These can produce hard masses that may cause ulceration of the overlying skin and extrusion of chalky material.

Radiographic features include eccentric nodular soft tissue swelling. Soft-tissue masses are especially suggestive of tophi when they have high density on radiographs due to microcalcifications, often related to chronic renal disease. Soft-tissue tophi may produce erosion of subjacent bone, including deposition in the olecranon bursa that may be associated with erosion of the olecranon.

Erosions are suggestive of gout if they are located at a distance from any joint. In many cases, though, they may be intra-articular and may be marginal in location, mimicking rheumatoid arthritis. However, other features are helpful for the diagnosis of gout: erosions are often large in size (>5 mm), they are frequently oriented along the long axis of the bone, they are characteristically surrounded by a sclerotic border due to the long duration of disease, and there may be an "overhanging edge" of new bone partially surrounding them. Also, there is commonly relative preservation of the joint space, and there is not extensive osteoporosis.

Sonography may demonstrate soft-tissue tophi before they are radiographically evident. They appear as hyperechoic or heterogeneous masses, sometimes with acoustic shadowing due to calcifications. They may demonstrate hyperemia on power Doppler evaluation. The double contour sign, which is a hyperechoic irregular band over the superficial margin of cartilage and the presence of hypo- to hyperechoic, inhomogeneous material surrounded by a small anechoic rim, may also be suggestive of gout. Sonography can also be used to guide aspiration of a joint.

Computed tomography may be helpful to confirm the high density of a soft-tissue tophus (often about 160 HU), which is less than the density of hydroxyapatite deposits in calcific tendinitis. MRI features may be misleading, as there may be hypointense masses within the synovium on T2-weighted images, mimicking pigmented villonodular synovitis.

Calcium Pyrophosphate Dihydrate (CPPD) Crystal Deposition Disease

CPPD crystal deposition disease is generally observed in middle-aged and elderly patients. It may be associated with two types of radiographic features, which are frequently combined: articular/periarticular calcification and arthropathy.

Calcification

Chondrocalcinosis is the presence of intra-articular calcium-containing salts, most commonly CPPD, within hyaline cartilage and/or fibrocartilage. Calcium within the fibrocartilage is characteristically somewhat irregular, as seen in the menisci of the knee or the triangular fibrocartilage of the wrist. Calcification of hyaline cartilage along an articular surface appears as a fine, linear radiodensity closely paralleling the subjacent cortical margin. Capsular, synovial, ligament, and tendon calcifications are less frequent.

Many affected persons are asymptomatic, but in others, intermittent acute attacks of arthritis resemble gout (pseudogout). The correct diagnosis is established by the identification of typical CPPD crystals in synovial fluid. Sonography may also be helpful by demonstrating multiple sparkling hyperechoic dots without acoustic shadows in the joint fluid that are very suggestive of CPPD crystals.

Pyrophosphate Arthropathy

The joints most commonly involved are the knee, the radiocarpal and midcarpal joints of the wrist, the MCP joints of the hand, the shoulder, and the hip. The joint changes that occur in this disorder resemble osteoarthritis, with joint-space narrowing, bone sclerosis, and subchondral cyst formation. The unusual distribution of these findings, the small size of the osteophytes contrasting with the severity of the arthropathy, and the presence of chondrocalcinosis allow a specific diagnosis to be made. Involvement of the MCP joints, particularly the second and third, is characteristic of this disorder. Hemochromatosis also affects the MCP joints in a similar fashion, but all MCP joints are characteristically affected, and there may be large "hook-like" osteophytes along the radial aspect of the metacarpal heads.

Diabetic Osteoarthropathy

Diabetic osteoarthropathy is confined almost exclusively to the ankle and foot. Calcification of the smaller arteries of the foot is a frequent and important clue to the presence of underlying diabetes but may not always be evident. Fractures or fracture-dislocations of the tarsal bones or metatarsals are particularly common manifestations of diabetic neuropathic disease. Often such fractures or dislocations are incidental findings on radiographs obtained for the evaluation of infection of the foot or complaints of swelling without a history of trauma. Less commonly, the neuropathic process appears to be initiated by a traumatic event that results in a fracture or dislocation. Computed tomography may be useful to assess the extent of microtraumatic changes of joint surfaces. MRI may demonstrate extensive abnormal signal intensity changes of bone that may mimic infection, but the distribution of arthropathy is typically widespread, contrasted with the localized nature of osteomyelitis associated with adjacent soft-tissue infection.

Acknowledgment. The authors acknowledge the major contribution of material to this chapter by Lee F. Rogers, M.D.

Suggested Reading

Aliabadi P, Nikpoor N, Alparslan L (2003) Imaging of neuropathic arthropathy. Semin Musculoskelet Radiol 7(3):217-225

Bennett DL (2004) Spondyloarthropathies: ankylosing spondylitis and psoriatic arthritis. Radiol Clin North Am 42(1):121-134

Bohndorf K, Imhof H, Pope TL (2001) Musculoskeletal Imaging: a concise multimodality approach. Thieme, New York, pp 292-377

Buchmann RF (2004) Imaging of articular disorders in children. Radiol Clin North Am 42:151-168

Cotton A (2005) Imagerie musculosquelettique - Pathologies générales. Masson, Paris, p 767

Greenspan A (2003) Erosive osteoarthritis. Semin Musculoskelet Radiol 7(2):155-159

Gupta KB (2004) Radiographic evaluation of osteoarthritis. Radiol Clin North Am 42(1):11-41

Klecker RJ, Weissman BN (2003) Imaging features of psoriatic arthritis and Reiter's syndrome. Semin Musculoskelet Radiol 7(2):115-126

Monu JU (2004) Gout: a clinical and radiologic review. Radiol Clin North Am 42(1):169-184

Steinbach LS (2004) Calcium pyrophosphate dihydrate and calcium hydroxyapatite crystal deposition diseases: imaging perspectives. Radiol Clin North Am 42(1):185-205

Tehranzadeh J (2004) Advanced imaging of early rheumatoid arthritis. Radiol Clin North Am 42(1): 89-107

Metabolic Bone Disease

Murali Sundaram

Diagnostic Radiology, Musculoskeletal Division, Cleveland Clinic Foundation, Cleveland, OH, USA

Introduction

Metabolic bone disease may result from genetic, endocrine, nutritional, or biochemical disorders, with variable and often inconsistent imaging findings. For the radiologist, the cornerstone of "metabolic bone disease" has been osteoporosis, osteomalacia, hyperparathyroidism, and Paget's disease. Over the past three decades, the diagnosis and therapy of these diseases has changed, influenced by biochemical discoveries, imaging advances, and epidemiology studies that together, in turn, have had a strong impact on current radiological practice.

Osteoporosis

Osteoporosis remains the most common metabolic abnormality of bone. It has been described as "a silent epidemic" affecting 1 in 2 women and 1 in 5 men older than 50 years of age during their lifetime [1]. It is defined as a systemic skeletal disease characterized by low bone mass and microarchitectural deterioration of bone, resulting in with little or no trauma [2]. Although long recognized as a quantitative abnormality of bone, it was the introduction of dual energy x-ray absorptiometry (DXA) in 1987 [3, 4] with its advantages of high precision, short scan times, low radiation dose, and stable calibration, that permitted quantification of osteoporosis (bone mineral density, BMD) in routine clinical practice in order to make the diagnosis and guide management. Prior to BMD measurements, the development of a fracture was the first sign of the presence of osteoporosis. With the routine clinical application of BMD measurements, the diagnosis can be made based taking into account low bone mass, bone fragility, and increased fracture risk.

Trabecular bone comprises 20% of the skeleton and is highly responsive to metabolic stimuli. Therefore, the site-specific assessment of trabecular bone alone is felt to be important for determining osteoporosis fracture risk and treatment response [5]. While DXA measures cortical and trabecular bone, considerable research effort is being devoted to the assessment of the micro-trabecular architecture by CT and MRI [5].

Vertebral compression fractures occur in 26% of women over 50 years of age [6]. The fractures are not always symptomatic, and most heal within a few weeks or months – although a minority does not respond to conservative measures [7]. Percutaneous vertebroplasty (PV) is now a widely used technique for the treatment of such patients, preventing the further loss of bone that frequently accompanies prolonged bed rest.

Osteogenesis Imperfecta (Type V)

In 2000, Glorieux and co-workers described a subtype of the congenital disease osteogenesis imperfecta (OI) with a propensity to such abundant hyperplastic callus formation after fracture that the lesions bore a strong resemblance to those of osteosarcoma. They designated this particular complication as type V OI and considered the hyperplastic exuberant callus formation to represent a new form of brittle bone disease [8]. This form of the disease with hyperplastic callus formation can also lead to significant long-term morbidity [9].

Female Athlete Triad

The female athlete triad comprises an eating disorder, such as anorexia nervosa, a menstrual disorder (amenorrhea or oligomenorrhea), and osteopenia/osteoporosis [10]. "The female athlete triad" becomes a diagnostic consideration for the radiologist when stress fractures and serous atrophy of bone marrow are identified on magnetic resonance imaging (MRI) [11]. Serous atrophy of bone marrow on MRI demonstrates abnormal low signal on T1-weighted images and high signal on T2-weighted or STIR images and in advanced cases may be associated with loss of subcutaneous fat and loss of fat in muscle septa. Stress fractures are usually an unequivocal finding on MRI but may be difficult to identify in the presence of serous marrow change because the typical edema pattern silhouetting a fracture in normal bone marrow is masked by a serous marrow [12].

Osteomalacia and Rickets

Classically, a deficiency of vitamin D, essential for the absorption of calcium, has been the major cause of rickets in children and of osteomalacia in adults. Both conditions reflect the absence of or delay in mineralization of growth cartilage or newly formed bone collagen. Perhaps not as widely recognized is the development of rickets/osteomalacia as a consequence of a low serum phosphate and normal serum calcium. Two such conditions are X-linked, hypophosphatemic rickets/osteomalacia and oncogenic osteomalacia. When present, the signs of rickets and osteomalacia in the low serum phosphate states are indistinguishable from those of those in classic hypocalcemic states. In the child, these signs are a widened growth plate, metaphyseal cupping, and fraying about joints. In the adult, Looser zones (a lucency that runs perpendicular to the cortex of bone indistinguishable from the frequently encountered stress fracture) are seen [13, 14]. However, there are several distinctive imaging signs that have been recently emphasized in these two conditions, along with clinical, genetic, and biochemical advances.

X-Linked Hypophosphatemic Osteomalacia

The condition is characterized by low tubular reabsorption of phosphate in the absence of secondary hyperparathyroidism. X-linked hypophosphatemia occurs in about 1 in 25,000 and is said to be the most common form of genetically induced rickets [15]. From an imaging standpoint, a curious and paradoxical finding in this condition is that, in addition to Looser zones and femoral bowing, there may be striking extraskeletal ossifications at sites of enthesis (mimicking a sero-negative spondylitis or fluorosis) and, occasionally, intraspinal ossifications [16, 17].

Oncogenic Osteomalacia

Oncogenic osteomalacia was first described by Prader et al. in 1959 [18]. It is a paraneoplastic syndrome in which a bone or soft-tissue tumor or tumor-like lesion induces hypophosphatemia and low vitamin D levels , which reverse when the inciting lesion is resected.

Imaging Considerations

As elusive as this diagnosis appears to be for the clinician, it is more so for the radiologist unaware of the critical biochemical abnormalities of hypophosphatemia and hyperphosphaturia. The radiologist may consider the diagnosis of oncogenic osteomalacia if radiographs demonstrate Looser's zones in adults or the classic signs of rickets in children in the absence of malnutrition or malabsorption. Once the presumptive clinical diagnosis of oncogenic osteomalacia is made, the search for the causative neoplasm begins. A recent review observed a range of 5 months to 14 years from the time of presenta-

tion to diagnosis [19]. Skeletal surveys and radioisotope bone scans have been the mainstays in the search for clinically inapparent neoplasm. More recently, whole-body MRI and [111]indium-labeled octreotide scanning have been employed [20, 21]. Whatever the imaging modality used, any discovered lesion, however innocuous, should be considered causative of the syndrome and removed [22]. Tumors responsible for this syndrome may arise equally in bone or soft tissue, with a predilection for the craniofacial region and extremities.

Renal Osteodystrophy

The connection between renal glomerular disease and bone disease was made a little over 100 years ago [23], and the term renal osteodystrophy, describing the musculoskeletal complications of chronic renal failure, was introduced in 1943 [24]. Renal osteodystrophy is the result of two major pathological processes that vary in severity: hyperparathyroidism, from an excess of parathyroid hormone, and rickets or osteomalacia, from a deficiency of 1,25-dihydrocholecalciferol (1, 25 DHCC), the renal hormone of vitamin D [25]. Dialysis and renal transplantation, the only life-sustaining and life-saving therapeutic options for chronic renal failure, modify the natural history of renal osteodystrophy, and thus hyperparathyroidism and osteomalacia. Worldwide, there are over 1 million patients on maintenance hemodialysis [26]. Since hyperparathyroidism is universal in patients with chronic renal failure, irrespective of imaging findings, it may be assumed that these patients have renal osteodystrophy. The development of a new disease state, amyloidosis, is a direct consequence of long-term dialysis in chronic renal failure patients. The problem is unresolved and on the rise, since patients are kept alive by dialysis for long periods of time while awaiting renal transplantation. Cameron referred to this as the "rise and rise of amyloidosis" [27]. Amyloid deposition is a consequence of β2 microglobulin, which is 30 to 50 times above normal in patients with chronic renal failure. The complication is almost universal in those who have been on dialysis for 15 years or longer and tends to become evident after 8 years [27]. The most common location of these deposits is the carpal tunnel. Because primary hyperparathyroidism is diagnosed at a biochemical level and more patients with renal failure are being sustained for longer periods of time on peritoneal or hemodialysis, brown tumors are now not uncommonly seen in poorly controlled patients on dialysis. Thus, in contradistinction to what was taught three decades ago, the practicing radiologist in the Western world is more likely to more often encounter brown tumors as a manifestation of secondary rather than primary hyperparathyroidism.

Destructive discovertebral disease is occasionally encountered in patients on long-term dialysis and has been termed "renal spondyloarthropathy". Its prevalence is unknown, and whether the destructive changes are due to amyloid or is multifactorial is uncertain. The most pressing diagnosis to be excluded is discitis or osteomyelitis. Often this is resolved by an aspiration. However, in some of these patients the abnormality has a short T2 on MRI and in this circumstance may be considered to represent renal spondyloarthropathy rather than a discitis or discovertebral osteomyelitis [28] thereby obviating a biopsy.

Paget's Disease

There has been a significant decline in the prevalence of Paget's disease both in severity and disease of young onset. Paget's disease remains mostly asymptomatic and is often an incidental radiographic finding. MRI is employed when sarcoma is suspected and for staging prior to biopsy. An unexpected MRI finding of uncomplicated Paget's disease is the diffuse preservation of marrow fat, irrespective of the phase of the disease, in the appendicular skeleton on T1-weighted sequences [29, 30]. This has been attributed to a re-population of fat within the marrow space. Osteolytic Paget's, the result of osteoclastic resorption, radiographically may mimic a malignant process. The presence of a marrow fat signal should suggest the correct diagnosis. MRI may also serve to identify the so-called pseudosarcoma of Paget's disease, which clinically presents as a soft-tissue mass with or without erosion of the underlying cortex. Distinction from a sarcoma may be difficult, but preservation of the fatty marrow signal speaks against a sarcoma.

References

1. Sambrook P, Cooper C (2006) Osteoporosis. Lancet 367:2010-2018
2. Anonymous (1993) Consensus development conference, diagnosis prophylaxis and treatment of osteoporosis. Am J Med 94:646-651
3. Genant HK, Engelke K, Fuerst T et al (1996) Noninvasive assessment of bone mineral and structure: state of the art. J Bone Miner Res 11:707-730
4. Baran DT, Faulkner KG, Genant HK et al (1997) Diagnosis and management of osteoporosis – guidelines for the utilization of bone densitometry. Calcif Tissue Int 61:433-440
5. Majumdar S (2008) Magnetic resonance imaging for osteoporosis. Perspectives. Skel Radiol 37:95-97
6. Melton LJ III (1997) Epidemiology of spinal osteoporosis. Spine 22(Suppl):S2-S11
7. Rapado A (1996) General management of vertebral fractures. Bone 18(Suppl):1915-1965
8. Glorieux FH, Rauch F, Plotkin H et al (2000) Type V osteogenesis imperfecta a new form of brittle bone disease. J Bone Miner Res 15:1650-1658
9. Cheung MS, Azouz EM, Glorieux FH, Rauch F (2008) Hyperplastic callus formation in osteogenesis imperfecta type V: follow up of three generation over ten years. Skeletal Radiol 37:465-467
10. Nattor A, Loucks AB, Manore MM et al (2008) American College of Sports Medicine Position Stand. The female athlete triad. Med Sci Sports Exerc 39:1867-1882
11. Vande Berg BC, Malghem J, Devuyst O et al (1994) Anorexia nervosa: correlation appearance between MR appearance of bone marrow and severity of disease. Radiology 193:859-864
12. Tins B, Cassar-Pullicino V (2006) Marrow changes in anorexia nervosa masking the presence of stress fractures on MR imaging. Skeletal Radiol 35:857-860
13. Harrison HE, Harrison HC (1995) Rickets then and now. J Pediatr 87:1144
14. Pitt MJ (1991) Rickets and osteomalacia are still around. Radiol Clin North Am 29:97-118
15. Weissman Y, Hochberg Z (1994) Genetic rickets and osteomalacia. Curr Ther Endocrinol Metab 5:492-495
16. Polisson RP, Martinez S, Khoury M et al (1985) Calcification of enthesis associated with x-linked hypophosphatemic osteomalacia. N Engl J Med 313:1-6
17. Adams JE, Davies M (1986) Intraspinal new bone formation and spinal cord compression in familial hypophosphatemic vitamin D resistant osteomalacia. Am J Med 61:1117-1129
18. Prader VA, Illig R, Uehlinger E, Stalder G (1959) Rachitis infolge Knochentumors. Helv Pediatr Acta 14:554-565
19. Siegel HJ, Rock MG, Inwards C, Sim FH (2002) Phospahturic mesenchymal tumor. Orthopedics 25:1279-1281
20. Avila NA, Skarulis M, Rubino DM, Doppmath JL (1996) Oncogenic osteomalacia: lesion detection by MR skeletal survey. AJR Am J Roentgenol 167:343-345
21. Seufert J, Ebert K, Muller J et al (2001) Brief report: octreotide therapy for tumor induced osteomalacia. N Engl J Med 345:1883-1888
22. Sundaram M, McCarthy EF (2000) Oncogenic osteomalacia. Skeletal Radiol 29:117-124
23. Lucas RC (1883) On a form of late rickets associated with albuminuria: rickets of adolescents. Lancet 1:993
24. Liu SH, Chu HI (1946) Studies of calcium and phosphorous metabolism with special reference to pathogenesis and effects of dihydrotachysterol and iron. Medicine 22:103
25. Parfitt AM (1976) The actions of parathyroid hormone on bone: relation to bone remodeling and turnover calcium homeostasis and metabolic bone disease. Metabolism 25:1157
26. Cameron JS (2002) Dialysis today and tomorrow: history of the treatment of renal failure by dialysis. Oxford University Press, Oxford, p 336
27. Cameron JS (2002) A history of the treatment of renal failure by dialysis. Oxford University Press, Oxford, p 263
28. Leone A, Sundaram M, Cerase A et al (2001) Destructive spondyloarthropathy of the cervical spine in long-term hemodialyzed patients: a five-year clinical radiological prospective study. Skeletal Radiol 30:431-441
29. Kaufmann GA, Sundaram M, McDonald DJ (1991) Magnetic resonance imaging in symptomatic Paget's disease. Skeletal Radiol 20:413-418
30. Sundaram M, Khanna G, El-Khoury G (2001) T1 weighted MR imaging for distinguishing large osteolysis of Paget's disease from sarcomatous degeneration. Skeletal Radiol 30:378-383

Metabolic Bone Diseases

Bruno Vande Berg, Frederic Lecouvet, Paolo Simoni, Jacques Malghem

Department of Radiology, Cliniques Universitaires Saint-Luc, Université Catholique de Louvain, Louvain Academy, Brussels, Belgium

Introduction

The current chapter provides an overview of the important imaging features observed in metabolic bone diseases [1, 2]. Common and uncommon imaging findings observed in insufficiency stress fractures are reviewed and illustrated.

Overview of Metabolic Bone Disorders

Normal Bone Metabolism

Bone is a specialized connective tissue made up of a matrix of collagen fibers, mucopolysaccharides, and inorganic crystalline mineral matrix (calcium hydroxyapatite) that is distributed along the length of the collagen fibers. Bone remains metabolically active throughout life (bone turnover), with bone being constantly resorbed by osteoclasts (osteoclastic activity) and accreted by osteoblasts (osteoblastic activity). Since bone turnover mainly takes place on bone surface, trabecular bone, which has a greater surface to volume ratio than compact bone, is consequently some eight times more metabolically active than cortical bone. The strength of bone is related not only to its hardness and other physical properties but also to its size, shape, and the architectural arrangement of compact and trabecular bone.

Bone formation and bone resorption are linked in a consistent sequence under normal circumstances. Precursor bone cells are activated at a particular skeletal site to form osteoclasts, which erode a flairly constant amount of bone. After a period of time, bone resorption ceases and osteoblasts are required to fill the eroded space with new bone tissue. This coupling of osteoblastic and osteoclastic activity constitutes the basal multicellular unit (BMU) of bone and is normally in balance, with the amount of bone eroded being replaced with an equal amount of new bone in about 3-4 months. At any one time, there are numerous BMUs throughout the skeleton at different stages of this cycle. The amount of bone in the skeleton at any moment is entirely dependent on the peak bone mass attained during puberty and adolescence and on the balance between bone resorption and formation. Bone turnover is under the influence of several factors, including age and hormones, but is also locally modified by many other factors, such as physical forces.

Osteoporosis

Definition

Osteoporosis, by far the most common metabolic disease in Western countries, is a systemic skeletal disease with quantitative abnormality of bone; this is in contrast to rickets/osteomalacia, in which there is a qualitative abnormality of bone (Fig. 1). Osteoporosis is characterized by a reduction in bone mass (amount of mineralized bone per volume unit) and by an altered trabecular structure due to a loss of trabeculae interconnectivity. Consequent-

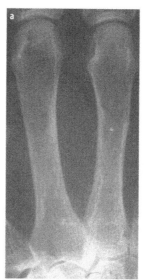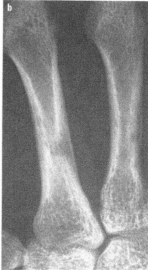

Fig. 1 a, b. Osteopenia and osteomalacia. **a** Osteopenia is characterized by quantitative bone abnormality with decreased bone density and cortical thinning (*arrow*). **b** Osteomalacia is characterized by qualitative bone abnormality with intracortical lucencies (*arrow*)

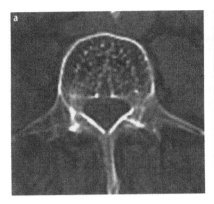
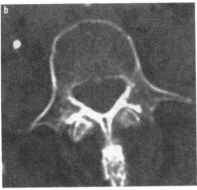

Fig. 2 a, b. Vertebral patterns of osteoporosis. **a** In senile osteoporosis, the vertical weight-bearing trabeculae can be thickened with a decrease in their number. **b** In steroid-associated osteoporosis, the number and thickness of all trabeculae are reduced (atrophic osteopenia)

ly, there is an increase in bone fragility (decrease in biomechanical strength) and susceptibility to fracture (insufficiency fractures) [3] (Fig. 2).

Prevalence of Osteoporosis

Osteoporosis is a serious public health problem; however, over the past 20 years, there have been significant advances in our knowledge of its epidemiology, pathophysiology, and treatment. In the Western world, osteoporosis is reported to affect 1 in 2 women and 1 in 5 men over the age of 50 years [4]. The risk of fracture increases with advancing age and progressive loss of bone mass and varies with the population being considered. The incidence of hip fracture has doubled over the past three decades and is predicted to continue to grow beyond what one would predicted from increased longevity. After hip of or vertebral fracture, mortality is about 20% greater than that expected. At 1 year after hip fracture, 40% of these patients are unable to walk independently, 60% have difficulty with one essential activity of life, 80% are restricted in other activities, and 27% will be admitted to a nursing home for the first time [4].

Clinical Presentation and Etiology

Generalized osteoporosis is a chronic disease with late clinical consequence (low trauma, insufficiency fractures) (Fig. 3). Vertebral fractures are the most common osteoporotic fracture. They occur as an acute event related to minor trauma or spontaneously and can be accompanied by pain, which generally resolves without treatment over 6-8 weeks. Vertebral fractures cause disability and limited spinal mobility and are associated with increased morbidity. They are powerful predictors of future fracture, with a 12% increased risk of a future vertebral fracture within 12 months if a single vertebral fracture is present (22% increased risk in the presence of multiple fractures) [2]. Consequently, the accurate identification and clear reporting of vertebral fracture by radiologists play a vital role in the diagnosis and appropriate management of patient with, or at risk of, osteoporosis. There is evidence that ver-

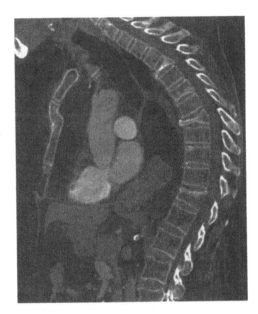

Fig. 3. Osteoporosis. Presence of multiple vertebral fractures with focal bone sclerosis superimposed on a background of hypertrophic osteoporosis. Note the sternal fracture associated with kyphosis

tebral fractures are under-reported (European Society of Skeletal Radiology, osteoporosis group and International osteoporosis foundation, www.osteofound.org).

Generalized osteoporosis is the end-stage of several diseases and can be primary or secondary (Tables 1, 2).

Imaging Findings in Osteoporosis

Radiography is relatively insensitive in detecting early bone loss (<30-40% loss of bone tissue). In addition, radiographic bone density is affected by patient characteristics and the radiographic parameters. The subjectivity of visual judgement of bone density on conventional radiographs supports the value of modern quantitative techniques, such as bone densitometry.

Table 1. Causes of primary osteoporosis

Idiopathic juvenile osteoporosis	Self-limited (2-4 year duration) form of osteoporosis in prepubertal children. Acute course of the disease with growth arrest and fractures. Mild to severe forms. Differential diagnosis: osteogenesis perfecta or other forms of juvenile osteoporosis, cortisolism and leukemia
Post-menopausal (type I) osteoporosis	Onset at the time of menopause but important bone loss during first 4 years after menopause, related to reduction in blood estrogen. Clinically significant in women 15-20 years after menopause. Fractures in bones with high trabecular:cortical ratio (vertebral bodies and distal forearm)
Senile (type 2) osteoporosis	Men and women ≥75 years of age, due to age-related bone loss (impaired bone formation associated with secondary hyperparathyroidism due to reduced calcium absorption from the intestine secondary to decreased renal production of the active form of vitamin D). Reduction in cortical and trabecular bone. Fractures in the vertebrae but also in bones with low trabecular:cortical ratio (tibia, humerus, and pelvis)
Osteogenesis imperfecta	Congenital disorders due to gene mutation associated with osteoporosis of variable severity. Blue sclerae and occasional dental involvement

Table 2. Causes of secondary osteoporosis

Endocrine	Glucocorticoid excess, estrogene/testosterone deficiency, hyperthyroidism, hyperparathyroidism
Nutritional	Intestinal malabsorption, chronic alcoholism, chronic liver disease, partial gastrectomy, vitamin C deficiency
Hereditary	Homocystineuria, Marfan syndrome, Ehler-Danlos syndrome
Hematologic	Sickle-cell disease, thalassemia, Gaucher disease, multiple myeloma
Others	Rheumatoid arthritis, hemochromatosis, long-term heparin therapy

The radiologic appearances of osteoporosis are essentially the same, irrespective of the cause (primary and secondary osteoporosis). The main radiographic features of generalized osteoporosis are decreased bone density and cortical thinning. A decrease in radiographic bone density, in the absence of fractures, is termed osteopenia and is due to resorption and thinning of trabeculae. The process initially affects the secondary (parallel to biomechanical forces) trabeculae; thus, the primary (perpendicular to biomechanical forces) trabeculae may appear more prominent as they are affected at a later stage.

Cortical thinning occurs as a result of endosteal, periosteal, or intracortical (cortical tunnelling) bone resorption. Endosteal resorption is the least specific radiographic finding because it may be evident in metabolic disorders, including osteoporosis, but also in marrow disorders. Intracortical tunnelling is more specific as it is mainly a feature of disorders in which there is rapid bone turnover, such as diffuse osteoporosis, and reflects sympathetic osteodystrophy. Subperiosteal resorption is the most specific finding, being diagnostic of hyperparathyroidism.

Osteoporosis remains occult on magnetic resonance imaging (MRI), although a relationship between trabecular bone density and marrow fat has been reported. The presence of multiple vertebral fractures with different ages (increased amount of fat in old fractures and marrow edema or infiltration in recent fractures) suggests increased bone fragility and, hence, osteoporosis.

Measurement of Osteoporosis

Several methods were previously used to standardize measurements of cortical thickness (radiogrametry), tra-

becular pattern (Singh index), and vertebral deformity (morphometry) from radiographs. These techniques lack accuracy and precision and have been replaced by several quantitative techniques, including dual-energy X-ray absorptiometry (DXA), quantitative computed tomography (QCT), and quantitative ultrasonography (QUS), all of which provide accurate and precise assessment of mineral bone density [2].

Rickets and Osteomalacia

Rickets and osteomalacia are similar metabolic bone disorders, each characterized by inadequate or delayed mineralization of osteoid in cortical and trabecular bone, in children and in adults, respectively [5].

Pseudofracture or Looser's zone is the radiological hallmark of osteomalacia, as it represents cortical fracture without a mineralized callus. Looser's zone corresponds to a linear cortical lucency frequently perpendicular to the cortex of the bone without periosteal reaction (Fig. 4). It typically involves the ribs, the superior and inferior pubic rami, and the inner margins of the proximal femora or lateral margin of the scapula. A widened physeal growth plate and metaphyseal cupping and fraying are the radiological signs of rickets that are best seen at rapidly growing ends of bone, such as the distal femur and radius or anterior ends of the ribs. Additional radiological findings of rickets/osteomalacia include bone deformities, osteopenia, and a coarsened pattern of cancellous bone [5].

There is no MRI hallmark of osteomalacia but the presence of multiple trabecular bone fractures with variable appearance at imaging (variable signal intensity on T2-weighted spin-echo (SE) images probably due the

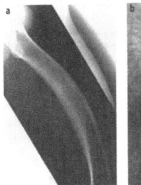
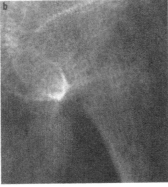

Fig. 4 a, b. Osteomalacia. **a** Lateral view of the femur demonstrates bone deformity with anterior bowing of the femoral shaft and cortical fracture. **b** Close-up radiograph from another patient with osteomalacia demonstrates pseudofracture or Looser's zone with cortical discontinuity and bone resorption

various ages of the fractures) in a background of normal bone marrow should suggest the disease [6, 7] (Fig. 5). Fractures in osteomalacia can show the nonspecific bone marrow edema pattern or a more linear pattern with an occasional double-line sign (probably due to the lack of adjacent edema). These fractures generally remain unchanged at short term follow-up MRI, as osteomalacia is a disease in which the healing process is deficient Typical cortical bone fractures or Looser's zones are barely visible at MRI as the cortical lesion is barely visible and the adjacent marrow and soft-tissue changes are discrete due to the chronicity of the lesion.

Renal Osteodystrophy and Hyperparathyroidism

The term renal osteodystrophy relates to all musculoskeletal manifestations of chronic renal failure [5]. Traditionally, renal osteodystrophy encompassed secondary hyperparathyroidism, osteomalacia, osteoporosis, and soft-tissue calcification. In fact, hyperparathyroidism and rickets, or osteomalacia, are the major pathologic processes of renal osteodystrophy. Primary hyperparathyroidism (generally related to the presence of a solitary adenoma in the parathyroid gland) and the classic radiographic changes of

hyperparathyroidism are largely historical because diagnosis and treatment are based on serum calcium and parathyroid hormone (PTH) levels.

The radiographic sign of hyperparathyroidism that may appear in the patient with chronic renal failure (as in primary hyperparathyroidism) are phalangeal resorption in the hands and/or exclusive phalangeal tuft resorption (Fig. 6). The hands are the earliest and most sensitive sites for the detection of hyperparathyroidism; other sites include the end of the clavicle, the sacroiliac joint, and other periosteal surfaces, such as the proximal humeri or proximal femora. Osteoclastoma, or brown tumor, occurs in renal osteodystrophy and, in fact, is encountered more frequently than in primary hyperparathyroidism, which is a rare condition. In the presence of brown tumors, there will almost always be phalangeal signs of hyperparathyroidism. Osteosclerosis may also be encountered in renal osteodystrophy and is commonly appreciated in vertebrae, pelvis, ribs, and the metaphyses of long tubular

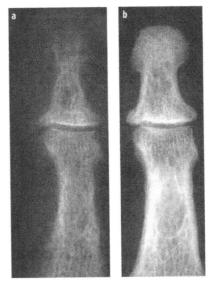

Fig. 6 a, b. a Radiographic signs of hyperparathyroidism include subperiosteal bone resorption and phalangeal tuft resorption. **b** After successful treatment, woven (primary) bone has reappeared

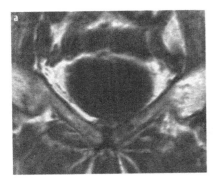
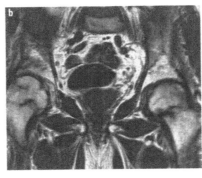

Fig. 5. Coronal T1-weighted images of the pelvis of a patient with osteomalacia demonstrates multiple trabecular bone fractures (*arrows*)

bones. In the vertebrae, sclerosis is frequently confined to the end-plates, producing a characteristic appearance of alternating bands of different densities (the so-called rugger jersey spine).

Marginal erosions at the periphery of articular surfaces in the peripheral joints have been reported with variable incidences. They are usually minor, progress slowly, and are not associated with a loss of joint space.

Soft-tissue calcifications may develop anywhere, in the vessels but also in the muscular or tendinous structures. Massive amorphous calcification can develop in the soft tissue around articulations and probably reflect poorly controlled renal osteodystrophy. The presence of chondrocalcinosis (knees and wrists) in patient younger than 50 years of age possibly reflects a hypercalcemic state but it should be kept in mind that hemochromatosis may also present with osteoporosis and chondrocalcinosis.

In mild hyperparathyroidism and renal osteodystrophy, DXA findings may be normal because the technique assesses the amount of trabecular bone. The most reliable site for measuring bone loss in primary hyperparathyroidism is the distal part of the forearm, which contains proportionately a large content of cortical bone (bone loss in hyperparathyroidism predominantly involves the outer compact bone).

Insufficiency Stress Fractures

Definitions of Bone Fractures

Fractures can be classified according to both the bone status before the fracture and the applied forces (Table 3). Traumatic fracture occurs as a response to an acute increase in biomechanical stress on normal bone. Fatigue fractures occur in response to a chronic repetitive increase in biomechanical stresses on normal bone. Insufficiency fracture occurs as a response to normal or slightly increased stress on diffusely weakened bones.

Medical imaging plays a crucial role in the diagnosis of insufficiency and pathological fractures because both conditions lack a suggestive clinical history [8-11]. Insufficiency stress fracture (ISF) of the cortical bone (femur, tibia, metatarsal bones) generally occurs in response to compression or traction stresses. ISF of the trabecular bone (vertebral body, long bone metaphysis, tarsal bone) generally occurs in response to compressive forces.

Radiographic Findings in Insufficiency Stress Fracture

The spectrum of radiographic findings in ISF depends on the cortical/trabecular bone ratio of the involved bone and on the age of the fracture (Table 4). The radiological diagnosis of ISF is difficult at an early stage (limited alterations) but also at a late stage (predominant healing-related changes). ISF of trabecular bone is barely seen on radiographs because of the lack of visibility of trabecular bone interruption and of significant bone deformation. At a later stage, radiographs display trabecular bone sclerosis that is typically linear and perpendicular to the dominant trabeculae. ISF of cortical bone can be recognized on plain films at an early stage if there is cortical bone discontinuity or bone deformity. After a few weeks, fractures become more obvious because of focal periosteal reactions, although the cortical discontinuity may be subtle.

Magnetic Resonance Imaging Findings in Insufficiency Stress Fracture

The MRI features of trabecular ISF include marrow edema or infiltration and intramedullary low signal intensity

Table 3. Classification of bone fractures

	Bone status	Applied forces	Clinical clues
Traumatic fracture	Normal	Increased	History
Fatigue fracture	Normal	Increased	History
Insufficiency fracture	Diffuse weakening	Normal	None
Pathological fracture	Focal weakening	Normal	None

Table 4. Radiologic appearance of trabecular and cortical insufficiency stress fractures (ISF)

Radiographs/computed tomography	Acute ISF	Chronic ISF	Healed ISF
Trabecular bone	Normal	Mild sclerosis	Normal
Cortical bone	Cortical interruption	Periosteal reaction	Cortical thickening
Pathological fracture	Focal weakening	Normal	None

Table 5. Magnetic resonance imaging (MRI) appearance of trabecular and cortical insufficiency stress fractures

MRI	Acute ISF	Chronic ISF	Healed ISF
Trabecular bone	Extensive edema	Band, edema	Normal
Cortical bone	Subtle marrow and soft-tissue edema	Subtle marrow and soft-tissue edema, periosteal callus	Normal

bands (impaction fractures) (Table 5). Marrow edema or infiltration could represent early marrow changes in response to increased biomechanical stress. Low signal intensity bands add specificity when present, because marrow infiltration or edema lacks specificity. Low signal intensity bands are best detected on T2-weighted SE, fat-saturated intermediate-weighted SE images, or enhanced T1-weighted SE images (in an unpredictable manner). Some features may be subtle with respect to marrow changes and include altered bone shape, cortical interruption, and periosteal reaction. The MRI features of cortical ISF are misleading because of the lack of obvious cortical bone fracture. Extensive infiltration of the adjacent medullary cavity or of the adjacent soft tissue is likewise deceptive. Bone scan is useful to exclude the possibility of a fracture. It is sensitive for the detection of ISF but generally lacks specificity.

Common Insufficiency Stress Fractures

Insufficiency Stress Fracture of the Vertebral Body

Vertebral fractures are the most common of the osteoporotic fractures. The anterior and central mid-portion of the vertebrae withstand compression forces less well than the posterior and outer ring elements of the vertebrae, re-sulting in wedge or endplate fractures or, less commonly, crush fractures. Good radiographic technique is required when imaging the spine, particularly in the lateral projection. The spine must be parallel to the radiographic table to prevent the vertebrae appearing to have a biconcave endplate, an artifact due to tilting of the vertebrae or to divergence of the X-ray beam (beam cam effect). Scheuermann's disease also causes vertebral body deformities. End-plate irregularity, most commonly in the thoracic spine and involving several adjacent vertebrae, generally enables the differentiation between vertebral fracture and growth-related bone deformities.

Typically, spinal ISF involves one or several vertebral bodies of the thoracolumbar junction and is not observed above the T4 level. Anterior wedge-shaped deformity is the most frequent pattern. On MRI, extensive bone-marrow edema that generally spares the posterior arch and the vertebral body opposite to the fracture vertebral end plate can be seen (differential diagnosis from disc-related marrow changes) (Fig. 7). The low signal bands are parallel to and located a few millimeters from the involved vertebral end plate.

Insufficiency Stress Fractures of the Pelvic Bones

Sites typically involved in ISF of the pelvic ring are the pubic and ischiatic rami, supra-acetabular area, and later-

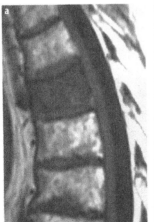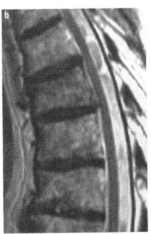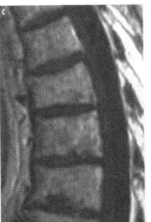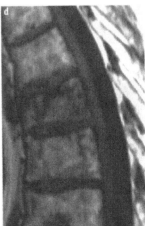

Fig. 7 a-d. Spontaneous insufficiency stress fracture (ISF) of a thoracic vertebral body. **a** T1-weighted image of the thoracic spine demonstrates a vertebral body with decreased signal intensity. **b** Corresponding T2-weighted and (**c**) enhanced T1-weighted spin-echo (SE) images demonstrate a return to normal signal intensity, suggestive of a benign fracture. **d** Follow-up T1-weighted SE image obtained 2 months later demonstrates partial and spontaneous regression of the lesion, with the appearance of intravertebral bands of low signal intensity

al aspects of the sacrum. The prevalence of these lesions is increased in patients who previously underwent radiation therapy (importance in the differential diagnosis of metastases). Radiographs are rarely diagnostic except in the pubic bones (cortical fracture). CT may contribute to the diagnosis by demonstrating cortical interruption or callus formation in trabecular bone (sacrum). MRI is the best imaging modality for sacral and supra-acetabular fractures. Fractures of the pubic bone are more difficult to recognize but adjacent muscle infiltration on STIR images is suggestive.

Insufficiency Stress Fracture of the Femoral Neck

Early recognition of femoral neck ISF is extremely important because of possible progression to displaced femoral neck fracture (if the cortex is involved). Plain films obtained early in the process may reveal cortical interruption with subtle periosteal reaction but are generally normal in trabecular bone fractures. MRI better displays associated marrow edema, showing intramedullary bands of low signal intensity (Fig. 8).

Insufficiency Stress Fractures of the Tarsal Bones

Lower-extremity ISF is frequent and involves the greater tuberosity of the calcaneus, the talar dome and neck, and the cuboid bone. Radiographs are generally normal (no deformity) except in cases involving the calcaneum (callus formation). MRI is diagnostic but confusion with acute reflex sympathetic dystrophy syndrome is possible. Bone scintigraphy may contribute to distinguishing between the two entities.

Uncommon Insufficiency Stress Fractures

Uncommon ISF can be related to characteristics intrinsic to the lesion (unusual topography or shape) or to patient characteristics (abnormal healing process).

Uncommon ISF Appearance due to Unusual Topography or Shape

Epiphyseal Insufficiency Fractures

Convex weight-bearing epiphyses, such as the femoral head, femoral condyles [12], and metatarsal heads [13] are typical sites of ISF (Fig. 9). Radiographs are generally normal but may show subtle subchondral sclerosis. MRI reveals extensive marrow edema and low signal intensity bands located a few millimeters from the subchondral bone plate, which is generally not deformed.

Untill the early 1990s, epiphyseal ISF remained underdiagnosed and epiphyseal osteonecrosis was the unique epiphyseal condition associated with metabolic bone disorders. The concept of transient epiphyseal bone lesions corresponding presumably to fractures emerged progressively and is now widely accepted [9]. There is also general agreement on the fact that some patterns of epiphyseal osteonecrosis, such as spontaneous osteonecrosis of the medial condyles (SONK), represent irreversible fracture or pseudoarthrosis rather than primary ischemic osteonecrosis [10, 12].

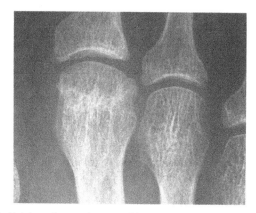

Fig. 9. Epiphyseal stress fracture of the second metatarsal head. Radiograph shows mild flattening and deformity of the epiphyseal contour (*arrow*) with linear sclerosis of the metatarsal head

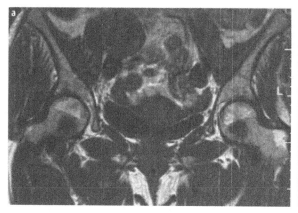

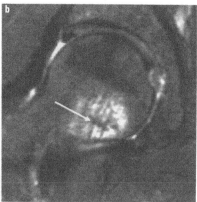

Fig. 8 a, b. Insufficiency stress fractures in a patients with recent renal transplant. **a** Coronal T1-weighted SE image of the pelvis demonstrates ill-delimited low signal intensity areas in both femoral necks. **b** Fat-saturated proton density image of the right femoral neck demonstrates nodular thickening of the weight-bearing trabeculae, which converge to form a line of low signal intensity (*arrow*)

Longitudinal Stress Fractures

Cortical ISF are generally perpendicular to the cortical shaft. Rarely, longitudinal ISF develop in the tibia but also in the femur or metatarsal bones [14, 15]. Cortical interruption is difficult to detect because it is parallel to the longitudinal axis of the bone. Axial CT images are important for the recognition of cortical discontinuity (underlining the importance of settings window for bone) [14]. The lesion may be confused with infection or tumor at MRI because of the longitudinal extent of marrow infiltration [15] (Fig. 10).

Uncommon ISF Appearance due to Abnormal Healing Processes

The healing process can be altered by various mechanisms (Table 6), which causes unusual features at imaging (Table 7). An imbalance in favor of bone destruction

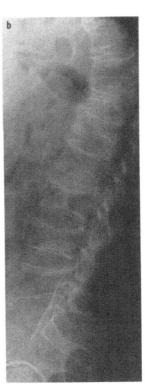
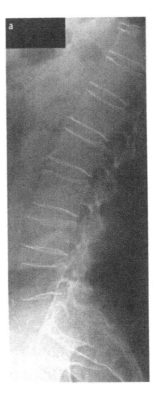

Fig. 11 a, b. Multiple vertebral fractures in a patient with osteoporosis and receiving long-term steroid therapy. **a** Initial lumbar spine radiograph demonstrates osteoporosis with L4 fracture. **b** A radiograph of the same area obtained 1 year later after an increase in steroid dosage demonstrates the appearance of multiple fractures and trabecular bone sclerosis

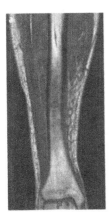
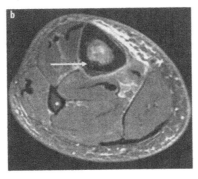

Fig. 10 a, b. Longitudinal ISF of the tibia. **a** Coronal T1-weighted images demonstrate marrow infiltration in the distal third of the tibia. **b** Transverse fat-saturated proton density weighted images demonstrates marrow and soft-tissue infiltration. Cortical discontinuity (*arrow*) is barely visible

Table 6. Causes of abnormal healing process

Local causes	Distraction stress (scaphoid) Persistent mechanical stress due to topography of the lesions (pubis, epiphysis, rib) or altered pain threshold (steroids, alcohol, neuropathy)
Regional causes	Radiation therapy, vascular disorders
Diffuse causes	Metabolic bone disease (osteomalacia, steroid or fluoride therapy)

Table 7. Unusual features of insufficiency stress fractures (ISF) related to altered healing process

Increased bone destruction (pubis bone, epiphysis, rib)

Increased callus formation

Increased number of fractures (steroid therapy, osteomalacia)

over bone reconstruction is observed in fractures that are submitted to repetitive persistent stress due to, e.g., reduced pain sensitivity (pelvic-ring fractures in patients receiving steroids) or in bones with altered metabolism (after radiation therapy) [16] (Fig. 11).

An imbalance in favor of bone sclerosis can be observed in chronic ISF in patients taking steroids. Steroid therapy results in a spectrum of changes that include a large number of spontaneous fractures with hypertrophic callus formation and unusual persistance of the lesions over time (Fig. 12). At MRI, these ISF show a wide spectrum of changes, ranging from marrow infiltration to focal lipomatosis in association with hypertrophic callus formation.

Conclusions

Metabolic disorders of the skeleton involve the mineralized components of the skeleton. Metabolic bone alterations can be depicted on radiographs and CT images but remain occult on MRI because the bone marrow is spared in the vast majority of these disorders.

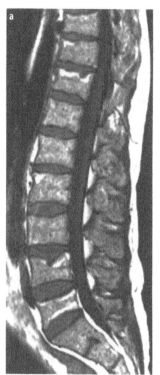
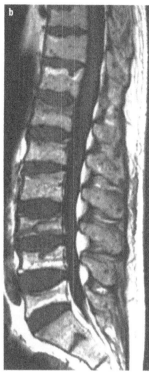
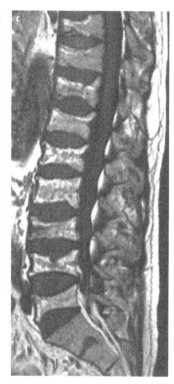

Fig. 12 a-c. Patient with multiple myeloma and chronic steroid treatment. **a** Initial T1-weighted MRI performed during treatment demonstrates multiple areas of increased signal intensity (similar to Modic II changes) in vertebrae with abnormal shape but without disc disease. **b** Eight months later, there are multiple fractures and bands of low signal intensity. **c** After 18 months, there is partial regression of focal marrow changes. Steroid-related vertebral fractures often show a very slow pace of change over time

Metabolic disorders of the skeleton affect all bone components histologically but involvement patterns may vary depending on the age of the patient (growing vs. the adult skeleton) as well as the type of bone (cortical vs. trabecular bone). The importance of cortical and trabecular bone in each individual bone (high trabecular/cortical ratio in vertebral bodies, ribs and pelvis; low trabecular/cortical ratio in long bones and extremities) may influence the radiographic patterns of metabolic bone diseases.

Medical imaging (X-ray, CT, bone scintigraphy, and MRI) plays a limited role in the detection and quantification of osteoporosis. It does, however, contribute to the work-up of symptomatic patients with suspected fractures and occasionally to the detection of patients at risk of vertebral fracture (old vertebral fractures). Accurate reporting of vertebral fracture is important.

Insufficiency stress fractures are characterized by a wide spectrum of marrow changes that are seen at MRI. Bone-marrow edema or infiltration is the most prominent feature of ISF of the trabecular bone at MRI, and the presence of low signal intensity bands (best seen on T2-weighted, fat-saturated intermediate-weighted, or enhanced T1-weighted images) adds specificity. In ISF of the cortical bone, cortical discontinuity is best appreciated on CT images rather than on MRI. Bone-marrow and adjacent soft-tissue edema or infiltration are subtle but occasionally misleading features in cortical fractures.

Uncommon ISF can be related to characteristics intrinsic to the lesion (unusual topography or shape) or to patient characteristics (abnormal healing process due to persistent mobility, radiation therapy, or osteomalacia and steroid therapy).

References

1. Resnik D, Niwayama G (1987) Diagnosis of bone and joint disorders, 2nd edn, vol. 4. WB Saunders, Philadelphia, pp 1983-1987, 2096-2099
2. Adams J (2008) Osteoporosis. In: Pope TL, Bloem HL, Beltran J, Morrison W (eds) Imaging of the musculoskeletal system. WB Saunders, Philadelphia, pp 1489-1508
3. Bouxsein ML, Karasik D (2006) Bone geometry and skeletal fragility. Curr Osteoporos Rep 4:49-56
4. Sambrook P, Cooper C (2006) Osteoporosis. Lancet 367:2010-2018
5. Sundaram M, Schils J (2008) Hyperparathyroidism, renal osteodystrophy, osteomalacia and rickets. In: Pope TL, Bloem HL, Beltran J, Morrison W (eds) Imaging of the musculoskeletal system. WB Saunders, Philadelphia, pp.1509-1523
6. Kanberoglu K, Kantarci F, Cebi D et al (2005) Magnetic resonance imaging in osteomalacic insufficiency fractures of the pelvis. Clin Radiol 601:105-111
7. Ohashi K, Ohnishi T, Ishikawa T et al (1999) Oncogenic osteomalacia presenting as bilateral stress fractures of the tibia. Skeletal Radiol 281:46-48
8. Soubrier M, Dubost JJ, Boisgard S et al (2003) Insufficiency fracture. A survey of 60 cases and review of the literature. Joint Bone Spine 703:209-218

9. Vande Berg BC, Malghem J, Goffin EJ et al (1994) Transient epiphyseal lesions in renal transplant recipients: presumed insufficiency stress fractures. Radiology 1912:403-407

10. Vande Berg BC, Malghem J, Lecouvet FE, Maldague B (2001) Magnetic resonance imaging and differential diagnosis of epiphyseal osteonecrosis. Semin Musculoskelet Radiol 51:57-67

11. Cabarrus MC, Ambekar A, Lu Y, Link TM (2008) MRI and CT of insufficiency fractures of the pelvis and the proximal femur. AJR Am J Roentgoenol 1914:995-1001

12. Lecouvet FE, Malghem J, Maldague BE, Vande Berg BC (2005) MR imaging of epiphyseal lesions of the knee: current concepts, challenges, and controversies. Radiol Clin North Am 434:655-672

13. Torriani M, Thomas BJ, Bredella MA, Ouellette H (2008) MRI of metatarsal head subchondral fractures in patients with forefoot pain. AJR Am J Roentgoenol 1903:570-575

14. Feydy A, Drapé J, Beret E et al (1998) Longitudinal stress fractures of the tibia: comparative study of CT and MR imaging. Eur Radiol 84:598-602

15. Craig JG, Widman D, van Holsbeeck M (2003) Longitudinal stress fracture: patterns of edema and the importance of the nutrient foramen. Skeletal Radiol 321:22-27

16. Kwon JW, Huh SJ, Yoon YC et al (2008) Pelvic bone complications after radiation therapy of uterine cervical cancer: evaluation with MRI. AJR Am J Roentgoenol 1914:987-994

Trauma of the Axial Skeleton

Victor N. Cassar-Pullicino[1], Lee F. Rogers[2]

[1] Department of Diagnostic Imaging, The Robert Jones and Agnes Hunt Orthopaedic and District Hospital NHS Trust, Oswestry, UK
[2] Radiology, University of Arizona School of Health Sciences, Tucson, AZ, USA

Introduction

Diagnostic imaging of spinal trauma has been revolutionized as findings obscured in the shadows of radiography have been brought to light by computed tomography (CT) and magnetic resonance imaging (MRI). CT illuminates much that was previously unseen and still more that was unsuspected. The cumulative impact of advances in imaging on the initial diagnosis and subsequent treatment of patients with spinal cord injury has been enormous.

Imaging Techniques

Radiography was long the mainstay of imaging the potentially injured spine but has now, in large measure, been replaced by CT, particularly multidetector CT (MD-CT). This technique yields routine, excellent, immediately available image reconstructions in both the coronal and sagittal planes. CT can be readily obtained in the multiple injured patient, without the need for his or her undue manipulation. CT has proven to be much more sensitive than radiography in the detection of spinal injuries, revealing fractures that are unapparent on radiographs and significantly more fractures in patients with fractures shown by radiography (Fig. 1). Thin-section axial slices are obtained and images are reconstructed in the coronal and sagittal planes. Examination of the cervical spine should extend from the base of the skull to the fourth thoracic vertebra, and the thoracic and lumbar spine must be similarly covered in their entirety. Once a significant fracture or dislocation of the spine has been identified, it is important to examine the remainder of the spine to exclude the presence of other spinal injuries. CT of the entire spine is performed to clear the spine in obtunded patients.

The principal limitation of CT is its inability to directly visualize the spinal cord and the supporting ligamentous structures of the spine. However, these limitations can now be overcome with the use of MRI, which is ideally suited to evaluate the status of these vital structures (Fig. 2). While not yet used routinely in the assessment of spinal injuries, MRI is done in those patients with neurologic deficits, to assess the status of the spinal cord and determine the source of the deficit. MRI is not acquired acutely but rather is delayed until the patient is clinically stable. An examination of the entire spine should be performed to exclude or identify the relatively commonly associated discontiguous spinal injuries that may be present in such patients. MRI is also obtained in selected cases to assess the status of spinal ligaments prior to surgical intervention.

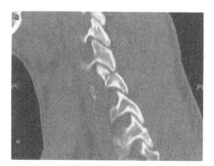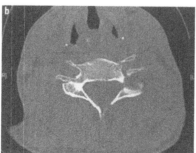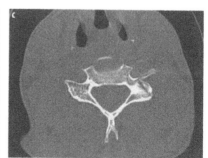

Fig. 1 a-c. Unifacetal fracture dislocation C5/6 showing extent of the fracture's involvement of the left lateral mass (**a**), foramen transversarium (**b**), and articular surface (**c**)

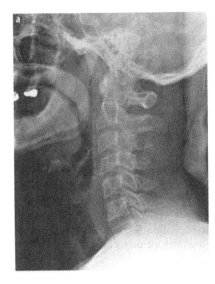

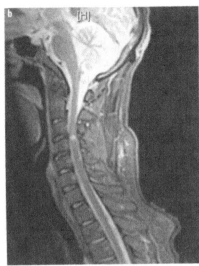

Fig. 2 a, b. Adult patient with spinal cord injury without radiographic abnormality (SCI-WORA). There was no evidence of radiographic injury (**a**) but spinal cord trauma at C3/4 is seen on MRI (**b**)

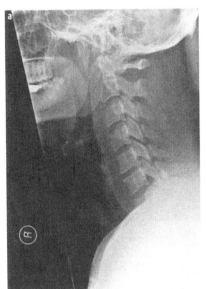

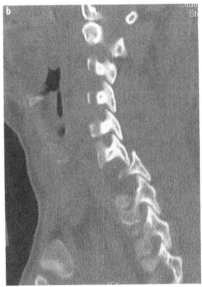

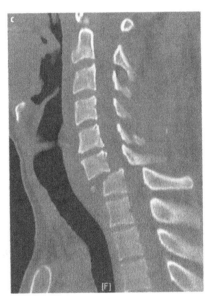

Fig. 3 a-c. Missed C6/7 bilateral facet dislocation on original radiographs (**a**). Note the widened pre-vertebral space and the failure to visualize the C7 level on lateral view. Injury is easily seen on sagittal CT reconstructions (**b, c**)

Common Sources of Diagnostic Error

Poorly performed radiographs of the spine remain a common cause of errors in the assessment of spinal trauma. This is particularly true for lateral views of the cervical spine that do not include all seven cervical vertebrae and underexposed radiographs of any portion of the spine (Fig. 3). Fractures and dislocations of the spine can also be easily overlooked on axial CT images. The conspicuity of injuries is greatly enhanced by coronal and sagittal reconstructions. The radiologist may fail to recognize the presence of spinal fractures in the mid- and upper thoracic spine as his or her attention is focused on excluding or identifying aortic injuries when interpreting CT or radiographs of the chest. This situation is compounded by the fact that both upper thoracic spinal fractures and aortic injuries may be associated with significant mediastinal hematomas.

Biomechanics of Spinal Injury

Denis' three-column concept of the spine is useful in understanding the creation of various spinal injuries and also helpful in the recognition of the various patterns of spinal injury when images of spinal fractures and dislocations are interpreted. The three-column concept states that the spine is considered to be made up of the anterior, middle, and posterior columns. The posterior column consists of the neural arch and intervening soft-tissue structures. The anterior column consists of the anterior longitudinal ligament, anterior annulus fibrosis, and anterior part of the vertebral body. The middle column consists of the posterior longitudinal ligament, posterior annulus fibrosis, and posterior part of the vertebral body. This column binds the anterior to the posterior column and serves as the fulcrum of motion between them.

The forces of spinal injury, flexion, extension, distraction, compression, shearing, and rotation, are multiple and therefore complex. The combination of flexion, compression, rotation, and shearing is particularly common. In general, compressive forces create fractures whereas rotational and shearing forces disrupt ligaments, resulting in dislocations. In most injuries a single force is dominant, and each force is associated with a relatively specific pattern of injury. Flexion is the most common force operative in spinal injury. In this case, the spine is arched anteriorly, pivoting about the fulcrum of the middle column, which results in compression in the vertebral body and tension within the neural arch posterior to the fulcrum. Extension forces do the opposite, resulting in tension anteriorly and compression posterior to the middle column. Compression is due to an axial load across the entire vertebra and involving all three columns, as in burst fractures. Distraction forces are those in which the vertebra is pulled in opposite directions in the axial plane, superiorly and inferiorly, as in chance fractures; they are the opposite of compression forces, In Chance fractures, the fulcrum of the forces is displaced anterior to the spine, classically to the seat belt in restrained automobile occupants or occasionally to the handlebars in motorcyclists.

Multiple-Level, Discontiguous Spinal Injury

Fractures are often encountered in contiguous adjacent vertebrae; thus, once a spinal fracture is identified, the radiologist should look closely at adjacent vertebrae for additional, often less obvious, fractures.

Additional spinal fractures or fracture dislocations may occur at discontiguous levels of the spine; for instance, fractures of C1 and C2 may be associated with fractures of the lower cervical spine; fractures of the thoracolumbar junction may be associated with fractures of the lower lumbar spine; and fractures and fracture dislocations of the mid-thoracic spine may be associated with fractures of either the cervical spine or the thoracolumbar junction. The reported incidence of second-level spinal fractures is dependent upon the means of examination: 5–7% by radiography, 15–17% by CT, and up to 50% by MRI. Fracture dislocations of the mid-thoracic spine are associated with the highest incidence of second-level discontiguous injuries, 2.5 to three times higher than at other levels.

Cervical Spine

What To Look For

The alignment of the vertebrae and height of the vertebral bodies should be closely observed. It should be kept in mind that the height of C4 and C5 can be normally less than that of adjacent vertebral bodies. Prevertebral soft-tissue swelling should be noted – the greater, the more worrisome. However, the width of the prevertebral soft tissues is quite variable (Fig. 4), and it is impossible to establish absolute values that consistently discriminate between normal and abnormal. Very serious injuries may be manifested by seemingly minor degrees of malalignment (Table 1). Therefore, each vertebra must be looked at individually in order to identify or exclude specific injuries that commonly occur at the locations described below.

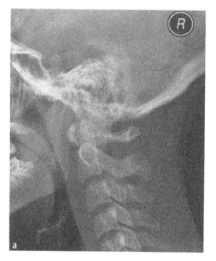

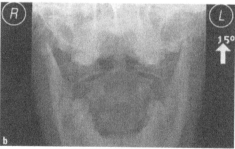

Fig. 4 a, b. Widened pre vertebral space in the upper cervical spine (**a**, lateral view) due to Jefferson's C1 fracture. Note the C1/C2 offset on the AP view (**b**)

Table 1. Factors suggestive of cervical instability

- Vertebral compression >25%
- Widened interspinous space or facet joints
- Subluxation >3.5 mm
- Kyphosis >11°
- Traumatic disc-space widening or narrowing

Specific Injuries

At the *atlas, C1 level*, Jefferson fractures, i.e., fractures of the anterior and posterior arches. are relatively common. They are noted by lateral offsets of articular facets of C1 upon C2 on open-mouth AP view and confirmed by CT. Isolated fractures of the neural arch must also be excluded.

Fractures of the *axis, C2 level* include Hangman's fracture, which consists of bilateral fractures of the neural arch and often located anterior to the inferior facet; they are caused by hyperextension of the head upon the neck, as occurs in a judicial hanging. They are easily seen on lateral view when symmetric but more difficult to see when asymmetric These fractures are best seen on CT, which may show extension of the fractures into the posterior aspect of the vertebral body. Hangman's fractures are commonly associated with a variable degree of dislocation of C2 upon C3 (Fig. 5).

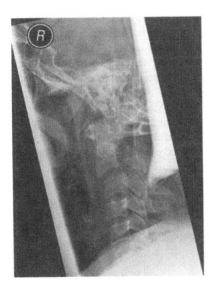

Fig. 5. Bilateral pedicular C2 fracture with C2/C3 disc injury (lateral view)

Dens fractures most commonly occur in the axial plane at the base of the dens. They are frequently undisplaced and difficult to appreciate on radiographs and axial CT images but are readily demonstrated on reconstructed CT images in the coronal and sagittal planes. Oblique fractures extend from the base of the dens into the body of C2, disrupting the ring of C2, and are best visualized by sagittal reconstruction CT.

Hyperextension tear drop fracture is a triangular, avulsion fracture of the anterior inferior margin of the C2 vertebral body caused by hyperextension of the head upon the neck. This may occasionally occur in association with a Hangman's fracture.

In the *lower cervical spine (C2–C7)*, anterior wedge compression fractures occur in the mid- to lower vertebrae. Note that the C4 and C5 vertebral bodies are often normally somewhat smaller and their vertebral body height is reduced compared to the adjacent vertebral bodies. This should not be misconstrued as a fracture. Burst fractures occasionally occur at C6 or C7; when a compressed vertebral body is seen at this level, the posterior aspect of the vertebral body should be examined closely for evidence of retropulsion of a fragment containing the posterior superior margin of the vertebral body into the spinal canal (Fig. 6).

Teardrop fracture is a specific form of the burst fracture in the cervical spine, being the cervical equivalent of the burst fracture encountered in the thoracolumbar spine. It is a fracture-dislocation consisting of a comminuted fracture of a vertebral body with a characteristic triangular or quadrilateral fragment from the anterior inferior margin of the vertebral body, the "teardrop." The injury is accompanied by a variable degree of posterior dislocation of the affected vertebra, widening of the interspinous distance, and disruption of the facet joints. Approximately 50% of these patients will have a vertical sagittal split in the vertebral body. Teardrop fractures are usually associated with spinal-cord injuries.

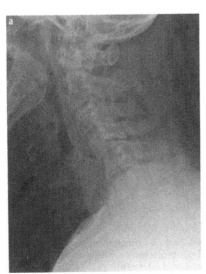
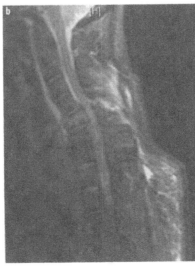

Fig. 6 a, b. C5 burst fracture with retropulsion and spinal-cord injury. Note the pre vertebral soft tissues swelling (**a**) and edema within vertebra and cord on MRI T2 sequence (**b**)

Facet locking is a specific form of fracture-dislocation of the cervical spine. Locking of the facets refers to displacement of the facet above a position anterior to the facet below, thus locking the facets. Locking may occur either unilaterally or bilaterally. The unilateral facet lock is the result of flexion, distraction, and rotation; it most commonly occurs at C5/C6 or C6/C7. In a unilateral facet lock, the vertebral body above is characteristically anteriorly displaced by 25% of the width of the vertebral body below. Bilateral locking of the facets characteristically results in anterior displacement of 50% or more of one vertebral body with respect to the other. Fractures of the facets commonly accompany these injuries. CT with images reconstructed in the sagittal plane clearly depicts these findings.

Thoracolumbar Spine

What To Look For

Manipulation of patients suspected of having spinal fractures should be kept to minimum to avoid inadvertent spinal-cord injury. These patients should be examined closely for evidence of malalignment, a certain sign of fracture-dislocation. The height and configuration of all vertebral bodies should be checked (Table 2). Once an anterior wedged compression fracture is identified, the precise nature of the fracture should be determined, i.e., simple compression, flexion-distraction, or burst fracture, as described below (Fig. 7).

Table 2. Radiographic indications of thoracolumbar spine instability

- Vertebral compression >50%
- Disruption of the posterior vertebral body line
- Widening of the interspinous and interpediculate spaces
- Widening of the facet joints
- Displaced vertebra (≥2 mm)
- Disc-space narrowing

Specific Injuries

Fractures and fracture dislocations of the upper thoracic spine can be difficult to identify on plain films because of the overlying mediastinal structures and mediastinal hematomas associated with vascular injuries as well as spinal injuries. Particular attention must be paid to the alignment of the vertebral bodies, as any degree of vertebral offset or malalignment is suspect and warrants a CT examination of the spine, including sagittal and coronal image reconstructions. In viewing CT images of the thoracic spine, one should pay particular attention to the status of the middle and posterior columns as well as that of the anterior aspect of the vertebral bodies before concluding that an injury is stable, i.e., limited to the anterior column (Fig. 8).

Simple (anterior wedged) compression fractures are the result of anterior flexion forces that compress the superior end plate of the vertebrae and reduce the anterior height of the vertebral body. There is often an irregular

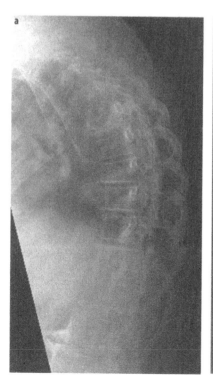 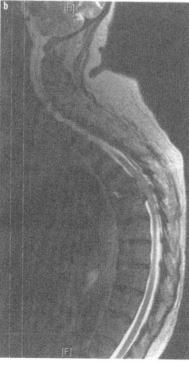

Fig. 7 a, b. T7 compression injury with vertebral involvement of the middle column (**a**) and cord injury (**b**)

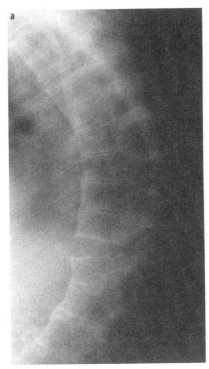
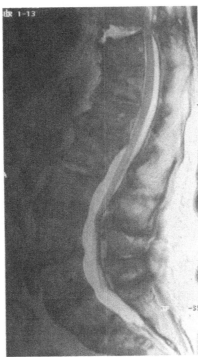
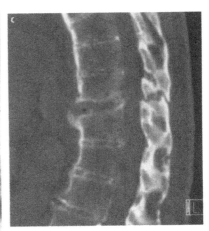

Fig. 8 a-c. Ankylosing spondylitis patient with a fracture in a fused spine involving the three columns at the T9/T10 level as seen on lateral (**a**), MRI T2 sequence (**b**), and CT reconstruction (**c**)

bulge at the anterior superior margin of the vertebral body. Less commonly, the inferior end plate is involved. In either circumstance the posterior wall of the vertebral body remains intact and the posterior height of the vertebra is maintained. The posterior elements and middle column remain intact as well.

Flexion-distraction fractures refer to fractures of the posterior elements that accompany the more severe compression fractures of the vertebral bodies; they are distinguished from simple wedge compression fractures. Flexion-distraction fractures are the result of simultaneous compression forces on the anterior column and tensile forces of distraction on the posterior column. This is created by extreme flexion of the spine focused on one vertebra. This fracture is identified by an anterior wedged vertebral body with the middle column intact – that is, the posterior vertebral body height is maintained – and a widening of the interspinous distance with variable fractures of the posterior elements.

Burst fractures are the result of compression forces across all three columns. These cause an anterior wedged deformity of the vertebral body with a characteristic triangular fragment from the posterior superior margin of the vertebral body retropulsed into the spinal canal. On CT, there is usually a vertical fracture in the sagittal plane of the vertebral body as well as a sagittal fracture at the junction of the spinous process and lamina. The latter is manifest on the AP radiograph by a widening of the interpediculate distance of the affected vertebra.

Chance fractures are also known as the seat belt fracture. In the usual flexion injury the compression forces are sustained by the anterior half of the vertebral body with the fulcrum in the middle column. In a person wearing a seatbelt, the fulcrum of the force is displaced anteriorly and lies at the seatbelt, such that the entire spine is posterior to the flexion axis and all of its components are subjected to tension stress. This results in disruption of the posterior ligaments or a transverse fracture of the posterior elements, and, at times, the vertebral body. There is characteristically little or no compression of the vertebral body (Fig. 9).

Conclusions

Spinal-cord injury carries with it substantial morbidity and mortality. The resources and expenditures required for the treatment and care of patients with spinal injuries are considerable. The primary objectives of the assessment and treatment of patients with potential spinal injury are to accurately exclude or correctly identify injuries, to preserve neurologic function when injuries are present, and to restore spinal stability in those so afflicted. Imaging plays an essential role in these endeavors.

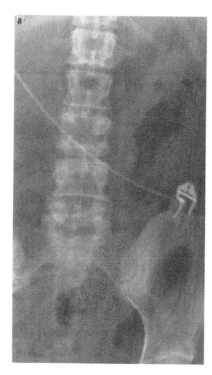 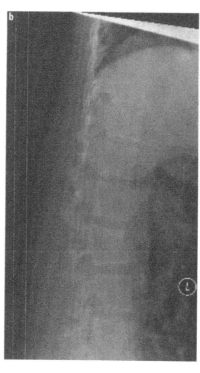

Fig. 9 a, b. Chance fracture at L3, showing a widened L2/L3 interspinous distance (**a**) and transverse fracture separating both pedicles at L3 as well as the posterior outline of the vertebra (**b**)

Suggested Reading

Cassar-Pullicino V, Imhof E (eds) (2006) Spinal trauma – An imaging approach. Thieme, New York Stuttgart

Roger LF (ed) (2001) Radiology of skeletal trauma. Churchill Livingston, Philadelphia

Trauma of the Appendicular Skeleton: Overuse-Related Injury

Mario Maas

Department of Radiology, Academic Medical Center, University of Amsterdam, Amsterdam, The Netherlands

Introduction

Acute traumatic injury of the appendicular skeleton requires fracture detection, classification, and then treatment, usually in an Emergency (Radiology) Department. Nearly every weekend, radiologists are confronted with various fracture types. In The Netherlands, the sudden reappearance in the winter of 2009 of below-freezing temperatures led to an enthusiastic increase in ice skating – with a dramatic increase in fractures, mainly of the wrist, in Dutch hospitals!

A not so well known entity is the sub-acute trauma, most typically caused by sports-related repetitive movements. This chapter will focus on these types of injury as a source of stress fractures, with the aim of increasing awareness amongst radiologists who deal with injured athletes.

Stress Fractures

These fractures are fatigue injuries of bone usually caused by changes in an athlete's training regimen. There has been a remarkable rise in the reported incidence of stress fractures in the past decades, most likely caused by increased levels of participation in sports in today's population. Also, the refinement of modern imaging technologies – with high magnetic field strength magnetic resonance imaging (MRI) using superb receiver coils; high-resolution multidetector-row computed tomography (CT); and high-frequency ultrasound – have allowed better delineation of these pathologies.

Nevertheless, at the same time there still is a need to increase radiologists' awareness especially concerning their pivotal role in dealing with stress fractures. Proper communication between the treating physician, physical therapist, and radiologist is needed to obtain a high index of suspicion for this easily overlooked entity.

Patients typically present with an insidious onset of pain over the affected region but without any form of trauma. First, pain is experienced during the provoking activity and relieved by rest. If the activity is continued at the same level, the persistent pain will eventually cause the athlete to cease that particular sport. Finally, pain is also experienced at rest. The incidence of bone stress injury varies with age, with the mean age being 19-30 years. Children are affected in ever greater numbers due to their increasing participation in rigorous training programs, but they are still the minority of such patients. The incidence in women is higher than in men, with a different distribution of bones affected. Stress fractures of the metatarsals and the pelvis are more common in women. The tibia is the most affected bone in both sexes.

Radiological Modalities

Radiographs are not reliable for the detection of stress fractures, as their sensitivity on initial examination is only 15-35%, which increases to 30-70% during follow-up. Thus, the radiologist should not be falsely reassured by radiographic assessment. However, radiographs are still the first step to rule out differentials, such as tumor, infection, or frank fracture.

What does a stress fracture look like? It presents in various ways. In cortical bone (e.g., tibia, navicular bone), a clear fracture line may be seen. More often, an endosteal or a periosteal callus is visible without a fracture line or there is a circumferential periosteal reaction with a visible fracture line through one cortex. More difficult is the detection of stress fractures in cancellous bone, e.g., calcaneal stress fractures. In cancellous bone, the stress fracture is usually seen as a focal linear area of sclerosis oriented perpendicular to the trabeculae. This appears only 3 or 4 weeks after the onset of pain. Of the tarsal bones, the calcaneus is the most affected, presenting as insidious-onset heel pain that is aggravated by running or jumping. Since timely diagnosis is essential for treatment and prognosis in this specific patient group, radiologists should not accept the results of a normal radiograph as the final answer.

Location is also an important variable in need of radiologists' attention. Most fractures are of low risk, yet specific anatomical locations host high-risk stress fractures; in other words, fractures that will not heal without surgery or are likely to evolve to delayed union, non-union, or displaced complete fractures. Stress fractures of these bones should be treated more aggressively. Examples include fractures located at the femoral neck (tension side = high risk, compression side = low risk), patella (transverse = high risk, longitudinal = low risk), and anterior tibial diaphysis. Also, tarsal navicular stress fractures need special attention because they are associated with the above mentioned high-risk complications. This is caused by poor vascularization at the most often affected middle third of the bone. Invariably, these fractures are linear and within the sagittal plane, implying that they are very difficult to see with plain radiography, which, in turn, delays their diagnosis. Indeed, not infrequently the navicular stress fracture is an incidental finding in an athlete with chronic anterior ankle/foot pain.

The state of the art second diagnostic step is MRI, as it has proven to be at least as sensitive as scintigraphy but with significantly higher specificity. The MRI protocol minimally consists of a basic set of sequences, namely STIR, T1-weighted, and T2-weighted images. With the use of these tools, MRI provides a reliable estimate of treatment time by dividing stress fractures into four grades. This grading system is important for prognostic purposes, in which radiologists can play a pivotal role. Grade 1 stress fractures show mild to moderate periosteal edema (high signal intensity) on STIR images but no marrow abnormalities. Grade 2 stress fractures show moderate to severe periosteal edema on STIR images with added marrow edema of high signal intensity on T2-weighted images. Grade 3 stress fractures show low-signal-intensity marrow edema on T1-weighted images while in grade 4 stress fractures a fracture line is clearly visible. The lower the grade, the better the prognosis and the more conservative the therapeutic approach. Accurate estimates of return to competition time is another benefit of MRI, which is likely to increase compliance of the athlete patient. To better depict the extent of the fracture, high-resolution MDCT with use of multiplanar reconstruction can be beneficial. This technique is favored by surgeons to better plan the therapeutic approach as it distinguishes between the need for conservative vs. surgical treatment.

From the above description it is clear that detecting stress fractures is best done using MRI, looking for bone marrow edema (BME). However, with the increased use of MRI in evaluating athletic injuries, new challenges have emerged. One of these is evaluating the significance of BME. The pattern of BME is very helpful in the classification of complex injuries and in understanding the mechanism of injury. However in the high-performance athlete BME very often is seen, without a clear correla-

tion as to pain or prognosis. Most often, there is a marked correlation with the specific sports biomechanics endured by the athlete. Evidence for this association was obtained in a MRI study of asymptomatic high-level collegiate basketball players; one of the most surprising findings was the number of those who had areas with BME. It is thought that bone is dynamic and responds to stress by hypertrophy and remodeling of bone trabeculae, with microfractures and medullary edema seen at histology. These findings may very well correspond to the BME visualized on MRI.

In summary, overuse-related injury of bone is very often seen on MRI. Stress-induced changes can be interpreted as a continuum, with the physiologic response to biomechanical load on the one end and stress fracture on the other. Correlation with the clinical situation is of utmost importance. Close collaboration between the radiologist, sports physician, orthopedic surgeon, and the athlete is the sine qua non of dealing with the injured athlete.

Suggested Reading

Arendt EA, Griffiths HJ (1997) The use of MR imaging in the assessment and clinical management of stress reactions of bone in high-performance athletes. Clin Sports Med 16:291-306

Berger FH, de Jonge MC, Maas M (2007) Stress fractures in the lower extremity. Eur J Radiol 62:16-26

Fredericson M, Bergman AG, Hoffman KL, Dillingham MS (1995) Tibial stress reaction in runners. Correlation of clinical symptoms and scintigraphy with a new magnetic resonance imaging grading system. Am J Sports Med 23:472-481

Groves AM, Cheow HK, Balan KK et al (2005) 16-Detector multislice CT in the detection of stress fractures: a comparison with skeletal scintigraphy. Clin Radiol 60:1100-1105

Hayes CW, Brigido MK, Jamadar DA, Propeck T (2000) Mechanism-based pattern approach to classification of complex injuries of the knee depicted at MR imaging. Radiographics 20:S121-S134

Kornaat PR, de Jonge MC, Maas M (2008) Bone marrow edema-like signal in the athlete. Eur J Radiol 67:49-53

Major NM, Helms CA (2002) MR imaging of the knee: findings in asymptomatic collegiate basketball players. AJR Am J Roentgenol 179:641-644

Sanders TG, Medynski MA, Feller JF, Lawhorn KW (2000) Bone contusion patterns of the knee at MR imaging: footprint of the mechanism of injury. Radiographics 2000 20:S135-S151

Schweitzer ME, White LM (1996) Does altered biomechanics cause marrow edema? Radiology 198:851-853

Sofka CM (2006) Imaging of stress fractures. Clin Sports Med 25:53-62, viii

Yao L, Johnson C, Gentili A et al (1998) Stress injuries of bone: analysis of MR imaging staging criteria. Acad Radiol 5:34-40

Imaging of Skeletal Trauma

Murray K. Dalinka

Penn Radiology, Hospital of the University of Pennsylvania, Philadelphia, PA, USA

Introduction

There have been major changes in the imaging of trauma in the last few years, primarily secondary to advances in magnetic resonance imaging (MRI) and the introduction of fast multislice CT. The use of cross-sectional imaging, however, is limited by availability, cost, and radiation exposure.

The imaging of skeletal trauma, as practiced in 2008, must take into account the following aspects.

1. The use of picture archiving and communication systems (PACS) has led to decreased turnaround time and has allowed clinicians to view images almost immediately; unfortunately, this has resulted in a marked decrease in direct consultation. The increased information gained from these consultations often provided more meaningful reports and were a learning experience for all involved.
2. Orthopedic surgeons and trauma physicians often feel that once the patient is in the CT gantry, obtaining images of additional body parts is quick and easy. This not infrequently results in the inappropriate use of computed tomography (CT) in patients whose standard radiographs are often diagnostic or in whom MRI is the study of choice. In the latter, case the negative CT may be followed by MRI, thus increasing the cost of the examination.
3. Many specialists refuse to examine a patient who has not been evaluated by CT or MRI.
4. Standard radiography in hospitalized trauma patients is often obtained at the bedside to exclude additional injuries; this is more expensive and less accurate.
5. In my opinion, the American College of Radiology's communications guidelines often create a burden for the busy radiologist, who has to contact the referring physician. Although this is sometimes necessary, it is often a disruptive, time-consuming task that not infrequently transmits information already known but not included in the consultation form. The name on the consultation form, particularly in a large teaching hospital, is not necessarily that of the physician who ordered the study and the contact information is often not correct.

This presentation is an overview of extremity trauma based upon illustrative case material, using radiography and, when necessary, CT and magnetic resonances images.

A few general caveats should be noted. Pertinent and specific clinical history should be included on the consultation form as this decreases the miss rate in subtle injuries by approximately 50% [1].

Errors in the radiologic evaluation of trauma may be secondary to incomplete studies or incorrect ordering of radiographs. Of course, errors may also be caused by incorrect interpretation or overlooking subtle abnormalities. In patients with severe trauma, examinations are often limited and the images may be marginal or suboptimal. Single views are often taken and sometimes large radiographs are obtained to image entire extremities rather than the specific area in question. In many trauma patients, this abbreviated examination may be necessary but additional radiographs of suspicious areas should be acquired following patient stabilization. Preferably, this should be done in the X-ray department and not at the bedside, with CT an adjunct rather than a replacement for conventional imaging. This is not true for spinal imaging, which is not the subject of this presentation.

Techniques

It is relatively standard to obtain two orthogonal views of an extremity which typically include the articulations proximal and distal. In large patients this may require additional images. The inclusion of the joint is not as important if joint involvement is suspected as in this case specific imaging of the joint in question should be performed. In the forearm or lower leg, the detection of a fracture should lead to a search for fracture of the paired bone or a dislocation of the proximal or distal joint. In the evaluation of a joint, at least one oblique view or supplementary views are often acquired. This is particularly common in the hand and wrist but often unnecessary in the shoulder or hip.

The use of CT has expanded markedly since the advent of fast multislice techniques but it is often performed unnecessarily at increased cost and radiation exposure. CT has been and is still frequently used to detect fractures in patients with "normal" X-rays; CT is also carried out in treatment planning, particularly in patients with intra-articular fractures and for the follow-up of fractures to detect early callus and union.

MRI is extremely accurate in the detection of fractures not seen on routine radiography and is particularly useful in detecting occult hip fractures as well as stress or insufficiency fractures. In the majority of cases, the diagnosis of stress fracture can be made on follow-up radiographs; this, of course, is much cheaper but requires waiting 10-21 days for definitive diagnosis Bone scanning is still used in some institutions for detecting stress fractures but if performed with SPECT scanning it is more expensive and less specific than MRI. Major soft-tissue injuries that occur in patients with fractures and which are often difficult to appreciate on routine radiographs may be detected with MRI, which is also unsurpassed in detecting injuries to tendons and muscle. In institutions with expertise, ultrasound can be used in the evaluation of many tendon and muscle injuries.

Injuries of the Upper Extremities

Shoulder

The most common shoulder injury in the elderly population is fracture of the surgical neck of the humerus. Neer [2] devised the well-accepted four segment classification of proximal humeral fractures, which is based upon the displacement of segments (humeral head, shaft, and greater and lesser tuberosities) rather than on number of fracture fragments. Stable, minimally displaced fractures account for 80-85% of these injuries; they have an excellent prognosis with conservative treatment. In patients with displaced fractures, the classification is thought to be helpful in determining treatment and results. Unfortunately, there is a high degree of intra- and inter-observer variation in classifying these fractures by routine radiography [3]. Neither CT [4] nor 3D radiographic analysis substantially increases intra- or inter-observer variation [5]. In patients with complex proximal humeral fractures, CT may reveal unsuspected abnormalities that may direct the choice of surgical procedure [6].

Fractures of the scapula in multiple-trauma patients have a high incidence of associated injury to the ipsilateral lung, shoulder girdle, neurovascular bundle, and ribs. CT is commonly performed in young patients with severe trauma and scapula fractures, to detect involvement of the glenoid. McAdams and colleagues [7] used CT in addition to radiographs in patients with scapular neck fractures and concluded that CT was of no value in these patients.

Anterior dislocation is the most common dislocation about the shoulder and it should not be confused with pseudosubluxation or "drooping shoulder" [8]. These dis-

locations are often associated with fractures of the greater tuberosity or compression fractures of the posterolateral aspect of the humeral head (Hill-Sachs deformity). Fractures of the anterior rim of the glenoid (bony Bankart deformity) may also be identified; these are best seen on axillary views of the shoulder. MRI is often obtained in patients with a history of anterior dislocation, particularly to determine the extent of injury to the glenoid labrum. It is typically performed prior to surgical repair or in patients with suspected labral injuries, with MRI often following intra-articular contrast injection.

Posterior dislocations of the shoulder are uncommon and are not infrequently overlooked on routine radiography. The history is often extremely helpful as they usually occur in patients with seizure disorders. The use of additional views, including the Grashey, axillary, or scapular-Y views, facilitates plain-film diagnosis. Compression fractures of the anteromedial aspect of the humeral head are commonly found in association with posterior dislocations, analogous to the Hill-Sachs defect seen with anterior dislocations. These compression deformities of the anteromedial aspect of the humeral head present as a trough in the humeral head and are often best seen on axillary images. When doubt exists concerning the presence of posterior dislocation, CT may be extremely valuable to determine that a dislocation is present and to assess associated fractures of the humeral head.

Acromioclavicular dislocations may be overlooked on radiographs of the shoulder as the acromioclavicular joint is overexposed on many shoulder radiographs. Changing the window levels on PACS systems or hot-lighting the radiograph is helpful. Note that there is considerable variation in the appearance of the acromioclavicular joint on routine radiography; thus, clinical history, weight-bearing views, and radiographs of the opposite side are helpful in avoiding misdiagnosis [9]. Stress radiographs may be helpful when initial images show no separation at the acromioclavicular joint. The most important aspect of the examination is to determine the integrity of the coracoclavicular ligaments, as disruption of these structures may require surgical therapy. The coracoclavicular distance may be assessed by comparison to the opposite side, with both sides included on a cross-wise AP image.

Sternoclavicular dislocations can be difficult to demonstrate on conventional imaging but are readily seen on CT examinations. Sternoclavicular dislocations may be anterior or posterior; of these, posterior dislocations may be associated with tracheal or vascular compression, and are very serious injuries. CT allows evaluation of the airway in addition to demonstrating the dislocation.

Elbow

Conventional radiographic imaging of the elbow should include AP, lateral, and oblique views. Displacement of the anterior and posterior fat pads is a reliable sign of intra-articular fluid; in the setting of trauma, the presence of displaced fat pads at the elbow should be considered presumptive evidence of intra-articular fracture. CT may reveal occult elbow fractures in children with effusions [10]. MRI may reveal bone marrow edema as well as fractures and does so without radiation exposure [11]; however, it is thought to have little bearing on patient treatment and outcome [12].

In the adult, the most common elbow fractures are those of the radial head or neck. Comminuted fractures of the radial neck associated with radial shortening and malalignment at the distal radioulnar joint is referred to as the Essex-Lopresti fracture.

Knowledge of the normal relationship of the humeral anterior cortex to the condyles is important in the detection of subtle supracondylar fractures, the most common elbow fracture in children. A line drawn along the anterior cortex of the humerus (anterior humeral line) should intersect the mid-third of the condyles; if the line intersects the anterior third of the condyle, a posteriorly displaced supracondylar fracture is likely present.

The most common dislocation of the elbow is posterior and is usually quite obvious clinically; it may be associated with a fracture of the ulnar coronoid process. A commonly missed elbow injury is the Monteggia fracture-dislocation, in which an angulated or displaced fracture of the proximal ulna is associated with dislocation of the radial head. A line drawn along the long axis of the radial neck should intersect the capitellum in every projection (radio-capitellar line), with overlap of the radial head on the capitellum on the AP image indicative of a dislocation.

Wrist

Radiographic examination of the wrist usually consists of three views: PA, lateral, and pronation oblique projections. Additional views, including angled views of the scaphoid (with ulnar deviation), a "clenched fist" view, and carpal tunnel views, may be helpful in specific situations.

An analytic approach to the diagnosis of wrist injuries was devised by Gilula [13], who focused primarily on conventional imaging findings of the carpal arcs, parallelism, and the overlap of articular surfaces. These criteria have withstood the test of time. Dislocation and fracture dislocations of the wrist fall into two major recognizable patterns: (1) lesser arc injuries, which are dislocations about the lunate, and (2) greater arc injuries, which are fractures about the vulnerable zone of the wrist [14]. Dislocations at the wrist include perilunate and lunate dislocations. Perilunate dislocations are frequently associated with fractures through the scaphoid waist (a trans-scaphoid perilunate dislocation). Virtually all perilunate dislocations are dorsal. Virtually all lunate dislocations, in contrast, are volar and are rarely seen in association with other fractures at the wrist.

Multidetector CT is used in the detection of carpal bone fractures in patients with negative or indeterminate plain films and for surgical planning [15]. In the wrist, the scaphoid is by far the bone most commonly fractured,

accounting for approximately 70% of all carpal bone fractures. A scaphoid fracture may be impossible to detect on conventional imaging but is often clinically suspected due to pain in the anatomic snuff box. These suspected fractures may be splinted for 10-14 days and then re-imaged. In the past, these patients were commonly examined with skeletal scintigraphy and CT [16]; however, if there is a strong suspicion and/or an immediate diagnosis is necessary, MRI is the procedure of choice. It may detect non-suspected injuries, including distal radial fractures, other carpal fractures, ligamentous injuries, and bone-marrow edema [17], and is cost effective in patients with negative X-rays in whom there is a strong clinical suspicion of a scaphoid fracture [18].

Isolated dislocations at the distal radioulnar joint are extremely difficult to diagnose because slight degrees of rotation of the wrist from the lateral projection may cause difficulty. When a question exists concerning the possibility of distal radioulnar dislocations, CT is the recommended technique for evaluation. Scans done in both pronation and supination are most helpful. The Galeazzi fracture is a fracture of the distal radial shaft associated with a dislocation at the distal radial ulnar joint (i.e., the reverse of the Monteggia fracture).

Hands

Conventional imaging of the hand should include PA, lateral, and pronation oblique views. In the digits, AP, lateral, and oblique projections of the digit in question should be obtained. The internal oblique view may detect fractures overlooked or significantly underestimated on standard views of the hands [19].

One of the more common injuries involving the hand is fracture of the distal portion of the fifth metacarpal, the "boxers fracture." While most of these fractures are identified on the PA radiograph, oblique and lateral radiographs are necessary to determine the degree of angulation. Fractures at the base of the thumb metacarpal are typically associated with a dislocation and proximal displacement of the metacarpal fragment, caused by the pull of the abductor pollicis longus muscle. The dorsal fragment almost always remains in place secondary to its strong attachments (Bennett's fracture); when these are comminuted, the fracture is termed a Rolando's fracture.

The so-called baseball finger or mallet finger is a fracture of the dorsal aspect of the base of the distal phalanx of the digit, almost always accompanied by flexion of the distal interphalangeal (DIP) joint. This injury may be purely tendinous and manifested only by flexion deformity at the DIP joint.

Volar plate fractures are quite common and are seen at the volar aspect of the base of the middle phalanx. They may be impossible to identify on PA radiographs but are usually evident on oblique or lateral images [20]. Dislocations at the interphalangeal joints may be seen in association with volar plate injuries; the dislocation may have been reduced prior to imaging.

A gamekeeper's (skier's) thumb is a disruption of the ulnar collateral ligament of the metacarpo-phalangeal joint. This is often accompanied by a fracture at the site of avulsion and may require stress views for evaluation when the injury is purely ligamentous. If the adductor aponeurosis is entrapped within the joint (Stenner lesion), surgery may be necessary. Ultrasound [21] and MRI have been advocated for the diagnosis of these injuries.

Carpometacarpal dislocations occur most commonly at the base of the fourth and fifth metacarpals, however, these may be difficult to recognize. The only radiographic sign on PA images may be overlap of the bases of the metacarpals on the hamate [22]. Dorsal chip fractures of the hamate may be seen on the lateral radiograph.

Injuries of the Lower Extremities

Hip

Fractures of the femoral neck may be displaced, with resultant shortening and external rotation of the lower extremity. Although these are readily diagnosed by conventional imaging, at times there is an apparent radiolucency in the femoral neck, suggesting that the fracture is pathologic. This appearance has been termed the pseudo-pathologic fracture. The area of lucency is due to rotation of the fracture fragments. When the radiographs are negative or equivocal and the clinical index of suspicion of hip fracture is high, particularly in the elderly, osteopenic patient, MRI can establish or exclude the diagnosis of fracture. In the absence of a hip fracture, MRI will often detect other abnormalities about the hip that are responsible for the symptoms [23].

Stress and insufficiency fractures about the hip are relatively common and may occur either in the young (fatigue fractures) or in the elderly with osteoporosis or other underlying disease (insufficiency fractures). Conventional imaging signs may be subtle or non-existent. Some patients will show vague bands of sclerosis extending across the femoral neck. Others will have no findings on conventional imaging and the presence of stress or insufficiency fracture may only be demonstrable on MRI.

In children and adolescents, avulsion fractures about the hip are not uncommon, particularly in athletes. The most common of these include avulsion fractures from the site of origin of the hamstring muscles (the ischial tuberosity), avulsions from the straight or reflected heads of the rectus femoris (seen at the anterior inferior iliac spine or in the supra-acetabular region), and avulsions of the lesser trochanter. These injuries may occur in the absence of a bone fragment. MRI is usually diagnostic in these cases.

The sports hernia is a relatively new diagnostic entity, accounting for approximately 5% of groin injuries. It is a chronic overuse injury secondary to an imbalance between the powerful adductor and weaker abdominal muscles across the symphysis pubis. The diagnosis can be made by MRI [24].

Knee

Routine imaging includes at least two views, AP and lateral. These may be supplemented by tangential views of the patella and tunnel views, particularly when joint effusions are demonstrable. In addition, oblique views may be helpful in detecting subtle fractures of the tibial plateau.

The presence of a knee-joint effusion following trauma to the knee but in the absence of a visible fracture is frequently secondary to ligamentous injury or a subtle intra-articular fracture. If a lipohemarthrosis is demonstrable on horizon-beam images, this is presumptive evidence for intra-articular fracture. In these cases, CT is often the most expeditious way to demonstrate these fractures; however, CT may not be able to detect other intra-articular abnormalities. For this reason, MRI may be the preferred approach as it can detect ligamentous injuries, meniscal tears, and chondral fractures as well as osseoous and osteochrondral fractures.

Avulsion of the lateral margin of the tibial plateau, the Segond fracture, occurs at the insertion of the lateral menisco-femoral ligament. This fracture, which can be demonstrated on conventional imaging, has an extremely high association with tears of the anterior cruciate ligament. When this fracture is identified, MRI will clearly demonstrate the ligamentous injury. Displaced fractures of the fibular head are often associated with cruciate ligament tears and frequently indicate associated posterior-lateral corner injuries [25].

In children and adolescents, Salter fractures are common in the distal femur but less common in the proximal tibia. In adolescent athletes, epiphyseal separations are more often seen than ligamentous injuries. Careful examination of the growth plate is warranted. Asymmetry in the width of the growth plate or small fracture fragments on the metaphyseal side of the growth plate should be sufficient to establish the diagnosis in most cases. MR may be a valuable technique when the nature of the injury is in question. It also allows evaluation of ligamentous structures about the knee.

Ankle and Hindfoot

Conventional imaging of the ankle should include AP, internal oblique ("mortise"), and lateral images. If a shift of the talus in the ankle mortise has occurred and no malleolar fracture is demonstrated, the entire length of the fibula should be examined in order to demonstrate proximal fibula fractures (Maisoneuve fracture). Pilon fractures represent comminuted fractures of the tibial plafond secondary to axial compression forces. There is typically a posterior tibial fragment that remains attached to the fibula, which is often used as a platform for repair. CT is very helpful in this evaluation [25].

Calcaneal fractures are commonly depressed and frequently involve either the posterior subtalar or calcaneocuboid joint. CT is typically employed in preoperative evaluation of these injuries. Isolated fractures of the anterior process of the calcaneus occur and must be distinguished from normal variants (accessory ossicles) in this location. They are often missed on conventional imaging and diagnosis often follows MRI performed for persistent ankle pain.

The Forefoot

The Lisfranc fracture-dislocation of the tarso-metatarsal joints is a frequent injury that is easily overlooked. Careful examination of the relationships of the metatarsal bases to the cuniforms is essential for diagnosis. Erect views are helpful for determining subtle subluxations and should be obtained if this fracture is suspected.

Avulsions of the base of the fifth metatarsal, at the point of insertion of the peroneus brevis muscle, should be distinguished from "dancer's fracture" or Jones' fracture. These occur near the base of the fifth metatarsal, approximately 2.5 cm distal to the base, in a relatively avascular area of the metatarsal and may go on to non-union.

Compartment Syndrome

Compartment syndrome represents a pathologic condition of skeletal muscle caused by increased interstitial pressure within a confined anatomic compartment that interferes with the circulation and function of the neurovascular components of the compartment. Diagnosis may be made clinically or by measuring intracompartmental pressure. Delay in diagnosis often leads to severe complications. The diagnosis can be made or suggested by MRI.

Conclusions

Fractures and dislocations in the appendicular skeleton are common and careful examination of the appropriate images obtained from each site is required for diagnosis. When aware of the common locations for fractures and dislocations, the radiologist is better prepared to make the diagnosis or to recommend additional imaging techniques. When doubt occurs based upon conventional imaging findings, CT and MRI will often be useful to establish the diagnosis or to exclude a fracture.

References

1. Berbaum, KS, El-Khoury GY, Franken EA et al (1988) Impact of clinical history on fracture detection with radiography. Radiology 168:507-511
2. Neer C (1970) Displaced proximal humeral fractures. J Bone Joint Surg 52-A(6):1077-1089
3. Siebenrock KA, Gerber C, Switzerland B (1993) The reproducibility of classification of fractures of the proximal end of the humerus. J Bone Joint Surg 75-A(12):1751-1754
4. Bernstein J, Adler LM, Blank JE et al (1996) Evaluation of the neer system of classification of proximal humeral fractures with computerized tomographic scans and plain radiographs. J Bone Joint Surg 78-A(9):1371-1375
5. Sjoden GO, Movin T, Aspelin P et al (1999) 3D-radiographic analysis does not improve the Neer and AO classifications of proximal humeral fractures. Acta Orthop Scand. 70(4):325-328
6. Castagno AA, Shuman WP, Kilcoyne RF et al (1987) Complex fractures of the proximal humerus: role of CT in treatment. Radiology 165:759-762
7. McAdams TR, Blevins FT, Martin TP, DeCoster TA (2002) The role of plain films and computer tomography in the evaluation of scapular neck fractures. J Orthop Trauma 16(1):7-10
8. Markham DE, Rowland J (1969) The shoulder joint – is it dislocated? Apparent dislocation of the shoulder joint. Clin Radiol 20:61-64
9. Keats TE, Pope TI (1988) The acromioclavicular joint: normal variation and the diagnosis of dislocation. Skel Radiol 17:159-162
10. Chapman V, Grottkau B, Albright M et al (2006) MDCT of the elbow in pediatric patients with posttraumatic elbow effusions. AJR Am J Roentgenol 187:812-817
11. Major NM, Crawford ST (2002) Elbow effusions in trauma in adults and children: Is there an occult fracture? AJR Am J Roentgenol 178:413-418
12. Griffith JF, Roebuck DJ, Cheng JCY et al (2001) Acute elbow trauma in children: Spectrum of injury revealed by MR Imaging not apparent on radiographs. AJR Am J Roentgenol 176:53-60
13. Gilula LA (1979) Carpal injuries: analytic approach and case exercises. AJR Am J Roentgenol 133:503-517
14. Johnson RP (1980) The acutely injured wrist and its residuals. Clin Orthop Rel Res 149:33-44
15. Kaewlai R, Avery LL, Asruni AV et al (2008) Multidetector CT of carpal injuries: anatomy, fractures, and fracture-dislocations. Radiographics 28:1771-1784
16. Groves AM, Cheow H, Balan K et al (2005) 16-MDCT in the detection of occult wrist fractures: a comparison with skeletal scintigraphy. AJR Am J Roentgenol 184:1470-1474
17. Brydie A, Raby N (2003) Early MRI in the management of clinical scaphoid fracture. Br J Radiol 76:296-299
18. Dorsay TA, Major NM, Helms CA (2001) Cost-effectiveness of immediate MR imaging versus traditional follow-up for revealing radiographically occult scaphoid fractures. AJR Am J Roentgenol 177:1257-1263
19. Street JM (1993) Radiographs of phalangeal fractures: importance of the internally rotated oblique projection for diagnosis. AJR Am J Roentgenol 160:575-576
20. Nance EP, Kaye JJ, Milek MA (1979) Volar plate fractures. Radiology 113:61-64
21. O'Callaghan BI, Kohut G, Hoogewoud HM (1994) Gamekeeper thumb: identification of the Stener lesion with US. Radiology 192:477-480
22. Fisher MR, Rogers LF, Hendrix RW (1983) Systematic approach to identifying fourth and fifth carpometacarpal joint dislocations. AJR Am J Roentgenol 140:319-324
23. Bogost GA, Lizerbram EK, Crues JV III (1995) MR Imaging in evaluation of suspected hip fracture: Frequency of unsuspected bone and soft-tissue injury. Radiology 1097:263-267
24. Omar IM, Zoga AC, Kavanagh EC et al (2008) Athletic pubalgia and "sports hernia": optimal MR imaging technique and findings. Radiographics 28:1415-1438
25. Gottsegen CJ, Eyer BA, White EA et al (2008) Avulsion fractures of the knee: imaging findings and clinical significance. Radiographics 28:1755-1770

Inflammatory Disorders of the Spine

Iain McCall

Department of Diagnostics Radiology, The Robert Jones and Agnes Hunt Orthopaedic and District Hospital NHS Trust, Oswestry, UK

Introduction

Inflammation in the spine may affect the ligaments, intervertebral disc, and synovial joints and result in osteitis of adjacent bone. The inflammation may subsequently cause mineralization and ossification of the ligaments and destruction of the joints, which in some conditions may also result in fusion. Ankylosing spondylitis (AS), psoriatic arthritis, non-specific spondylitis, and enteropathic spondylitis are inflammatory spondyloarthropathies that primarily affect the ligaments. Rheumatoid arthritis primarily affects the synovium. Rare disorders that primarily affect bone include SAPHO syndrome and chronic recurrent multifocal osteomyelitis; although these are also inflammatory disorders, they will not be considered in this review.

Etiology

The etiology of the inflammatory spondyloarthropathies is unknown. There is a hereditary component that varies in importance between the different conditions comprising this group. Human leukocyte antigen (HLA)-B27 is present in 90% of patients suffering from AS but only in 50% of patients with reactive arthritis, and 20% of patients with psoriasis. The human immunodeficiency virus (HIV) may be an underlying predisposing factor for reactive arthritis and psoriatic arthritis. Psoriatic spondyloarthropathy seems to be an autoimmune disorder that is multifactorial, T-cell-dependent, and mediated, at least in part, by tumor necrosis factor (TNF). It accounts for almost 20% of seronegative spondyloarthropathies.

Reactive arthritis (Reiter's disease) occurs after infection with specific organisms associated with diarrheal illness or urogenital infection. Enteric organisms include *Campylobacter*, *Salmonella*, *Shigella*, and *Yersinia* whereas most cases subsequent to urogenital disease are caused by *Chlamydia trachomatis*. The majority of individuals with symptomatic disease are either HLA-B27-positive or are infected with HIV, although the presence of HLA-B27 is not necessary for the diagnosis.

Prevalence

Ankylosing spondylitis affects young adults, with a peak age of onset between 20 and 30 years although patients with juvenile AS become symptomatic at or before the age of 16 years and 80% of patients develop the first symptoms before their third decade of life. The prevalence of AS is 0.1-1.4%, depending on ethnicity, prevalence of HLA-B27, selection of patients for evaluation, and the screening criteria used for diagnosis [1]. The prevalence in central Europe has been reported to be 0.3-0.5% [2]. Men are more often affected with AS than women, the ratio being approximately 3:1. The condition is more common in persons of Euro-Caucasian origin; 4-13% of this population is positive for HLA-B27 whereas HLA-B27 positivity in black Africans is rare.

The prevalence of reactive arthritis is particularly variable as it is highly dependent on the diagnostic criteria and mild cases may never be recorded. Reactive arthritis that is *Chlamydia*-associated is most commonly seen in males whereas reactive arthritis associated with enteric infection has an equal sex distribution. Clinical manifestation is most common in individuals between 20 and 40 years. Among those who are HIV-infected, the incidence of reactive arthritis is at least ten times greater than in the general population.

The incidence of psoriasis in males and females is similar and peaks in a slightly older population, between 30 and 50 years. There is also ethnic variation, but 1-6% of the population of Western Europe suffers some degree of clinical psoriasis and up to15% of these patients may develop some degree of psoriatic arthritis.

Pathology

The pathology of the spinal inflammation differs depending on whether it is ligament-based or synovial. The inflammatory site in AS is the enthesis, where the collagen of the ligament or intervertebral disc enters bone directly. The cause of the inflammation is the generation of cytokines, which result in edema, bone erosion, disorganization of bone and ligament structure, and, finally, ossification of the ligament and osteitis in the bone interface.

Histological analysis of samples obtained from sites of enthesitis shows a macrophage-predominant cellular infiltrate, consistent with the fact that TNF-α, a pro-inflammatory cytokine produced by macrophages, has been shown to play a key role in inflammatory spondyloarthropathies [3].

Clinical Features

The key feature of inflammatory spondyloarthropathy is inflammatory back pain that is worse at night and in the early morning. AS also presents with early-morning stiffness that is eased by movement and exercise. The onset is usually insidious and with relapsing attacks of pain, which initially involve the lower back but eventually migrate up the vertebral column. As the disease progresses, stiffness becomes the predominant symptom, with an increase in thoracic kyphosis and cervical movement. The proximal joints may also be affected particularly the hip knee and shoulder.

The current criteria for the diagnosis of AS, the modified New York criteria, require the presence of at least one of the following clinical features: low back pain and stiffness of >3 months duration that improves with exercise but is not relieved by rest, limitation of motion of the lumbar spine in both the sagittal and coronal planes, and limitation of chest expansion relative to normal values combined with radiographic evidence of either bilateral grade 2 or unilateral grade 3 sacroiliitis [4]. However fulfilment of these criteria results in a delay in diagnosis, due also to the low sensitivity of the radiographic diagnosis of sacroiliitis. Hence, there is a need for new diagnostic criteria, particularly regarding early-stage disease [5].

Symptoms of reactive arthritis usually develop around 4 weeks following the gastrointestinal or urinary infection, although a triggering infection is identified only in up to 60% of patients. The predominant feature is an asymmetric lower-limb-predominant oligoarthritis. This may be associated with conjunctivitis, which in a few cases may progress to uveitis and, in patients with urogenital infection, urethritis (seen in up to 30% of patients). Inflammatory markers are frequently elevated. Heel pain is a common presenting feature due to enthesitis of the Achilles tendon and plantar aponeurosis. Dactylitis, resulting from inflammation of the entheses and synovial linings of an entire digit, producing a sausage finger, may occur. The peripheral arthritis predominantly involves large joints of the lower extremity and often only a single joint with erythema, swelling, and joint effusion. The enteric form appears to affect the upper limb more frequently than the *Chlamydia*-associated form. Low back pain is a frequent symptom that may be asymmetric and refer to the buttocks.

In psoriatic spondyloarthropathy, the dermatological changes include erythematous macules with silvery-white scale; nail changes and sterile pustules are also present.

Sacroiliitis

The demonstration of sacroiliitis is a fundamental part of establishing the diagnosis of AS but is also relevant to the other spondyloarthropathies. In AS, it is bilateral but in psoriatic spondylitis and reactive arthritis it may be bilateral or unilateral. The initial diagnostic imaging should be radiographic despite its relatively high false-negative rate in early disease. The standard examination of the lumbar spine must include the whole of the sacroiliac joints; this is usually performed as lateral and anteroposterior (AP) projections. However, the sacroiliac joints are divergent in the AP projection taken at an angle of approximately 10°; therefore, an additional posteroanterior (PA) projection may be more helpful. Lumbar lordosis may also affect the visualization. An additional angulation of 15-25° cephalad for the AP projection and caudad for the PA projection will improve visualization of the inferior sacroiliac joint. The radiographic features are those of erosions, which may be difficult to detect initially; sclerosis of the subchondral bone on either side of the joint; and bony bridging, which marks the beginning of ankylosis (Fig. 1a). The

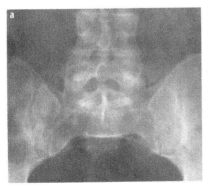 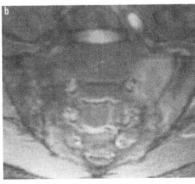

Fig. 1 a, b. a Radiographs of the sacroiliac joints show irregularity of the articular surface with some pseudo-widening and sclerosis of the adjacent sub-chondral bone. **b** Magnetic resonance (MR) STIR sequence shows high signal in the ala of the sacrum and on both sides of the lower part of the joints due to inflammatory changes and bone edema

initial appearance may be a loss of sharpness of the outline of the joint, which then becomes irregular due to the erosions; these may also appear to produce local widening of the joint (Fig. 1). The sclerosis involves both the inferior and middle portion of the joint and is often more pronounced on the iliac side. The loss of sharpness may also be due to the early ossification across the joint, which will eventually progress to complete ankylosis. Radiographic sacroiliac changes have been graded as part of the modified New York criteria:
– Grade 0, no abnormality
– Grade 1, suspicious changes
– Grade 2, sclerosis with some erosions
– Grade 3, severe erosions, pseudo-widening of the joint space, and partial ankylosis
– Grade 4, complete ankylosis

Radiological evidence of sacroiliitis is seen in up to 30% of patients with reactive arthritis and half of the patients with psoriatic spondyloarthropathy. In reactive arthritis, it is asymmetric but usually bilateral although it maybe unilateral in the early stages of the disease and later in the disease it may become symmetric. In psoriatic arthritis it is usually unilateral but may be bilateral. Ankylosis is a late feature. The identification of sacroiliitis on radiographs has only modest sensitivity and specificity [6].

The late development of radiological changes in AS patients often results in a delay in diagnosis, which may be avoided by the use of magnetic resonance imaging (MRI). Pericartilage osteitis is an important feature of AS that is well-demonstrated by MRI as bone marrow edema. T1-weighted spin echo sequences may be performed to examine the articular cartilage for the presence of erosions while T2-weighted sequences with fat suppression or STIR sequences demonstrate the increased signal of bone edema (Fig. 1b), which will also be seen as reduced signal on T1. In chronic sacroiliitis or fused sacroiliac joints, the subchondral bone may show a high signal on T1 due to the increased yellow marrow often associated with osteoporosis of adjacent bone with fused joints. The extent of the edema may vary and may be in localised foci or parallel to the joint line. Early signs of inflammation on MRI have been consistently found in the inferior iliac portion of the joint [7], whereas the synovial part is confined in normal sacroiliac joints [8]. If there is adjacent para-articular sclerosis, it may appear as a rim of high signal around the endosteal edge of the low signal on both T1- and T2-visualized sclerosis. The use of dynamic post-contrast imaging with Gd-DTPA has been advocated, as in active disease there is a linear rise in the signal at the point of maximal enhancement in the joint cartilage and periarticular tissue in the first 1-2 min. Acute sacroiliitis was demonstrated in all 15 patients with possible early AS who had normal sacroiliac joints on radiography while all controls were normal [9]. However, contrast enhancement is only required if the STIR sequence is equivocal.

Computed tomography (CT) defines the parallel articular surface of the synovial part of the sacroiliac joint compared to the contour irregularities of the fibrous part. The joint space is clearly visible and erosions, particularly on the iliac side, as well as subchondral sclerosis and early bony bridging are easily detected. Nonetheless, the sensitivity of CT in the detection of acute inflammatory lesions is poor compared to MRI. CT is valuable to differentiate intra-articular bony bridging from diffuse idiopathic skeletal hyperostosis or advanced degenerative disease with bony bridges. However, abnormal findings on CT are frequently detected in the sacroiliac joints of asymptomatic normal controls [10].

Bone scintigraphy using single photon emission computed tomography (SPECT) was previously employed to diagnose active sacroiliitis, but the lack of specificity was a major drawback and quantitative measurements have not improved this situation. A recent study has concluded that scintigraphy plays no role in the diagnosis of acute sacroiliitis [11].

Axial Skeleton

Ankylosing Spondylitis

The primary site of pathology is the enthesis, where the longitudinal ligaments and the annulus fibrosis collagen merge directly with bone. The osteitis caused by the inflammatory process leads to bone edema and subsequently to ossification of the ligaments. The synovial joints are also affected by inflammation, with erosions followed by bone production and ankylosis.

The initial examination of the spine has traditionally been radiographic. The radiological features of enthesitis and localized osteitis are erosion of the enthesis and localized sclerosis (Fig. 2). This results in focal loss of the margins of the vertebral endplates and apparent squaring of the anterior and, to a lesser extent, the posterior surfaces of the vertebral body. The anterior lesion has been

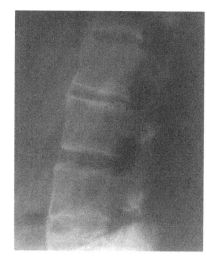

Fig. 2. Lateral radiograph of the lumbar spine showing a combination of marginal erosions, focal sclerosis, squaring of the anterior vertebral body, and syndesmophytes of two levels

called the Romanus lesion A rim of sclerosis develops on the vertebral side of the enthesis, referred to as the "shiny corner sign" (Fig. 2). Romanus lesions tend to resolve, with resultant syndesmophyte formation. The syndesmophyte is the characteristic feature of AS and is due to ossification of the longitudinal ligament, which runs parallel to the line of the vertebral edge and annular surface and develops from the corner of the vertebra (Fig. 2). This may initially appear at a single disc level but can eventually involve multiple segments, producing a bamboo spine. Ossification of the longitudinal ligaments of the posterior elements and interspinous ligaments also takes place. In addition, in the fused spine, there may be dystrophic calcification of the intervertebral discs.

Radiographic scoring methods have been developed for evaluation of the inflammatory changes in the spine. The modified Stoke ankylosing spondylitis score (mSASSS) is based on an analysis of the anterior cervical and lumbar vertebral spinal unit, which is graded as: 0 normal, 1 erosions/squaring/sclerosis, 2 syndesmophytes, 3 total bone bridging. The mSASSS has been found to be the most sensitive to change, which is the main focus of interest in clinical trials [12], and syndesmophytes have proven to be the best predictors of radiographic progression [13].

Erosion or destruction of the subdiscal bone may become extensive and resemble a spondylodiscitis, referred to as an Anderson type B lesion. The degree of vertebral destruction is usually mild but there is often extensive bone sclerosis (Fig. 6a) and in longstanding cases the endplates may be completely destroyed. These lesions are due to increased mobility at a level between fused segments or from posterior-element pseudarthrosis in solidly fused spines. Risk factors, including osteoporosis, marked thoracolumbar kyphosis, and minor trauma, are associated with renewed onset of pain in patients who have previously become pain-free. Care should therefore be undertaken in reviewing the status of a posterior-element fusion.

In reactive spondyloarthropathy, radiographs of the spine may demonstrate asymmetric, coarse, thick paravertebral ossifications that are non-marginal and originate away from the vertebral-body endplates. They are most commonly seen in the lower thoracic and upper lumbar spine. Erosion of the longitudinal ligament annulus fibrosis complex, the Romanus lesion, is uncommon in reactive spondyloarthropathy. The appearances may be difficult to differentiate from diffuse idiopathic skeletal hyperostosis, although this is usually asymptomatic and affects an older population. In psoriatic spondyloarthropathy, there is a predilection for the upper lumbar spine but any level, including the cervical spine, may be involved. The typical feature is non-marginal syndesmophytes but marginal syndesmophytes may also be seen. Paravertebral ossification, which is usually large, non-uniform, and asymmetric (Fig. 3), is a characteristic feature but is seen at a late stage of the disease; nonetheless, it provides differentiation from

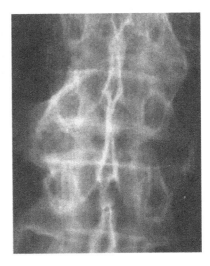

Fig. 3. Radiograph of paravertebral ossification in psoriasis, which is thick, merges with the vertebral wall, and is asymmetric

AS. Romanus lesions are a feature of psoriatic spondyloarthropathy and discovertebral destruction may occur. The radiographic spinal features of Reiter's disease and psoriasis may be identical but the peripheral inflammation involves the lower limb including the heels and the larger joints are also affected.

Peripheral joint involvement is present in psoriatic arthropathy and characteristically affects the distal interphalangeal joints with erosions, layered periosteal reaction in the shafts of the tubular bones, ossification at the margins of the joints, non-delineation of the subchondral plate, joint-space narrowing, and sclerosis of bone. These features are asymmetric and polyarticular, affecting both hands and feet.

The Role of MRI

Magnetic resonance imaging is now the initial investigation in the majority of cases of back pain and has proven to be the most sensitive diagnostic tool for discovertebral inflammation. Inflammatory changes are most commonly present in the lower thoracic spine so that this area should be included in any MRI examination for AS [14]. Romanus lesions are identified most clearly in the sagittal plane and are characterized by the presence of a triangular edema pattern at the corners of the vertebral endplates, with low signal on T1-weighted images (Fig. 4a) and high signal on STIR and T2-FS sequences (Fig. 4b). The vertebral body may appear squared anteriorly and small erosions producing focal defects may be visible. In chronic lesions, the edema pattern may disappear and be replaced by yellow marrow at the enthesis and adjacent vertebral body, with a high signal on T1 and low signal on STIR and T2-FS sequences. Where fusion is extensive, multiple triangular fat accumulations are seen and high signal may be present in the intervertebral discs on T1 due to the presence of fine calcification. A scoring

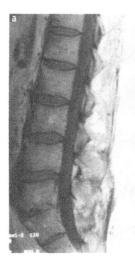
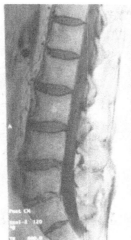
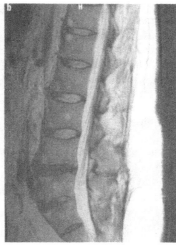

Fig. 4 a, b. Sagittal MR study of the lumbar spine demonstrates anterior endplate erosions and adjacent vertebral inflammatory response with bone marrow edema pattern, which is low signal on T1-weighted sequence (**a**) and which enhances following Gd-DTPA injection (**a**) and high signal on STIR (**b**)

system for the spinal changes seen on MRI has been developed based on the acute and chronic pathologic features. Marginal erosions and edema are the key criteria [15] and have been subsequently validated in a multi-center study [16]. The scoring system helps to evaluate the progress of treatment with TNF-α inhibitors and may also predict the likely improvement in clinical score for those treated [17].

Following contrast medium injection there is enhancement of acute lesions and the erosions may be more clearly defined (Fig. 4a). However, comparative studies with STIR sequences have found little advantage, as both have high intra- and inter-observer reliability and more-active lesions are seen on STIR. Dynamic Gd-DTPA studies may be more selective and specific; they also provide complementary information in some cases or in cases of continued doubt [18].

Syndesmophytes are not well-demonstrated by MRI due to the low signal of the normal longitudinal ligament and annulus, but involvement of the costovertebral and facet joints is readily seen on the axial studies, which show joint-line erosion adjacent bone edema, effusions, and eventually fusion. Sagittal MRI studies should be sufficiently wide to include the facet and costovertebral joints, to ensure that inflammatory lesions are not overlooked.

Anderson type A lesions resemble Schmorl's nodes and have a rim of edema in the vertebral body, which is of low signal on T1-weighted sequences (Fig. 5a) and of high signal on T2-weighted sequences (Fig. 5b). These lesions will enhance after contrast injection.

The changes induced by Anderson type B lesions are well-demonstrated on CT and MRI. CT demonstrates the sclerosis and the state of the posterior elements (Fig. 6b); the pseudarthrosis will be easily identified on sagittal reconstructions. MRI shows the irregular destruction of the endplates and extensive vertebral-body edema but with limited visualization of paravertebral inflamed soft tissue

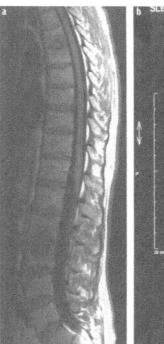
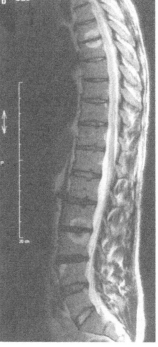

Fig. 5 a, b. MR demonstrates Anderson type A endplate erosions with extensive surrounding edema at two levels, in addition to a marginal erosion anteriorly on the T1 (**a**) and T2 (**b**) sequences

(Fig. 6c, d). Posterior-element pseudarthroses are highlighted as low signal across the lamina on T1-weighted sequences, with adjacent edema seen on STIR.

Complications

The main spinal complications of AS are osteoporosis, trauma, and, rarely, cauda equina.

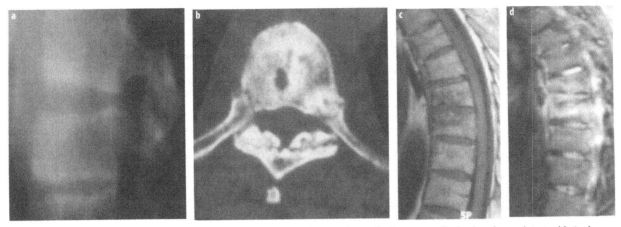

Fig. 6 a-d. Lateral radiograph of the thoracic spine demonstrates endplate erosion and adjacent vertebral sclerosis consistent with Anderson type B lesion (**a**). Careful scrutiny of the posterior elements demonstrates the pseudarthrosis (**a**). CT confirms the erosions and sclerosis of the facets and costovertebral joints (**b**). Sagittal T1 (**c**) and STIR (**d**) MR sequences demonstrate the adjacent vertebral edema without any soft-tissue component, which differentiates it from infection

Fig. 7 a, b. Sagittal computed tomography reconstruction demonstrates the chalkstick fracture through the disc anteriorly and the posterior elements with angulation (**a**). The sagittal T2 sequence shows that the cord is not compressed or edematous (**b**)

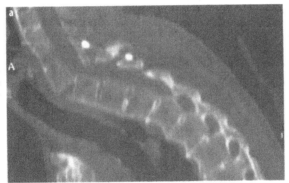

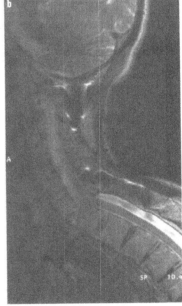

Osteoporosis increases in prevalence with patient age, disease duration, severity of the spinal involvement, and peripheral arthritis. It may result in vertebral compression fractures and also increases the chance of pseudarthrosis and trauma. The degree of osteoporosis may be evident on radiographs but can be measured by dual-energy X-ray absorptiometry (DEXA) or quantitative computed tomography (QCT). On MRI, vertebral marrow signal is increased on the T1 sequences due to the osteoporosis.

Fractures of the cervical spine in particular may occur after minor trauma to the head and neck. The typical ap-

pearance on plain radiographs is of a chalkstick break across either the disc or the vertebral body and the posterior elements. These fractures are best evaluated by CT, with the full extent of the fracture well-demonstrated using both axial and reconstructed sagittal and coronal reconstructions (Fig. 7a). MRI is essential to assess whether there has been associated cord injury (Fig. 7b), whether edema or hemorrhage is present, and the extent of either one. It will also demonstrate the presence of hematoma.

Cauda equina is seen as an enlarged spinal canal with thecal diverticular erosion of the lamina and adherent nerve roots.

References

1. Lawrence RC, Helmick CG, Arnett FC et al (1998) Estimates of prevalence of arthritis and selected musculoskeletal disorders in the United States. Arthritis Rheum 41:778-799
2. Braun J, Sieper J (2007) Ankylosing spondylitis. Lancet 369:1379-1390
3. McGonagle D, Marzo-Ortega H, O'Connor P et al (2002) Histological assessment of the early enthesitis lesion in spondyloarthropathy. Ann Rheum Dis 61:534-537
4. Van der Linden S, Valkenburg HA, Cats A (1984) Evaluation of diagnostic criteria for ankylosing spondylitis. A proposal for modification of the New York criteria. Arthritis Rheum 27:361-368
5. Rudwaleit M, Khan MA, Sieper J (2005) The challenge of diagnosis and classification in early ankylosing spodylitis. Do we need new criteria? Commentary. Arthritis Rheum 52:1000-1008
6. Van Tubergen A, Heuft Dorenbosch L, Schulpen G et al (2003) Radiographic assessment of sacroiliitis by radiologists and rheumatologists: does training improve quality? Ann Rheum Dis 62:519-525
7. Bollow M, Hermann KG, Biedermann T et al (2005) Very early spondyloarthritis: where the inflammation in the sacroiliac joints starts. Ann Rheum Dis 64:1644-1646
8. Puhakka KB, Melsen F, Jurik AG et al (2004) MR imaging of the normal sacroiliac joint with correlation to histology. Skeletal Radiol 33:15-28
9. Braun J, Bollow M, Eggens U et al (1994) Use of dynamic magnetic resonance imaging with fast imaging in the detection of early and advanced sacroiliitis in spondyloarthropathy patients. Arthritis Rheum 37:1039-1045
10. Vogler JB, Brown WH, Helms CA, Genant HK (1984) The normal sacroiliac joint: a CT study of asymptomatic patients. Radiology 151:433-437
11. Song IH, Carrasco J, Rudwaleit M, Sieper J (2008) The diagnostic value of scintigraphy in assessing sacroiliitis in ankylosing spondylitis – a systematic literature search. Ann Rheum Dis doi:10.1136/ard.2007.083089
12. Wanders AJ, Landewe RB, Spoorenberg A et al (2004) What is the most appropriate radiologic scoring method for ankylosing spondylitis? A comparison of the available methods based on the Outcome Measures in Rheumatology Clinical Trials Filter. Arthritis Rheum 50:2622-2632
13. Baraliakos X, Listing J, Rudwaleit M et al (2007) Progression of radiographic damage in patients with ankylosing spondylitis: A randomised clinical trial. Ann Rheum Dis 66:910-915
14. Baraliakos X, Landewe R, Hermann KG et al (2005) Inflammation in ankylosing spondylitis. A systematic description of the extent and frequency of acute spinal changes using magnetic resonance imaging. Ann Rheum Dis 64:730-734
15. Braun J, Baraliakos X, Golder W et al (2003) Magnetic resonance imaging examinations of the spine in patients with ankylosing spondylitis, before and after successful therapy with infiximab: evaluation of a new scoring system. Arthritis Rheum 48:1126-1136
16. Lucas C, Braun J, van der Heijde D et al (2007) ASAS/OMERACT MRI in AS working group scoring inflammatory activity of the spine by magnetic resonance imaging in ankylosing spondylitis: a multireader experiment. J Rheumatol 34:862-870
17. Rudwaleit M, Schwarzlose S, Hilgert ES et al (2008) Magnetic resonance imaging (MRI) in predicting a major clinical response to anti TNF-α treatment in ankylosing spondylitis. Ann Rheum Dis 67:1276-1281
18. Baraliakos X, Hermann KGA, Landewe R et al (2005) Assessment of acute spinal inflammation in patients with ankylosing spondylitis by magnetic resonance imaging(MRI): a systematic comparison between contrast enhanced T1 and short tau recovery (STIR) sequences. Ann Rheum Dis 64:1141-1144

Mimickers of Inflammatory Diseases of the Spine

Frieda Feldman

Musculoskeletal Radiology, Columbia University College of Physicians and Surgeons, New York, NY, USA

This chapter emphasizes commonly encountered, etiologically unrelated patho-anatomic changes that may simulate primary inflammatory diseases of the spine. Such "pseudoinflammations" are important to recognize, since inappropriate treatment or intervention may follow their misinterpretation as an infection.

Magnetic resonance imaging (MRI) is the commonest initial study ordered by referring physicians and radiologists to clarify symptoms related to the spine in general and infection in particular. However, commonly accepted MRI-based criteria for identifying "inflammatory" lesions, including infections and non-inflammatory entities such as spondylosclerosis, osteoarthrosis, and Schmorl's nodes, may share similar imaging features with resultant difficulty in confidently distinguishing them. Although widely considered the modality of choice for detecting early inflammation, the specificity of MRI lags behind its high sensitivity, despite improving technology and the use of creative fluid-sensitive sequences supplemented by contrast agent. MRI findings, therefore, remain essentially non-specific.

Bone-marrow edema, a "classic" MRI criterion for inflammation may, in fact, be "reactive" rather than a "definitive" sign of intrinsic infection. Similarly, diffuse or focal soft-tissue prominence, in the guise of an enhancing "mass", may be sterile, non-infected and due to "reactive edema". The latter may occur in the spine or its neighboring constituents, including discs, tendons, ligaments, muscles, and pre-vertebral soft tissues, which may all serve as "crystal depositories" [1-4].

While calcium pyrophosphate dihydrate (CPPD) deposition is the most common irritant, others, in order of frequency, hydroxyapatite, calcium carbonate, phosphate, and oxylate, may also be associated with various metabolic and non-metabolic disorders, such as hemochromatosis, rheumatoid arthritis, neuroarthropathy, and ochronosis, all of which may involve the spine (Fig. 1) [5, 6].

The significance of these sometimes subtle calcifications, particularly in the spine, has not been accorded adequate attention. Perhaps this is due to their poor conspicuity, particularly on MRI, where they may be barely perceptible or entirely inapparent, even when suspected.

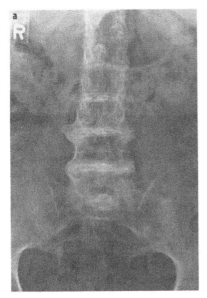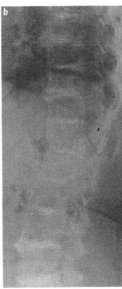

Fig. 1 a, b. Anteroposterior (**a**) and lateral (**b**) views of the thoracolumbar spine in a 50-year-old man with ochronosis, back pain, and "wafer like" calcifications in the discs and the inner margins of the annulus due to hydroxyapatite crystal deposits (X-ray diffraction analysis) in brittle, degenerated intervertebral cartilage with prior abnormal pigment accumulation due to deficient homogentisic oxidase. Compromised right and ankylosed left sacroiliac joints mimic seronegative spondylitis

Conversely, if noted, they are usually not considered causative factors for co-existent, occasionally severe symptoms [5]. They are rather regarded as "ancillary" findings even when readily recognized and not as often held responsible for clinical complaints in the spine as they are in the knees, shoulders and wrists, in descending order of frequency. The ability of MRI to depict early edema may be the most efficient means of directly defining elusive, but secondary inflammatory effects. However, since they are not well established by MRI, cause and effect relationships between bone and soft-tissue edema due to "crystal incitement" are difficult to establish in individual patients. Large deposits are more successfully depicted on radiographs and computed tomography (CT), although their physiologic effects are not.

Usually unwarranted biopsy may also be unrevealing since all "crystal culprits" cannot be distinguished on light microscopy. Moreover, neuropathologists may not be as familiar as surgical pathologists or rheumatologists with the special stains needed for the definitive identification of the lesions in question. Radiologists may initially suggest such corroboration in the face of high indices of suspicion. Conversely, autopsy specimens often reveal the responsible agents, but, unfortunately "after the fact" (Fig. 2) [7, 8].

Another systemic entity, collagen vascular disease, may sometimes be severely involved with crystal deposits. Nevertheless, despite their common presence in other anatomic loci, such as the skin, lungs, and viscera, they are not as readily related to the spine even when considerable. Conversely, larger, more obvious conglomerates evident on radiographs and CT are non-specifically labeled "tumoral calcinosis", which is a solely descriptive term. However, tumoral calcinosis most often results from several systemic aberrations that must be excluded, including primary or secondary hyperparathyroidism and renal disease, which, unlike "idiopathic" tumoral calcinosis, are usually associated with early abnormal laboratory findings. Renal disease is a common cause of tumoral calcinosis, with and without dialysis, but a relatively recently recognized association is a destructive spondyloarthropathy that closely simulates infection [9] (Fig. 3). Prior imaging studies, including radiographs, along with clinical and laboratory data, are essential for accurate diagnosis. Amyloid deposits in the spine and viscera, secondary to other conditions, including renal disease and chronic osteomyelitis at any site, may also mimic infection (Fig. 4).

Seronegative spondylitis, an independent inflammatory process of still uncertain origin, may also be misconstrued as a primary infection [10].While the latter may occur in seronegative spondylitis, an often unsuspected complication, occult fracture, is another example of a "pseudo-inflammation". The restrictive ankylosis commonly accompanying advanced seronegative spondylitis is usually relatively asymptomatic, but sudden or inadvertent movement or minor stress when superimposed on rigid skeletons along with osteoporosis of disuse all promote fragility. Infection, however, is more often clinically considered the likely source of pain. The initially subtle, non-displaced fracture, its predilection for the posterior elements at the site of severest kyphosis, and pre-existent, often florid, bone formation all combine to delay discovery. Unappreciated fractures may propagate anteriorly to involve vertebral body cortices and intervertebral discs with eventual pseudoarthrosis formation. Chronic "grinding and grating" of irregular apposing surfaces and reactive sclerosis contribute to a complex of changes mis-

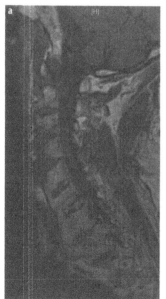
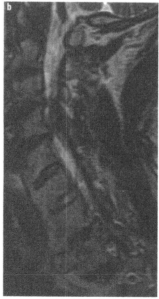

Fig. 2 a, b. A 60-year-old woman with neck pain, Sagittal (**a**) T1-weighted and (**b**) T1-weighted fat-saturated off-center magnetic resonance images show diffuse osteophyte formation, most markedly at the C3-C4, C4-C5 levels, and increased signal intensity due to crystal deposition in relatively preserved C5-C6 and C6-C7 discs. Note incidental DISH. Heterotopic bone blends with C5-T1 anterior vertebral cortices

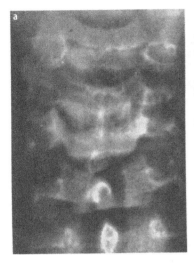

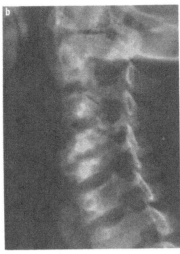

Fig. 3 a, b. Anteroposterior (a) and oblique (b) radiographs of the cervical spine in a 53-year-old woman on dialysis, with end-stage renal disease. The images reveal reactive sclerosis, narrowing, irregularity, of apposing C4-C5 surfaces. The images, unchanged in appearance for several years, are consistent with dialysis arthropathy due to calcium pyrophosphate dihydrate deposition disease

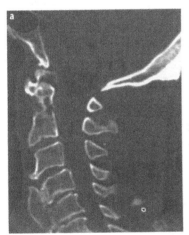

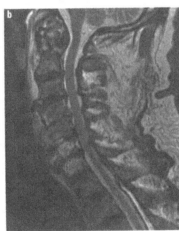

Fig. 4 a, b. a CT sagittal reconstruction: Lucencies in the odontoid process and anterior C1 arch with focal and prevertebral soft-tissue prominence and incidental DISH involving the anterior C5 and C6 vertebra. b Sagittal T2-weighted image of the cervical spine. The images show an inhomogeneous signal in the odontoid process and anterior C1 arch, a surrounding focal mass, and increased signal intensity in the C5-C6 disc and prevertebral soft tissues due to chronic renal disease. In addition, C1-C2 amyloid deposits and prevertebral "reactive" edema in the soft tissues due to calcium pyrophosphate dihydrate deposition disease are seen. Incidental DISH involves the C4 and C5 anterior vertebra

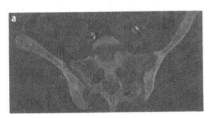
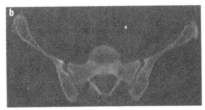
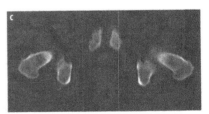

Fig. 5 a-c. A 40-year-old patient with subperiosteal bone resorption in the sacroiliac margins due to secondary hyperparathyroidism; on CT imaging, these changes mimic those of inflammatory seronegative spondylitis (a-c). Note the distinguishing features, as seen in a young male patient: same changes as in (c) symphysis pubis, thin, indistinct cortices, lytic lesions throughout compatible with cysts and/or brown tumors, and vascular calcification

construed as infection by the unwary. A high index of suspicion for this source of acute or chronic pain in this population must be maintained. The sacro-iliac joints, particularly on CT in primary or secondary hyperparathyroidism, may also be misconstrued as the site of an inflammatory process mimicking seronegative spondylitis due to subperiosteal bone resorption in the former (Figs. 5, 6).

Axial neuroarthropathy, as exemplified by the "Charcot spine", may similarly mimic infection and is particularly problematic [11-13]. The marked disorganization associated with tertiary luetic disease may exist with or without infection, with distinguishing characteristics difficult to pinpoint by pathologists and by the various imaging modalities. Detailed information as to when and if classic trauma occurred or, more importantly, was

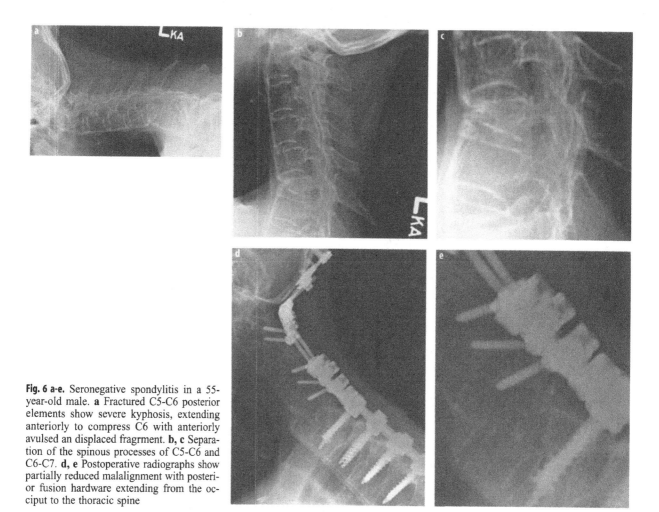

Fig. 6 a-e. Seronegative spondylitis in a 55-year-old male. **a** Fractured C5-C6 posterior elements show severe kyphosis, extending anteriorly to compress C6 with anteriorly avulsed an displaced fragrment. **b, c** Separation of the spinous processes of C5-C6 and C6-C7. **d, e** Postoperative radiographs show partially reduced malalignment with posterior fusion hardware extending from the occiput to the thoracic spine

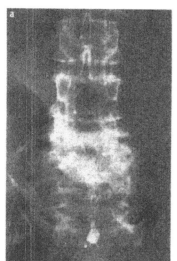

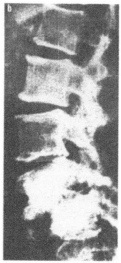

Fig. 7 a, b. Anteroposterior (**a**) and lateral (**b**) radiographic views of a 60-year-old male with tertiary syphilis who had slight pain with no change in 30 years. The patient was provided with a brace

appreciated by the patient are clues to a neuropathic etiology, particularly in a setting of compromised sensitivity. Laboratory markers for luetic disease, ESR, C-reactive protein, and fever will confirm an appropriate diagnosis. Deceivingly, however, pain, albeit diminished may still be present (Fig. 7). Rather than calcifications, focal or diffuse spinal ossifications, including ossification of the posterior longitudinal ligaments (OPLL), ossification of the anterior longitudinal ligaments (OALL), and disseminated idiopathic sclerosing hyperostosis (DISH), while usually occurring independently may co-exist or be attributed to seronegative spondylitis [14-18] (Figs. 8, 9).

"Modic changes", irregular, apposing vertebral body articulations with increased or decreased signal on either or both T1-weighted and fluid-sensitive sequences are another MRI "pitfall". Varying signal intensities, rather than edema, have been related to the degenerative changes of spondylosis and fatty replacement of normal erythropoietic vertebral marrow. They may, however, be asymptomatic [19-21] (Fig. 10).

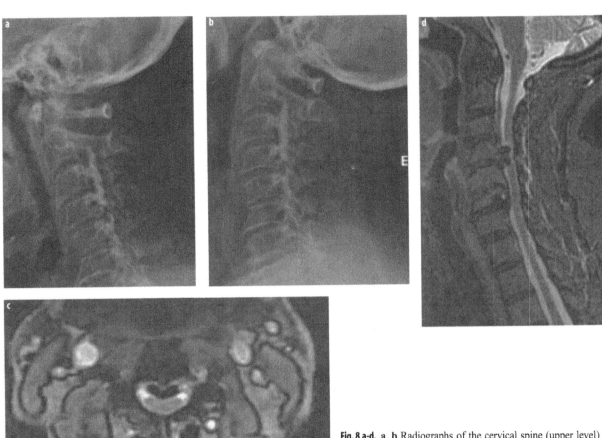

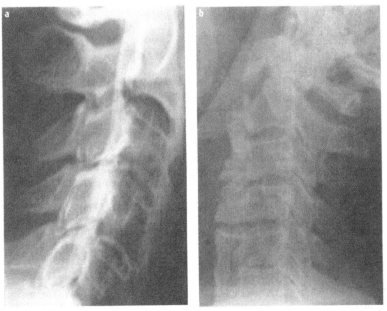

Fig. 8 a-d. a, b Radiographs of the cervical spine (upper level) in a 53-year-old woman with parathesias and a "stiff" neck. The ossified posterior longitudinal ligament limits flexion and extension. **c, d** Axial and off-center sagittal fluid-sensitive MRI shows the compressed spinal cord, C6 posteroinferior Schmorl's node and osteoarthrosis

Fig. 9 a, b. a Ossification of both the posterior and the anterior longitudinal ligaments; **b** right DISH with relatively preserved discs in another patient

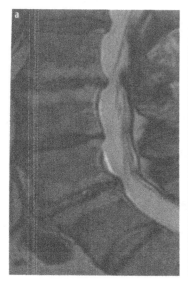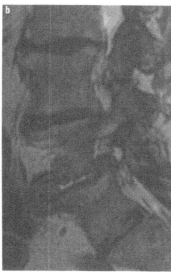

Fig. 10 a, b. Sagittal T2-weighted MRI without fat saturation. **a** Multiple posterior disc "bulges" and narrowed intervertebral spaces, compatible with osteoarthrosis. Modic changes are seen at L2-L3 and L4-L5 with hyperintense signal intensity irregular apposing endplates most prominent at L2-L3. Focally punctate increased signal intensity at L3-L4 disc compatible with crystal deposition. **b** Detail of crystal deposition at L4-L5 disc

Benign, often innocuous Schmorl's nodes, unassociated with other vertebral pathology including fracture, are occasionally confused with inflammation or neoplasia since they may display increased signal on fluid-sensitive MRI sequences obtained with or without contrast. Recognition of the physiologic enhancement of these nodes is important since it may occur or coexist with metastatic involvement of segments of the same or other vertebra [22-25].

Although they are almost universally present and often multiple, many Schmorl's nodes are not apparent on radiographs. They are best seen on MRI at multiple sites on both T1-weighted and fluid-sensitive sequences, where they are usually focal with a familiar "horseshoe pattern". The latter is also evident on CT, which reveals the often sharp, often sclerotic rims of these nodes to better advantage. While these findings tend to refute intrinsic pathology, adjacent malignant deposits in the same vertebrae may obscure the node's distinctive margins or invade it with or without a pathologic fracture. Metastatic foci at other levels do not always solve the problem since vertebrectomy, for the treatment of solitary vertebral neoplastic involvement, is often employed. Two additional important "pseudoinflammations", one common, the other rare, may also be mistaken for seronegative spondylitis. The first, "osteitis" condensans ilii, is a prime offender. Its name is a "triple misnomer" and deceiving in itself, but it may present in a number of ways. It may solely involve one ilium, bordering the sacroiliac joint on one or both sides; the ilium and sacrum on one sides; or both iliac bones and sacrum on both sides, but all variants have well-defined joints. The condition may also be associated with "osteitis pubis", another misnomer.

All manifestations, misconstrued as infections for years, are commoner in women and ascribed to fractures due to pelvic stress in conjunction with multiple births. Residual ligamentous laxity with ensuing chronic instability results in a similar complex of findings about the symphasis pubis. Similar stigmata may be seen in males with "osteitis pubis", attributed to surgical trauma due to prolonged application of suprapubic retractors. Hypoparathyroidism is a rare source of confusion with seronegative spondylitis due to similarly associated back pain and bony ankylosis, particularly of the sacro-iliac joints as well as ossification and florid calcification in soft tissues at multiple sites. The seronegative spondylitides are more often associated with ligaments or tendons and heterotopic bone formation, with calcifications not as widely distributed, e.g., in brain. Laboratory and clinical examination will aid in identifying this rare metabolic disease [26-29].

References

1. Resnick D, Pineda C (1984) Vertebral involvement in calcium pyrophosphate dehydrate crystal deposition disease. Radiographic pathological correlation. Radiology 153:55-60
2. Willoughby DA, Dunn CJ, Yamamotos S et al (1994) calcium pyrophosphate-induced pleurisy in rats; a new model of acute inflammation. Agents Actions 43:221-224
3. Brown TR, Quinn SF, D'Agustino AN (1991) Deposition of calcium pyrophosphate dihydrate crystals in the ligamentum flavum: evaluation with MR imaging and CT. Radiology 178:871-873
4. Zunkeler B, Schelper R, Menezes AH(1996) Periodontoid calcium pyrophosphate dihydrate deposition disease: "pseudogout" mass lesions of the craniocervical junction. J Neurosurg 85:803-809
5. Wells CR, Morgello S, Dicarlo E (1991) Cervical myelopathy due to calcium pyrophosphate dihydrate deposition disease. J Neurol Neurosurg Psychiatry 54:658-659
6. Bywaters EG, Hamilton EB,William SR (1971) The spine in idiopathic haemochromatosis. Ann Rheum Dis 30:453-465

7. Cheng XG, Rrys P, Nils Jet al (1996) Radiologic prevalence of lumbar intervertebral calcification in the elderly: an autopsy study. Skeletal Radiol 25:231-235

8. WittchowR, LandasS, Schelper (1991) Correlative light microscopy,scanning electron microscopy and energy dispersive spectroscopy of pseudogout presenting as spinal masses. Am J Clin Pathol 95:274

9. Natio M, Ogata K, Nakamoto M et al (1992) Destructive spondylarthropathy during long-term hemodialysis. Skeletal Radiol 19:43

10. Jevtic V, Kos-Golja M, Mc Call I (2000) Marginal erosive discovertebal romanus lesions in ankylosing spondylitis demonstrated by contrast enhanced Gd-DTPA magnetic resonace imaging. Skeletal Radiol 29:27-33

11. Feldman F, Johnson AM, Walter JF (1974) Acute axial neuroarthropathy. Radiology 111:1-16

12. Frewin DB, Downey JA, Feldman F et al (1973) Neuropathic arthropathy: a report of two cases. Aust NZ J Med 3:587-592

13. Wagner SC, Schweitzer ME, Morrison WB et al (2000) Can imaging findings help differentiate spinal neuropathic arthropathy from disk space infection? Initial experience. Radiology 214:693-699

14. Otani K, Aihara T, Tanaka A et al (1986) Ossification of the ligamentum flavum of the thoracic spine in adult kyphosis. Int Orthop 10:135-139

15. Resnick D, Niwayama G (1976) radiographic and pathologic features of spinal involvement in diffuse idiopathic skeletal hyperostosis (DISH). Radiology 119:559-568

16. Resnick D, Guerra J, Robinson CA et al (1978) Association of diffuse idiopathic skeletal hyperostosis (DISH) and calcification and ossification of the posterior longitudinal ligament. AJR Am J Roentgenol 131:1049-1053

17. Olivieri I, D'Angelo S, Cutro MS et al (2007) Diffuse idiopathic skeletal hyperostosis may give the typical postural abnormalities of advanced ankylosing spondylitis. Rheumatology 46:1709-1711

18. Mizuno J, Nakagawa H, Song J (2005) Symtomatic ossification of the anterior longitudinal ligament with stenosis of the cervical spine. Bone Joint Surg 87-B:1375-1379

19. Modic MT, Masaryk TJ, Ross JS et al (1988) Imaging of degenerative disc disease. Radiology 168:177-186

20. Chung CB, Van de Berg BC, Tavernier T et al (2004) End plate marrow change in the asymptomatic lumbosacral spine. Skeletal Radiol 33:399-404

21. Chanchairujira K, Chung CB, Kim JY et al (2004) Intervertebral disk calcification of the spine in an elderly population: radiographic prevalence location, and distribution and correlation with spinal degeneration. Radiology 230:499-503

22. Hamanishi C, Kawabata T, Yosli T et al (1994) Schmorl's nodes on magnetic renasonce imaging: their incidence and clinical relevance. Spine 19:450-453

23. Stabler A, Bellan M, Weiss M et al (1997) MR imaging of enhancing intraosseous disk herniation(Schmorl's nodes). AJR Am J Roentgenol 168:933-938

24. Pfirrman CWA, Resnick D (2001) Schmorl nodes of the thoracic lumbar spine: radiographic-pathologic study of prevalence, characterization, and correlation with degenerative changes of 1,650 spinal levels in 100 cadavers. Radiology 219:368-374

25. Hmanishi C, Kawabata T, Yosil T et al (1994) Schmorl's nodes on magnetic resonance imaging: their incidence and clinical relevance. Spine 19:450-453

26. Adams JE, Davies M (1977) Paravertebral and peripheral ligamentous ossification: an unusual association of hypoparathyroidism. Postgrad Med J 53:167-72

27. De CarvalhoA, Jurik AG,Illum F (1986) Case Report 335. Skeletal Radiol 15:52-55

28. Lambert RGW, Becker EJ (1989) Diffuse skeletal hyperostosis in idiopathic hypoparathyroidism. Clinical Radiology 40:212-215

29. Korkmaz C (2005) Hypoparathyroidism simulating ankylosing spondylitis. Joint Bone Spine 72:89-97

Degenerative Diseases of the Spine

Axel Stäbler

Radiology Munich Harlaching, Orthopaedic Clinic Munich Harlaching, Munich, Germany

Introduction

Degenerative diseases of the spine consist of various processes that depend on the anatomically involved portion. Thus, there may be degeneration of the intervertebral disc and endplates or of the intervertebral joints. Activated intervertebral or facet-joint osteoarthrosis may become symptomatic due to an increased stimulation of sensitive nerve endings by synovitis and fibrovascular tissue. Facet joint osteoarthrosis can also be responsible for central spinal canal stenosis and stenosis of the recess or narrowing of the neuroforamen. Degeneration of the intervertebral disc can result in annular tears and disc herniation, with compromise or compression of the nerve roots. Dehydration and disintegration of the disc tissue leads to increased segmental mobility. In some patients, instability with symptomatic osteochondrosis (activated erosive intervertebral osteochondrosis) develops.

In intervertebral osteochondrosis, in addition to erosions, Schmorl's nodes, representing herniations of nucleus pulposus through the vertebral endplate into the trabecular bone, can occur.

Erosive Intervertebral Osteochondrosis

Degeneration of the intervertebral discs is part of the normal aging process. Spine radiograms of 70-year-old individuals show a reduction in the height of at least one intervertebral disc space and osteophytic lipping in almost all of them [1, 2]. Magnetic resonance imaging (MRI) studies have shown a high prevalence of degeneratively affected lumbar discs of people without back pain [3], and all degrees of disc degeneration can be found in asymptomatic populations [4]. Some cases of intervertebral disc degeneration are accompanied by band-like/hemispherical medullary bone edema in the adjacent vertebrae (Fig. 1). If this becomes chronic, it may lead to fatty degeneration of the medullary cavity [5]. Also, a band-like vascularity in the disc space at the discovertebral junction can be found in this type of disc degeneration [6]. As bony changes and spurs at the endplates are absent or only moderately developed, segmental instability plays a causative role in the development of erosive intervertebral osteochondrosis.

Patients with activated erosive intervertebral osteochondrosis suffer from localized back pain, often accom-

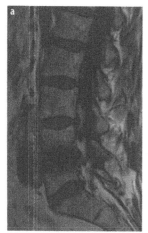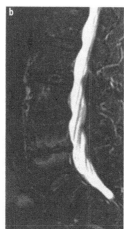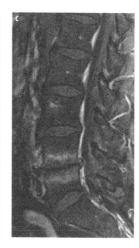

Fig. 1 a-c. Activated erosive intervertebral osteochondrosis. T1-weighted image with irregular destruction of the endplates (**a**). On STIR image, a band-like bone marrow edema is seen adjacent to the affected endplates (**b**), which exhibit uptake of contrast material on this T1-weighted fat-saturated image (**c**)

panied by pseudoradicular pain into the legs but seldom reaching the lower leg. In the majority of patients, MRI shows a band-like or hemispherical bone marrow edema adjacent to the affected endplates, pronounced at one side, and/or a band-like enhancement of disc tissue following gadolinium administration. On spine radiograms, bony spurs are minor and point away from the affected disc segment ("traction spur") or are absent.

The intervertebral discs of neonates and infants are well-vascularized [7-9]. The vessels enter the disc from the ossification center of the vertebra and from the longitudinal ligaments. Therefore, the intervertebral discs of children up to the age of 18 months to 2 years show early enhancement after gadolinium administration [10]. These vessels rapidly obliterate in childhood; from the age of about 13 years on, no vessels are found in discs on pathological examination [7-9]. The disc tissue of adults is free of vessels and therefore exhibits no early vascularity-related contrast material enhancement. In some patients, however, disc degeneration is followed by the ingrowth of vascularized granulation tissue, resulting in secondary vascularization of the disc material [7, 9].

As soon as radial tears reach the outer part of the annulus fibrosus and the longitudinal ligaments, vascularized granulation tissue can invade both the tear and the adjacent disc. Ross demonstrated that tears of the annulus fibrosus could be diagnosed using gadolinium diethyltriaminepentaacetic acid (Gd-DTPA) [11]. A punctate uptake in the outer part of the annulus indicates the presence of a circumscribed annulus defect, which may not necessarily be symptomatic. Although healing by scar tissue formation is possible, disc degeneration frequently progresses to complete disintegration of the disc. In advanced cases, the disc tissue is replaced by a highly vascularized granulation tissue [8, 9]. Later on, scars develop and vascularity is reduced.

Mechanical instability plays the most important role in the development of activated erosive intervertebral osteo-chondrosis. Segments without translatory movement >2 mm can be instable at surgery. When bony contact at the corresponding endplates is present, already minor movements in these segments can irritate the endplates, resulting in localized pain.

In disc degeneration, there may be erosions of the adjacent vertebral endplates. However, the peripheral cortical bone of the vertebra is visible in disc degeneration and, frequently, sclerosis is found. This imaging feature can help to differentiate disc degeneration from disc infection.

Disc Herniation

Disc herniation, also referred to as "disc prolapse", is defined as dislocation of nucleus pulposus material through a defect of the annulus fibrous (annular tear) beyond the outer part of the annulus fibrosus (Fig. 2) [12]. The process of disc herniation develops over time and different stages are described; these are not always present at distinct periods in the evolution of a disc hernia.

Beginning at about age 15 years, the annulus fibrosus shows oval or irregular areas of mucoid degeneration. When these become larger, small circular tears in the annulus fibrosus may result. The normal fibrous structure disappears and the lamellae may hyalinize [8, 9]. Circular tears do not communicate with the nucleus pulposus. At age ~20 years, the circular tears may progress to radial tears that extend from the nucleus pulposus to the outer areas of the annulus fibrosus. According to the site of mucoid degeneration, radial tears are located posteriorly or dorsolaterally in the lower lumbar segments and anteriorly in the thoracic segments. Annular tears or "high intensity annulus fibrosus lesions" are bright on T2-weighted images and are a precursor of disc herniation in most patients.

A dislocation of nucleus pulposus material into an annular tear within the disc is called "intradiscal disc her-

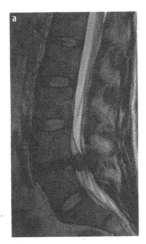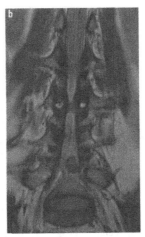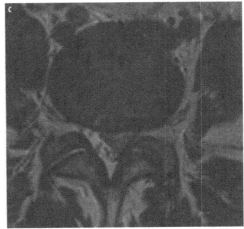

Fig. 2 a-c. Patient with left-sided radiculopathy. On this T2-weighted image, a large disc herniation is present on the left side at L4/5 (**a**), with compression of the L5 nerve root seen also on coronal proton-density-weighted (**b**) and axial T2-weighted (**c**) images

nia". This process often leads to a bulging or protrusion of disc material into the periphery, sometimes overriding the bony boarder of the ring apophysis. If no disc material is found outside the level of the annulus fibrosus, the phenomenon is called "disc protrusion" or "bulging disc". A reduction of disc height almost always creates a circular bulging of the disc, a status not to be confused with a herniated disc.

When disc material is found above or below the level of the endplates on sagittal MRI or sagittal multidetector-row computed tomography (MDCT) mutiplanar reconstructions, the criteria of a disc herniation are fulfilled, with disc material present beyond the outer fibers of the annulus fibrosus. Sometimes, the appearance of a herniated disc material mimics that of a disc protrusion, and the outer contour may not show any concavity on axial images. Such cases qualify as disc hernia because disc material of higher signal intensity is found outside and "on top" of the Sharpey's fibers, which define the outer part of the annulus fibrosus.

The location of a disc hernia is described as central (medial), paracentral (mediolateral), lateral, foraminal, or extraforaminal. If disc material has become dislocated above or below the level of the endplate, disc herniation is described as having migrated upward or downward. If the migrated disc material has lost its connection to the disc of origin, the disc fragment is a "sequestrated disc". The direction of migration or sequestration (upwards, downwards) is determined by the location of the annular tear. Tears at the fibro-osseous junction of the lower endplate create upwards migration, tears at the upper endplate open the pathway for downwards migration [13].

Mandatory for reporting a herniated disc is precise knowledge of the patient's symptoms, the involved site, and the exact nerve root that are affected. Only findings that correlate with the patient's symptoms are relevant.

Spinal Stenosis

Lumbar or cervical spinal stenosis may be congenital or acquired by degenerative constriction of the neural canal, leading to spinal cord, nerve root, or cauda equina compression [14]. Clinical presentation is described as neurogenic claudication or painful radiculopathy. Physical signs include sensory loss, weakness, and reflex attenuation. Typically, the patients are middle-aged or elderly. MRI of the spine and electrodiagnostic tests (EMG) are the most informative diagnostic modalities [15].

Measurement of the bony spinal canal is of minor help in the determination of the clinical significance of a narrowing of the spinal canal. At every segmental level, two pairs of nerve roots exit the spinal canal, reducing the cross-sectional area needed for nerve tissue to pass unaffected through the spinal canal downwards. Therefore, the necessary space varies from level to level and increases with ascending lumbar spine levels. The most important MRI criterion for judging the severity of spinal canal stenosis is the amount of residual subarachnoid space, as seen on axial T2-weighted images (Fig. 3).

It is of practical value to group patients with spinal stenosis into those with relative spinal canal stenosis, with some residual subarachnoid space, and those with high-grade central spinal canal stenosis, without preservation of the subarachnoid space. Lumbar spinal stenosis is aggravated by hyperlordosis. In a patient who uses a foot pad to reduce lumbar lordosis, the significance of a spinal stenosis may be underestimated. The presence of fluid in the joint space of degenerated facet joints is an indicator of possible dynamic worsening of spinal stenosis, as seen on MRI studies of patients in supine position.

Findings that correlate with the severity and clinical relevance of spinal canal stenosis on MRI are relative elongation of the cauda equina either above or, rarely, below the stenotic segment. Also, there may be swelling and

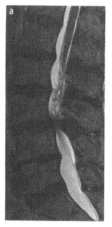
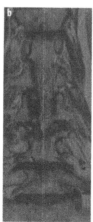
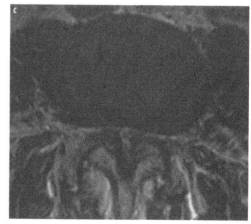

Fig. 3 a-c. High-grade spinal stenosis at the L3/4 level as seen on a T2-weighted image (**a**). There is relative elongation of the cauda equina fibers above the stenotic segment, also visible on this proton-density-weighted coronal image (**b**). On the axial T2-weighted image, no signal from cerebral spinal fluid is visible (**c**)

edema of the nerve roots at the level of narrowing. In some patients, there may be uptake of gadolinium contrast material in the nerve roots, which indicates high-grade spinal stenosis. This represents a negative prognostic sign for recovery from symptoms related to spinal stenosis following decompression surgery. Conservative management often is successful, at least for a period of time, but surgical decompression is indicated in refractory cases.

Intraosseous Disc Herniation (Schmorl's Nodes)

Schmorl's nodes are herniations of nucleus pulposus into the trabecular bone through the vertebral endplate [16]. They are the most common non-intervertebral disc abnormality on MRI in people without back pain and are found in 19% of the population [3]. There is controversy about the clinical significance of Schmorl's nodes [17]. They are mostly found incidentally on lateral chest films in patients without a history of previous trauma, but they can also be related to trauma with axial loading. Only 5-35% of all Schmorl's nodes can be detected on conventional radiographs [18, 19]. In human cadaver studies, the prevalence of Schmorl's nodes is reported to be 36-79% [20]. It has been suggested that these herniations develop through congenitally weak points in the cartilaginous disc plates, left by the attrition of blood vessels and small defects from notochord remnants. Schmorl's nodes are frequently encountered in young adolescents before growth has ended and in patients over age 50, when osteopenia increases in frequency.

After its herniation into the trabecular bone, avascular nucleus pulposus material can become vascularized. This vascularity can be demonstrated by means of MRI following intravenous administration of gadopentetate dimeglumine. Cartilaginous nucleus pulposus hernias can become inflammatory, which probably leads to back pain (Fig. 4) [21].

In a very few cases, Schmorl's nodes may be symptomatic. Using MRI, Hamanishi et al. [19] found Schmorl's nodes in 9.4% of 106 asymptomatic patients. However, in 400 patients with pain in the lumbar spine, the prevalence of Schmorl's nodes was 19%. Several cases of symptomatic Schmorl's nodes have been reported [22-25]. For example, limbus vertebrae, an entity similar to Schmorl's hernia, may develop in childhood and can be symptomatic or asymptomatic [26]. The sizes of the enhancing Schmorl's nodes and concomitant edema within the adjacent bone marrow were recognized as correlating with the probability of localized symptoms over the affected segment [6]. Martel et al. [27] found that large Schmorl's nodes (15-20 mm) are frequently symptomatic. Vascularity is a secondary process that follows displacement of nucleus pulposus material, because the normal nucleus pulposus of adults is without blood or lymph vessels. It may be a normal attempt to heal intraosseous cartilaginous hernias and is not necessarily accompanied by back pain. However, enhancing Schmorl's nodes are larger and more often accompanied by bone marrow edema in patients with back pain than in those without. Enhancing Schmorl's nodes should not be confused with tumor or infection.

As the prevalence of Schmorl's nodes decreases with age from youth to adulthood, healing may be possible. Therefore proliferative processes must take place in the area of intraosseous herniation. In the peripheral regions of Schmorl's nodes, where the vertebral bodies are in contact with the node, the growth of cartilage has frequently been observed. After intraosseous herniation, the ingrowth of vessels takes place from the adjacent bone

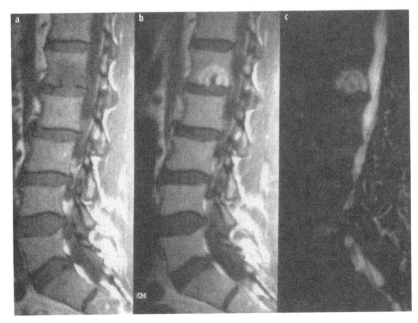

Fig. 4 a-c. Vascularized Schmorl's node. The intraosseous hernia has low signal on T1-weighted image (**a**) with marked enhancement following gadolinium administration (**b**) and bright signal on STIR image (**c**)

marrow into the periphery of the node, progressing to the center of the node. In 30% of enhancing hernias, a bone marrow reaction with high signal intensity on T2-weighted or STIR images surrounding the intraosseous hernia is present [28]. The frequency of bone marrow edema depends on the size of a vascularized Schmorl's node, as the mean diameter of a node without bone marrow edema is smaller than that of a hernia with bone marrow edema.

References

1. Powell MC, Wilson M, Szypryt P et al (1986) Prevalence of lumbar disk degeneration observed by magnetic resonance in symptomless women. Lancet 2:1366-1367
2. Resnick D (1985) Degenerative disease of the vertebral column. Radiology 156:3-14
3. Jensen MC, Brant-Zawadzki MN, Obuchowski N et al (1994) Magnetic resonance imaging of the lumbar spine in people without back pain. N Engl J Med 331:69-73
4. Buirski G, Silberstein M (1993) The symptomatic lumbar disk in patients with low-back pain. Spine 18:1808-1811
5. Modic MT, Steinberg PM, Ross JS et al (1988) Degenerative disk disease: assessment of changes in vertebral body marrow with MR imaging. Radiology 166:193-199
6. Stäbler A, Weiss M, Scheidler J et al (1996) Degenerative disk vascularization on MRI: correlation with clinical and histopathologic findings. Skeletal Radiol 25:119-126
7. Böhmig R (1930) Die Blutgefäßversorgung der Wirbelbandscheiben, das Verhalten des intervertebralen Chordasegments und die Bedeutung beider für die Bandscheibendegeneration. Arch klin Chir 158:374-424
8. Hassler O (1970) The human intervertebral disc. Acta Orthop Scand 40:765-772
9. Hirsch C, Schajkowicz F (1952) Studies on structural changes in the lumbar annulus fibrosus. Acta Orthop Scand 22:184-231
10. Sze G, Bravo S, Baierl P, Shimkin PM (1991) Developing spinal column: Gadolinium-enhanced MR imaging. Radiology 180:497-502
11. Ross JS, Modic MT, Massaryk TJ (1990) Tears of the anulus fibrosus: assessment with Gd-DTPA-enhanced MR imaging. AJR Am J Roentgenol 154:159-162
12. Milette PC (2000) Classification, diagnostic imaging, and imaging characterization of a lumbar herniated disk. Radiol Clin North Am 38:1267-1292
13. Fardon DF, Milette PC (2001) Combined Task Forces of the North American Spine Society, American Society of Spine Radiology, and American Society of Neuroradiology. Nomenclature and classification of lumbar disc pathology. Recommendations of the Combined task Forces of the North American Spine Society, American Society of Spine Radiology, and American Society of Neuroradiology. Spine 26:E93-E113
14. Modic MT, Ross JS (2007) Lumbar degenerative disk disease. Radiology 245:43-61
15. Chad DA (2007) Lumbar spinal stenosis. Neurol Clin 25:407-418
16. Schmorl G (1928) Über Knorpelknötchen an den Wirbelbandscheiben. Fortsch Röntgenstr 38:265-279
17. Schmorl G (1930) Die Pathogenese der juvenilen Kyphose. Fortsch Röntgenstr 41:359-383
18. 13. Malmivaara A, Videman T, Kuosma E, Troup JD (1987) Plain radiographic, discographic, and directo bservations of Schmorl's nodes in the thoracolumbar junctional region of the cadaveric spine. Spine 12:453-457
19. Hamanishi C, Kawabata T, Yosii T, Tanaka S (1994) Schmorl's nodes on magnetic resonance imaging. Their incidence and clinical relevance. Spine 19:450-453
22. Kornberg M (1988) MRI diagnosis of traumatic Schmorl's node. A case report. Spine 13:934-935
20. Hilton RC, Ball J, Benn RT (1976) Vertebral endplate lesions (Schmorl's nodes) in the dorsolumbar spine. Ann Rheum Dis 35:127-132
23. Lipson SJ, Fox DA, Sosman JL (1985) Symptomatic intravertebral disc herniation (Schmorl's node) in the cervical spine. Ann Rheum Dis 44:857-859
21. McCarron RF, Wimpee MW, Hudkins PG, Laros GS (1987) The inflammatory effect of nucleus pulposus: a possible element in the pathogenesis of low-back pain. Spine 12:760-764
24. McCall IW, Park WM, O'Brien JP, Seal V (1985) Acute traumatic intraosseous disc herniation. Spine 10:134-137
25. Smith DM (1976) Acute back pain associated with a calcified Schmorl's node: a case report. Clin Orthop 117:193-196
26. Henales V, Hervas JA, Lopez P et al (1993) Intervertebral disc herniations (limbus vertebrae) in pediatric patients: report of 15 cases. Pediatr Radiol 23:608-610
27. Martel W, Seeger JF, Wicks JD, Washburn RL (1976) Traumatic lesions of the discovertebral junction in the lumbar spine. AJR 127:457-464
28. Stäbler A, Bellan M, Weiss M et al (1997) MR imaging of enhancing intraosseous disk herniation (Schmorl's nodes). AJR Am J Roentgenol 8:933-938

The Degenerative Spine

Nicolas Theumann

Service de Radiologie, Centre Hospitalier Universitaire Vaudois (CHUV), Lausanne, Switzerland

Introduction

Back pain is an important problem that affects two-thirds of adults at some time in their lives. One of the leading causes of functional incapacity is spinal degeneration, which is a common source of chronic disability in the working population. Traditionally, disk degeneration has been linked to mechanical loading. Disk failure is more common in areas of the back subject to the heaviest mechanical stresses, such as the lower lumbar region. It has been suggested that mechanical factors produce endplate damage [1]. The disk is metabolically active, and its metabolism is dependent on the diffusion of fluid, either from the marrow across the subchondral bone and cartilaginous endplate or through the annulus fibrosus from the surrounding blood vessels. Morphological changes in the vertebral bone and cartilaginous endplate, which occur with advancing age or degeneration, can interfere with normal disk nutrition and further the degenerative process [2]. As degeneration progresses, structures of the disk become increasingly disarranged such that greater stresses are placed on the annulus and facet joint. In addition to mechanical and nutritional causes, a genetic predisposition has been suggested by studies in which animals consistently develop degenerative disk disease at an early age. as well as reports of familial osteoarthitis and lumbar-canal stenosis in humans [3].

Abnormalities of collagen are most often cited in connection with a genetic influence in degenerative disk disease. Type II collagen, often referred to as the major collagen, is the most abundant collagen of cartilaginous tissues. It forms heterotopic fibrils with the less-abundant minor collagens type IX and XI. Diseases that cause mutations in type II and XI collagens have has been demonstrated in a number of chondrodystrophies. Multiple epiphyseal dysplasia, associated with a disease in which there is a mutation in collagen IX, leads to important, pathological alterations in structural components such as the annulus fibrosus, nucleus pulposus, and hyaline cartilage of the endplate [2].

In this chapter, an overview of the spectrum of degenerative disease of the spine is provided. Special emphasis is directed to the magnetic resonance imaging (MRI) ap- pearance of degenerative spine disorders, since MRI has become the standard of reference regarding the evaluation of patients with back pain with or without neurological deficit [4, 5].

Anatomical Considerations

The disco-vertebral joint is a three-joint complex, consisting of the endplate-disk-endplate joint of the anterior column and the two facet joints of the posterior column, supported by ligaments and muscles groups. There is also a layer of cartilaginous endplate. Numerous vascular channels diffuse nutriments and, during imaging, contrast medium through the endplates into the disk.

The annulus fibrosus can be divided into outer and inner components or rings. The outer rings contain the densest fibrous lamella, which displays low signal intensity on T2-weighted MRI due to the absence of ground substance. The cells in the outer ring of the annulus are almost exclusively fibroblasts while those in the inner ring are predominantly chondrocytes, accounting for its high signal intensity on T2-weighted images.

The second component of the intervertebral disk is the nucleus fibrosus, which consists of collagen and hydrophilic proteoglycans. The disk usually lacks either innervation or vascularity whereas the anterior and posterior ligaments, facet joints, vertebral endplates, and peripheral layer of the annulus fibrosus are innervated. Therefore, the disk is not usually a source of pain, although disk degeneration may lead to pain by stretching of the ligamentous tissue or due to nerve compression or inflammation.

Disk Degeneration

The term "degeneration" includes any or all of the following: real or apparent desiccation, fibrosis, narrowing of the disk space, diffused bulging of the annulus, extensive fissuring, and mucinous degeneration of the annulus. With aging, the nucleus pulposus becomes dehydrated. Increases in the amounts of collagen and decreases in the glycosaminoglycan content are believed to be responsible for the decreased water content. A radial or type III tear plays a role in disk degeneration since it concerns the entire annulus fibrosus and correlates with shrinkage and disorganization of the nucleus [6]. Hydration and annular integrity seem to be important for the disk to absorb and transmit compressive loads to the vertebral column. As the disk ages and degenerates, it progressively loses these capacities.

The degenerative and age-related changes in the nucleus pulposus and annulus fibrosus are well-depicted with MRI. These changes are evident as a loss of signal intensity [7], since T2 signal intensity reveals regions of high glycosaminoglycan percentage rather than absolute water content [8].

MRI is also the most important method for the clinical assessment of disk degeneration. A proposed classification for lumbar intervertebral disk degeneration uses five grades to describe the different stages that characterize this process [9]. The grading system is based on MRI signal intensity, disk structure, the distinction between nucleus and annulus, and disk height (Fig. 1). This classification has shown reasonable intra- and inter-observer agreement and has proven to be very useful in daily practice.

When the disk loses its annular integrity, it begins to expand outward, resulting in a variety of morphological abnormalities. Currently, the most widely accepted terms to describe disk abnormalities are: normal, bulging, protrusion, extrusion, and sequestration [10]. A disk is considered normal when it does not reach beyond the border of the adjacent vertebral bodies. Bulging is defined as cir-

cumferential, symmetric disk extension around the posterior vertebral border. The annulus fibrosus remains intact. Protrusion is the focal or asymmetric extension of the border between the disk and the vertebral bodies, with the disk origin broader than any other dimension of the protrusion. In extrusion, there is more extreme extension of the disk beyond the vertebral border, with the base of the disk of origin being narrower than the diameter of the extruding material; there is also a connection between this material and the disk of origin (Fig. 2). Sequestration is defined as a free disk fragment that is distinct from the disk and which has intermediate signal intensity on T1-weighted images and increased signal intensity on T2-weighted images.

This system for classifying disk abnormalities does not include the term "disk herniation," which is defined as the displacement of disk material beyond the normal margin of the intervertebral disk space [11]. The herniated material may include the nucleus pulposus, cartilage, fragmented apophysal bone, or fragmented annular tissues. Some authors use the term "disk herniation" to refer to combined protrusion and extrusion [11].

Annular tears, although properly called annular fissures, are separations between the annular fibers, avulsion of fibers from their vertebral-body attachment, or breakthrough fibers that extend radially, transversally, or concentrically and involve one or many layers of the annular lamellae. Although annular disruption is a known sequela of degeneration and is often associated with it, its role as a causal agent of disk degeneration has yet to be established.

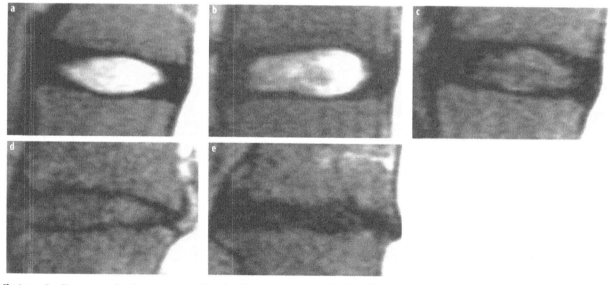

Fig. 1 a-e. Grading system for the assessment of lumbar disc degeneration. **a** Grade I: The structure of the disc is homogeneous, with a bright hyperintense white signal intensity and normal disc height. **b** Grade II: The structure of the disc is inhomogeneous, with a hyperintense white signal. The distinction between nucleus and annulus is clear, and the disc height is normal, with or without horizontal gray bands. **c** Grade III: The structure of the disc is inhomogeneous, with an intermediate gray signal intensity. The distinction between nucleus and annulus is unclear, and the disc height is normal or slightly decreased. **d** Grade IV: The structure of the disc is inhomogeneous, with a hypointense dark-gray signal intensity. The distinction between nucleus and annulus is lost, and the disc height is normal or moderately decreased. **e** Grade V: The structure of the disc is inhomogeneous, with a hypointense black signal intensity. The distinction between nucleus and annulus is lost, and the disc space is collapsed. Grading is based on the results of T2-weighted mid-sagittal (repetition time 5000 ms; echo time 130 ms) fast-spin-echo images. (From [9])

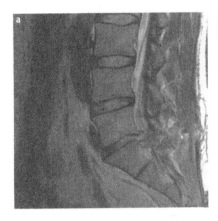

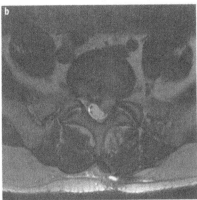

Fig. 2 a, b. T2-weighted images in the sagittal (**a**) and axial (**b**) planes demonstrate disk extrusion at the L5/S1 disk level with compression of the left-sided S1 nerve root

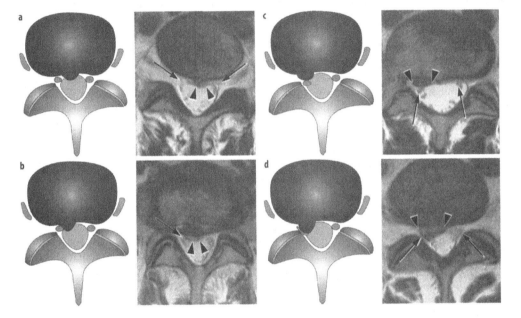

Fig. 3 a-d. a Diagrammatic (*left*) and transverse T2-weighted fast-spin-echo (repetition time 4000 ms; echo time 122 ms) MR (*right*) images show no compromise of the nerve root. A normal epidural fat layer (*black arrowheads*) is visible between the nerve root (*arrows*) and the disk material (*white arrowheads*). **b** Diagrammatic (*left*) and transverse T2-weighted fast spin-echo (repetition time 4000 ms; echo time 122 ms) MR (*right*) images show contact of disk material (*arrowheads*) with the right nerve root (*arrow*). No epidural fat layer is visible between the nerve root and the disk material. The nerve root is in the normal position and is not dorsally deviated. **c** Diagrammatic (*left*) and transverse T2-weighted fast spin-echo (repetition time 4000 ms; echo time 122 ms) MR (*right*) images show dorsal deviation of the right nerve root (*arrow*), caused by contact with disk material (*arrowheads*). **d** Diagrammatic (*left*) and transverse T2-weighted spin-echo (repetition time 4000 ms; echo time 122 ms) MR (*right*) images show compression of the right nerve root (*arrow*) between disk material (*arrowheads*) and the wall of the spinal canal. The nerve root appears flattened and is indistinguishable from disk material. (From [15])

A radiolucent collection (vacuum disk phenomena), representing gas, occurs at sites of negative pressure produced by the abnormal space [12]. The vacuum phenomenon within the degenerated disk is seen on spin-echo images as areas of signal void [13]. Whereas gas within the disk is common in degenerative disease, spinal infection may rarely be accompanied by intra-discal or intra-osseous gas [14] Calcifications have also been described by MRI as regions of decreased or absent signal intensity. For concentrations of calcium particles up to 30% by weight, the signal intensity on standard T1-weighted images increases but subsequently decreases [2].

When reporting imaging findings in patients with back pain, the clinician must not only report the morphology, location, and site of the disk abnormality but also describe the relationship between the disk and the nerve root. Pfirrmann recently proposed a new MRI-based grading system to assess the compromised lumbar nerve root caused by disk herniation [15]. The relationship between the disk and the nerve root is as follows: no contact, contact of the disk with the nerve root with deviation of the nerve root, nerve root deviation, or nerve root compression (Fig. 3). Although the grading system is primarily based on the assessment of axial images, sagittal images are also useful, in particular to detect a compromised nerve root within the narrowed neural foramina.

Degenerative Marrow Changes

There is a relationship between the vertebral body, endplate, annulus, and disk in the degenerative spine. Signal-intensity changes in the marrow of the vertebral body, adjacent to the endplate of degenerated disks, are a common observation on magnetic resonance images. Modic et al. [5, 16], defined three different types of endplate abnormalities according to the signal abnormality of the adjacent bone marrow: In type I (inflammatory type), compared to fatty bone marrow, the signal intensity is lower on T1-weighted images and higher on T2-weighted images. Histopathologic sections of disks with type I changes show disruption and fissuring of the endplate and vascuralized fibrous tissues within the adjacent marrow, prolonging T1 and T2. In type II changes, there is increased signal intensity on T1-weighted images and iso- or slightly hypersignal on T2-weighted images. Disks with type II changes also have evidence of endplate disruption, with yellow (lipid) marrow replacement in the adjacent vertebral body resulting in a shorter T1. Type III changes present as decreased signal intensity on both T1- and T2-weighted images and correlate with extensive bony sclerosis on plain radiographs. This reflects the absence of marrow in areas with advanced sclerosis.

Degenerative Facet Disease

Disk degeneration and a lost of disk-space height increase stresses on the facet joints, with cranio-caudal luxation resulting in arthrosis and ostoeophytosis. Facet arthrosis can cause narrowing of the central canal, lateral recesses, and foramina and is an important component of lumbar stenosis (Fig. 4). However, it has been pro-posed that facet arthrosis may occur independently and can be a source of symptoms on its own [17]. The mechanism of pain can be related to nerve-root compression from degenerative changes of the facets or by direct irritation of pain fibers from the innervated synovial line and joint capsule [18].

Functional Sequelae

Degenerative disk disease can lead to potential complications as alignment abnormalities, intervertebral disk displacement, and spinal stenosis. Segmental instability can result from degenerative changes, involving the intervertebral disk, vertebral bodies, and facet joints, that impairs the usual pattern of spinal movement, thus producing irregular, excessive, or restricted motion. Spondylolisthesis results when one vertebral body becomes displaced relative to the next-most inferior vertebral body. The most frequent type is related primarily to degenerative changes of the apophyseal joints and is most common at the L4 and L5 vertebral level [2]. Predilection for degenerative spondylolisthesis at this level is thought to be related to the more sagittal orientation of the facet joint, which makes it increasingly prone to anterior displacement.

Stenosis of the Spinal Canal

Stenosis has been defined as a narrowing of the spinal canal, nerve root canals, or intervertebral foramina [19]. Among the many types of spinal stenosis, congenital developmental stenosis (IJ, idiopathic achondroplasia, osteopetrosis) and acquired stenosis are the two main groups. Developmental stenosis can be exacerbated by superimposed acquired degenerative changes. In the acquired type, there is no association between the severity of pain and the degree of stenosis. The most common symptoms are sensory disturbances in the legs, low back pain, neurogenic claudication, weakness, and relief of

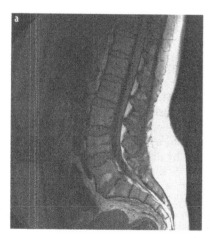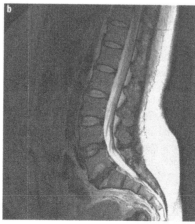

Fig. 4 a, b. Sagittal (a) T1-weighted and T2-weighted (b) images demonstrate endplate changes (Modic type II) at the L5/S1 disk level

pain by bending forward [2]. The imaging changes are, in general, more extensive than expected from the clinical findings. The degree of stenosis is not static and extension worsens the degree of central and foraminal stenosis while flexion appears to improve it by an average of 10% [2]. Segmental instability, which can cause static and dynamic stenosis, is considered a cause of low back pain but is poorly defined [20].

The measurement of the cross-sectional area of the dural sac by CT or MRI is probably the most reliable technique for assessment of the width of the spinal canal at the lumbar level. If the area of the dural sac is a 75 mm^2, the likelihood of stenosis is high. A loss of high-signal-intensity cerebrospinal fluid (CSF) around the nerve roots or cord on T2-weighted axial images is also valuable for evaluating clinically irrelevant spinal stenosis. Unfortunately, this does not appear to be a reliable prognostic imaging finding with respect to a correlation with surgical success or to identifying those patients who would benefit from surgery [21]. Axial images are also useful to diagnose stenosis at the lateral recess. The lateral recesses are bordered posteriorly by the superior articular facet, laterally by the pedicule, and anteriorly by the lateral vertebral body and disk. Lumbar lateral recess stenosis occurs when the hypertrophic superior facet encroaches on the recess, often in combination with narrowing due to a bulging disk and osteophytes. When the epidural fat surrounding the nerve root within the foramen is obliterated, as seen on sagittal T1-weighted scans, marked encroachment is present.

Magnetic Resonance Imaging Methods

An evaluation of the signal-intensity changes associated with degenerative disk disease is obtained with T1 and T2 imaging methods. Recovery or fat-suppressed T2-weighted images have been added by many groups because it is believed that they are more sensitive to marrow and soft-tissue changes. Due to the better signal to noise ratio and improved resolution, our group has added T1-weighted imaging with fat suppression and gadolinium IV injection in order to better visualize soft-tissue changes around the joints and in the epidural space.

Other new techniques have been developed for spine imaging when a routine evaluation of degenerative disk disease yields ambiguous results. These techniques are more physiologic and functional than strict anatomical imaging [22]. Dynamic imaging can be obtained in an upright open MR system that allows flexion and extension imaging or by axial loading in the supine position by mean of a harness attached to a non-magnetic, adjustable compression foot plate [23, 24]. Dynamic MRI has been used to evaluate the occurrence of occult herniation, which may not be visible or is less visible when the patient is supine, to measure motion between spinal segments and to determine the canal or foraminal diameter under axial loading. In one study [25] of 200 patients with clinical symptoms of spinal stenosis, there were on-

ly five cases in which the neurosurgeons involved in the clinical evaluation changed their treatment decision from conservative to decompressive surgery. In daily practice, the additional machine time and patient discomfort associated with other methods is not always an advantage, considering the small subset of patients that may benefit from this type of evaluation.

MR neurography using high-resolution T1 imaging for anatomical detail and fat suppressed T2-weighted imaging to show abnormal nerve hyperintensity. This technique was used in one study, in which piriformis syndrome with muscle asymmetry and sciatic nerve hyperintensity, which can be specific in this syndrome, was demonstrated [26].

The apparent diffusion coefficient (ADC) in the normal degenerative intervertebral disk has been studied. The results suggested that impaired blood flow plays an important role in disk degeneration [27, 28]. Diffusion tensor imaging has been evaluated as well but has yet to be used in clinical applications.

Intravenous contrast enhancement is another approach to assess diffusion into the intervertebral disk. A normal disk slowly enhances after contrast material injection, which in animal models may be as much as 36% [2]. A degenerative disk with decreased glycosaminoglycan content has a more intense and rapid enhancement [29].

Correlations Between Clinical and Imaging Findings

Anatomical areas of the spine can serve at sites of pain generation through intrinsic or acquired innervation. The mechanisms for this process often act in combination and include: (a) instability, with associated disk degeneration, facet hypertrophy or arthropathy; (b) mechanical compression of nerve by bone, ligament, or disk material; and (c) biochemical mediators of inflammation and/or pain [2].

It is important to emphasize that disk degeneration is not painful and in fact has a very high prevalence in the asymptomatic population. In addition, imaging findings of degenerative disk disease do not help to predict subsequent symptom development over time [30]. In the classic concept of nerve dysfunction or pain with a mechanical compression or deformity of the nerve roots, it is assumed that there is displacement and effacement of neural tissue by disk herniation. Similar mechanical compression or traction mechanisms may be involved with the instability associated with stenosis. Venous stasis edema as well as intraneural and perineural fibrosis also play a role in nerve root dysfunction. There are more complex situations, in which patients complain of incapacity from back pain but there is no morphological abnormality. This has lent credence to the concept of the disk as a pain generator, with disk tissue assumed to produce an inflammatory response. New assay techniques have demonstrated chemical radiculitis, related to nuclear material and glycoprotein, as potent irritants of nerve tissue [31]. Disk cells are also capable of expressing other proinflammatory substances, such as tumor necrosis factor (TNF)-α, which can produce radicular morphological abnormalities similar to those seen with nucleus pulposus application [32]. A wide variety of inflammatory agents are capable of penetrating the site of herniation, including those from migratory macrophages or via direct stimulation by chondrocytes. The presence of many other molecules has also been demonstrated in degenerated or herniated disks and may play additional roles in the inflammatory reaction. These substances include intercellular adhesion molecules-1, fibroblast growth factors, and vascular endothelial growth factor [2].

The very high importance of imaging findings must be kept in mind in the evaluation of patients with back pain. Important strides in imaging have been made with respect to obtaining accurate morphological information as well as information regarding cellular and biochemical alterations. Any study aimed at elucidating the natural history of degenerative disk disease, the prognostic value of imaging, or its effect on therapeutic decision-making will be confounded by the high prevalence of morphological changes in the asymptomatic population [33, 34]. Indeed, more than 25% of asymptomatic patients demonstrate disk herniation and the majority have evidence of additional degenerative disk disease. These findings are not only non predictive at the moment but prospective. In a 7-year follow-up of the Borenstein study [30], the original MRI findings were not predictive for the development or duration of low back pain. One study showed that the only substantial morphological difference between symptomatic patients and asymptomatic volunteers was the presence of neural compromise (83 vs. 22%) [35]. Thus, in explaining the origin of pain in degenerative disk disease, neural compromise may have a more important role than the morphological extension of disk material beyond the intervertebral space.

In a study of symptomatic patients, the prevalence of disk herniation in patients with low back pain and those with radiculopathy at presentation was similar [36], but the prevalence was higher (60%) than in asymptomatic volunteers (25%). In general, one-third of patients with disk herniation at presentation have significant resolution or disappearance by 6 weeks and two-thirds by 6 months [36]. Neither the type, size, and location of the herniation at presentation nor the changes in the herniation site and type over time correlated with outcome. In fact, the presence of a herniation at MRI was a positive prognostic finding. As noted above, the lack of prognostic value also appears to apply to the conservative management of spinal stenosis.

Some studies have shown a high correlation between the presence of a hyperintensity zone (HIZ), indicating annular tears, and pain concordant with the usual symptoms at discography. However, the high prevalence of HIZ in asymptomatic volunteers, as reported by Weisshaupt et al. [37], indicated that these results should be interpreted with care. A recent study of the natural history of HIZ has shown that it often remains unchanged for several years and there was no correlation between resolution or an increase in the severity of HIZ and changes in symptoms.

Degenerative marrow changes may also vary over time. In all three types, there is always evidence of associative degenerative disk disease at the level of involvement. Type I changes may revert to normal or convert to type II with time, suggesting stabilization of the degenerative process. Type II changes tend to be more stable but may convert to type I or a mixed combination of type I and type II. When changes do occur in type II marrow, there is usually evidence of additional or accelerated degeneration or a superimposed process such as infection or trauma.

The clinical importance of marrow changes associated with degenerative disk disease remains unclear. Type I changes seems to be associated with unusual stresse or macro- or micro-instability. Discography in degenerative marrow changes suggests that those of type I are invariably associated with a painful disk [38]. Surgical studies have indicated that patients with type I marrow changes who undergo fusion for low back pain do better than those with endplate changes or type II pattern [39]. The hypothesis is that type I degenerative marrow changes are related to or serve as an indicator of some degree of instability. Thus, type I changes may not only be an important criterion for surgery but the disappearance of type I changes may be indicative of successful fusion and stabilization. Type I marrow changes can convert to a normal marrow, with normal signal intensity, as can type II changes, both with good clinical results.

References

1. Adams MA, Freeman BJ, Morrison HP et al (2000) Mechanical initiation of intervertebral disc degeneration. Spine 25:1625-1636
2. Modic MT, Ross JS (2007) Lumbar degenerative disk disease. Radiology 245:43-61
3. Kresina TF, Malemud CJ, Moskowitz RW (1986) Analysis of osteoarthritic cartilage using monoclonal antibodies reactive with rabbit proteoglycan. Arthritis Rheum 29:863-871
4. Kent DL, Haynor DR, Longstreth WT Jr et al (1994) The clinical efficacy of magnetic resonance imaging in neuroimaging. Ann Intern Med 120:856-871
5. Modic MT, Masaryk TJ, Ross JS et al (1988) Imaging of degenerative disk disease. Radiology 168:177-186
6. Yu SW, Haughton VM, Ho PS et al (1988) Progressive and regressive changes in the nucleus pulposus. Part II. The adult. Radiology 169:93-97
7. Modic MT, Pavlicek W, Weinstein MA et al (1984) Magnetic resonance imaging of intervertebral disk disease. Clinical and pulse sequence considerations. Radiology 152:103-111
8. Majors A, McDevitt C, Silgalis I et al (1994) A correlative analysis of T2, ADC and MT radio with water, hydroxyproline and GAG content in excised human intervertebral disk. Orthopedic Research Society, New Orleans, pp 116-120
9. Pfirrmann CW, Metzdorf A, Zanetti M et al (2001) Magnetic resonance classification of lumbar intervertebral disc degeneration. Spine 26:1873-1878

10. Fardon DF, Milette PC (2001) Nomenclature and classification of lumbar disc pathology. Recommendations of the Combined task Forces of the North American Spine Society, American Society of Spine Radiology, and American Society of Neuroradiology. Spine 26:E93-E113

11. Weisshaupt D, McCall I (2005) Degenerative diseases of the spine. In: Hodler J, Schulthess GK von, Zollikofer CL (eds) In: Musculoskeletal diseases diagnostic imaging and interventional techniques, IDKD 2005. Springer, Berlin Heidelbeg New-York, pp 132-137

12. Knutsson F (1942) The vacuum phenomenon in the intervertebral discs. Acta Radiol 23:173-179

13. Grenier N, Grossman RI, Schiebler ML et al (1987) Degenerative lumbar disk disease: pitfalls and usefulness of MR imaging in detection of vacuum phenomenon. Radiology 164:861-865

14. Bielecki DK, Sartoris D, Resnick D et al (1986) Intraosseous and intradiscal gas in association with spinal infection:report of three cases. AJR Am J Roentgenol 147:83-86

15. Pfirrmann CW, Dora C, Schmid MR et al (2004) MR image-based grading of lumbar nerve root compromise due to disk herniation: reliability study with surgical correlation. Radiology 230:583-588

16. Modic MT, Steinberg PM, Ross JS et al (1988) Degenerative disk disease: assessment of changes in vertebral body marrow with MR imaging. Radiology 166:193-199

17. Harris RI, Macnab I (1954) Structural changes in the lumbar intervertebral discs; their relationship to low back pain and sciatica. J Bone Joint Surg Br 36-B:304-322

18. Schellinger D, Wener L, Ragsdale BD et al (1987) Facet joint disorders and their role in the production of back pain and sciatica. Radiographics 7:923-944

19. Arnoldi CC, Brodsky AE, Cauchoix J et al (1976) Lumbar spinal stenosis and nerve root entrapment syndromes. Definition and classification. Clin Orthop Relat Res 4-5

20. Inufusa A, An HS, Lim TH et al (1996) Anatomic changes of the spinal canal and intervertebral foramen associated with flexion-extension movement. Spine 21:2412-2420

21. ECRI (2001) Treatment of degenerative lumbar spinal stenosis. I. Evidence report. Agency for Healthcare Research and Quality publication no. 01-E048 32. ECRI, Plymouth Meeting, PA

22. Haughton V (2004) Medical imaging of intervertebral disc degeneration: current status of imaging. Spine 29:2751-2756

23. Danielson B, Wllen J (2001) Axially loaded magnetic resonance image of the lumbar spine in asymptomatic individuals. Spine 26:2601-2606

24. Jinkins JR, Dworkin JS, Damadian RV (2005) Upright, weight-bearing, dynamic-kinetic MRI of the spine: initial results. Eur Radiol 15:1815-1825

25. Hiwatashi A, Danielson B, Moritani T et al (2004) Axial loading during MR maging can influence treatment decision for symptomatic spinal stenosis. AJNR Am J Neuroradiol 25:170-174

26. Filler AG, Haynes J, Jordan SE et al (2005) Sciatica of nondisc origin and piriformis syndrome: diagnosis by magnetic resonance neurography and interventional magnetic resonance imaging with outcome study of resulting treatment. J Neurosurg Spine 2:99-115

27. Kealey SM, Aho T, Delong D et al (2005) Assessment of apparent diffusion coefficient in normal and degenerated intervertebral lumbar disks: initial experience. Radiology 235:569-574

28. Kerttula L, Kurunlahti M, Jauhiainen J et al (2001) Apparent diffusion coefficients and T2 relaxation time measurements to evaluate disc degeneration. A quantitative MR study of young patients with previous vertebral fracture. Acta Radiol 42:585-591

29. Ibrahim MA, Haughton VM, Hyde JS (1995) Effect of disk maturation on diffusion of low-molecular-weight gadolinium complexes: an experimental study in rabbits. AJNR Am J Neuroradiol 16:1307-1311

30. Borenstein DG, O'Mara JW, Jr., Boden SD et al (2001) The value of magnetic resonance imaging of the lumbar spine to predict low-back pain in asymptomatic subjects :a seven-year follow-up study. J Bone Joint Surg Am 83A:1306-1311

31. Marshall LL, Trethewie ER, Curtain CC (1977) Chemical radiculitis. A clinical, physiological and immunological study. Clin Orthop Relat Res 61-67

32. Igarashi T, Kikuchi S, Shubayev V et al (2000) 2000 Volvo Award winner in basic science studies: exogenous tumor necrosis factor-alpha mimics nucleus pulposus-induced neuropathology. Molecular, histologic, and behavioral comparisons in rats. Spine 25:2975-2980

33. Jensen MC, Brant-Zawadzki MN, Obuchowski N et al (1994) Magnetic resonance imaging of the lumbar spine in people without back pain. N Engl J Med 331:69-73

34. Weishaupt D, Zanetti M, Hodler J et al (2001) Painful lumbar disk derangement: relevance of endplate abnormalities at MR imaging. Radiology 218:420-427

35. Boos N, Rieder R, Schade V et al (1995) 1995 Volvo Award in clinical sciences. The diagnostic accuracy of magnetic resonance imaging, work perception, and psychosocial factors in identifying symptomatic disc herniations. Spine 20:2613-2625

36. Modic MT, Obuchowski NA, Ross JS et al (2005) Acute low back pain and radiculopathy: MR imaging findings and their prognostic role and effect on outcome. Radiology 237:597-604

37. Weishaupt D, Zanetti M, Hodler J et al (1998) MR imaging of the lumbar spine: prevalence of intervertebral disk extrusion and sequestration, nerve root compression, end plate abnormalities, and osteoarthritis of the facet joints in asymptomatic volunteers. Radiology 209:661-666

38. Sandhu HS, Sanchez-Caso LP, Parvataneni HK et al (2000) Association between findings of provocative discography and vertebral endplate signal changes as seen on MRI. J Spinal Disord 13:438-443

39. Vital JM, Gille O, Pointillart V et al (2003) Course of Modic 1 six months after lumbar posterior osteosynthesis. Spine 28:715-720; discussion 721

Imaging of Musculoskeletal Infections

Theodore T. Miller[1], Mark E. Schweitzer[2]

[1] Department of Radiology and Imaging, Hospital for Special Surgery, New York, NY, USA
[2] Department of Diagnostic Imaging, The Ottawa Hospital, Ottawa, Ontario, Canada

Introduction

Evaluation of clinically suspected infection is a common imaging task, in which many factors have to be taken into consideration, such as the pathogen (bacteria, mycobacteria, fungus, or virus), the location of the suspected infection (bone, soft tissue, joint, or disc space), the age of the patient (infant, child, adult), the time course of the infection (acute, subacute, chronic), and whether there are any underlying complicating factors (e.g., infarct or other bone disease, joint replacement in the area of clinical concern, or diabetic arthropathy). Radiography, computed tomography (CT), sonography, scintigraphy, and magnetic resonance imaging (MRI) all have roles and varying usefulness in the imaging evaluation.

Acute Osteomyelitis

Pyogenic

Osteomyelitis is an infection of the medullary cavity of bone. It may occur as a result of hematogenous spread, contiguous spread from an adjacent site of infection, or direct inoculation, such as iatrogenic or traumatic (including penetrating trauma such as bullets and open fractures). The most common pathway is hematogenous spread, and in children and adults the most common site of infection in a long bone is the metaphysis. This is due to sluggish flow in the metaphyseal end-arterioles, which allows the deposition of organisms [1]. In infants up to approximately 18 months of age, the most common site in a long bone is the epiphysis, because transphyseal vessels allow the blood-borne organisms to cross the growth plate from the metaphysis into the epiphysis.

Plain radiographs should be the starting point for any imaging evaluation of suspected infection. The earliest radiographic changes are soft-tissue swelling and blurring of adjacent fat planes, which may take several days to become apparent after the onset of infection [2]. Approximately 10 days post- onset, the radiographs may demonstrate lysis of the medullary trabeculae, focal loss of cortex, and periosteal reaction [3] (Fig. 1). If the radi-

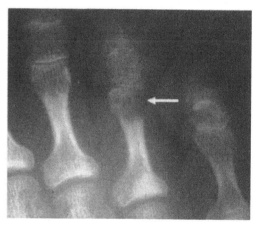

Fig. 1. Osteomyelitis. Antero-posterior (AP) radiograph of the toes shows focal trabecular and cortical lysis involving the head of the 4th proximal phalanx (*arrow*)

ographs are normal or equivocal, more advanced imaging may be required – most commonly, MRI and nuclear scintigraphy. The general advantages of MRI over scintigraphy are its superb anatomic detail, including the ability to evaluate both bone and adjacent soft tissue, and its quicker performance.

The earliest finding of acute osteomyelitis on MRI is alteration of the normal marrow signal intensity, which can be seen as early as a few days after the onset of infection. Due to the inflammatory edema, which is the hallmark of acute infection, the signal intensity of marrow becomes low to intermediate on T1-weighted sequences and high on fat-suppressed T2-weighted sequences (Fig. 2). The margins of the area of abnormal signal intensity are usually ill-defined. Periosteal reaction and adjacent soft-tissue edema subsequently occur and will become apparent on MRI sooner than on radiographs.

The negative predictive value of MRI for excluding osteomyelitis is 100%; that is, if the marrow is completely normal on all pulse sequences, then infection can be reliably excluded. Its positive predictive value, i.e., its ac-

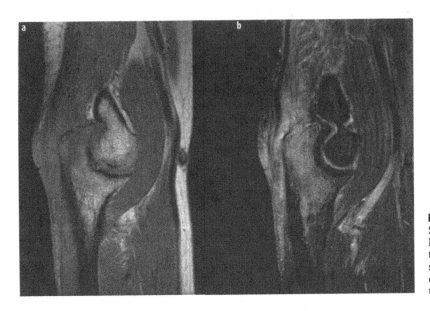

Fig. 2 a, b. Osteomyelitis of the olecranon. **a** Sagittal T1-weighted image shows ill-defined low-signal-intensity marrow edema within the olecranon. **b** Corresponding sagittal fat-suppressed fast spin echo T2-weighted sequence shows high-signal-intensity edema in the marrow and surrounding soft tissue

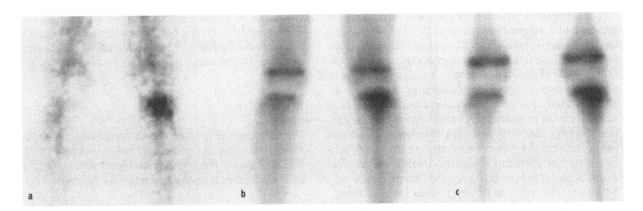

Fig. 3 a-c. Three-phase bone scan of osteomyelitis shows increased radiotracer uptake in the proximal tibia on the flow phase (**a**), blood-pool phase (**b**), and bone phase (**c**). (Courtesy of C. Palestro)

curacy for determining osteomyelitis if abnormal signal intensity is present in the marrow, is not as good because of other causes of edema, such as neuropathic arthropathy and "reactive marrow edema." The latter is a non-infectious edema occurring in marrow adjacent to a site of soft-tissue infection or even adjacent to another site of osteomyelitis [4]. Its exact pathogenesis is unknown but it is thought to be due to vasogenic hyperemia. The signal intensity of reactive marrow edema can mimic that of osteomyelitis and it can enhance with gadolinium contrast agents, similar to osteomyelitis, thus causing false-positive interpretations.

Several different scintigraphic methods using various radiopharmaceuticals are also available for the evaluation of osteomyelitis [5]. The traditional method of scintigraphic evaluation has been the three-phase bone scan us-

ing 99m-technetium-MDP. A positive examination will show increased uptake in all three phases, being particularly hottest in the bone phase at 4 h (the third phase) (Fig. 3), and will persist on 24-h delayed bone-phase images. An advantage of this method over MRI is its ability to image the entire body in patients with suspected multifocal osteomyelitis. Disadvantages include exposure to ionizing radiation, lack of anatomic detail, and false-positive studies due to uptake by other bone abnormalities. False-negative bone scans can result from poor blood supply to the infected site or bony lysis without a compensatory bone reaction.

In an attempt to increase the accuracy of bone scanning, it has been combined with gallium-67 scanning, since this isotope is also a bone agent. Decreased gallium uptake relative to Tc mitigates against osteomyelitis, while increased gallium uptake suggests infection. Another scintigraphic method is white-cell imaging, in which neutrophils are linked either to 111-indium (111In) or to 99m-technetium (99mTc). A disadvantage of this technique is that the white-cell tracer will accumulate in areas of normal red marrow in addition to areas of neutrophil uptake. Therefore, in order to improve the accuracy of the technique it has been combined with ^{99}mTc-sulfur-colloid scanning, in which a positive scan is demonstrated by increased uptake of white-cell tracer compared to the sulfur colloid. A white-cell study is not useful in nonbacterial or chronic infections since the inflammatory response is not neutrophilic.

Computed tomography and sonography can also evaluate acute osteomyelitis. Features of acute osteomyelitis on CT are increased density of the normal fatty medullary canal, as it is replaced by the infectious edema; blurring of fat planes, and, eventually, periosteal reaction and loss of cortex [3, 6]. CT is also excellent for the evaluation of soft tissue gas. Although CT may show these changes earlier than plain radiographs, it is less preferable than MRI because of decreased soft-tissue contrast compared to MRI as well as exposure to ionizing radiation in children.

The sonographic criterion for acute osteomyelitis is the presence of a subperiosteal abscess [7] (Fig. 4). Advantages of sonography are that it is rapidly performed, does not use ionizing radiation, and does not require the sedation of small children. Sonography can also be helpful in anatomic regions that are complicated by orthopedic instrumentation or in patients who have a contraindication to MRI. However, sonography cannot image past the cortex of a bone, and therefore early osteomyelitis that has not yet produced a subperiosteal abscess may be falsely interpreted as normal. Conversely, a soft-tissue abscess that is adjacent to bone but is not truly subperiosteal may be falsely interpreted as positive. Power Doppler sonography will eventually show hyperemia around the periosteal abscess, but may not do so in the first several days of its occurrence [8].

Tuberculosis

Tuberculous osteomyelitis has a much more prolonged and insidious time course than pyogenic infection, running on the order of months. It is hematogenous in etiology, but only about one-third of patients have concurrent pulmonary involvement.

Radiographically, the tuberculous lesion of long bones is lytic, with minimal if any periosteal reaction, and these lesions occur at the end of the bone or in the metaphyseal region [9] (Fig. 5). Tuberculosis of the short tubular bones of the hands and feet (tuberculous dactylitis) has a different appearance, called spina ventosa, consisting of bony expansion and prominent periosteal reaction. Spina ventosa is more common in children than in adults and may have multifocal involvement in up to one-third of patients.

Tuberculous osteomyelitis may have an associated soft-tissue abscess, typically larger than that associated with pyogenic infections [10]; the tuberculous abscess is considered "cold" because it is usually well-defined and lacks the surrounding inflammatory edema of pyogenic abscesses that blur the adjacent soft-tissue planes. Both CT and MRI can show both the bony involvement and cold abscess, but bone scan is falsely negative in as many as one-third of patients because of the lack of bony response to the infection. White-cell imaging is not helpful since the inflammatory response is histiocytic, not neutrophilic.

Fungus

Fungal osteomyelitis, due to such organisms as histoplasmosis, blastomycosis, and coccidioidomycosis, is of variable appearance, potentially resembling pyogenic or tuberculous infection. It has a predilection for the ends of bone.

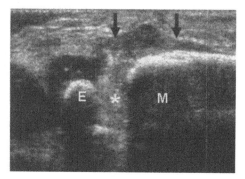

Fig. 4. Ultrasound of osteomyelitis. Longitudinal sonogram of the proximal tibia in a child shows a subperiosteal abcess (*arrows*), tracking into and causing widening of the physis (*asterisk*). *M,* Metaphysis; *E,* epiphysis

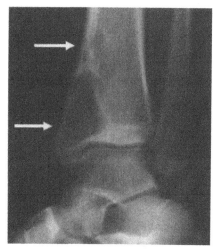

Fig. 5. Tuberculous osteomyelitis. Oblique radiograph of the ankle shows an irregularly shaped lytic lesion involving the distal aspect of the tibia (*arrows*). Note that there is no adjacent periosteal reaction

Chronic Recurrent Multifocal Osteomyelitis

Chronic recurrent multifocal osteomyelitis (CRMO), despite its name, is a non-infectious inflammatory disorder of bone. Its etiology is unknown but may be a post-infectious autoimmune response. Biopsies have occasionally demonstrated *Staphylococcus epidermidis* and *Propionibacterium acne*, but these organisms may be merely contaminants and not causative. The disease has some features in common with the synovitis, acne, pustulosis, hyperostosis, and osteitis (SAPHO) syndrome, and the two diseases may be variants of the same underlying disease [11]. CRMO typically affects children or young adults, is more common in girls, and can have a prolonged, albeit self-limited course. During clinical exacerbation the erythrocyte sedimentation rate is elevated, but the C-reactive protein level and white blood cell count may be normal. Histologically, there is a chronic rather than an acute inflammatory response. It is discussed in this chapter because its imaging appearances are similar to those of pyogenic osteomyelitis.

CRMO affects both tubular bones and flat bones, especially the clavicle. In tubular bones, the metaphysis is affected and the lesions appear radiographically as focal trabecular lysis with periosteal reaction [12, 13]. There is variability in the size of the metaphyseal lesions and degree of periosteal response, which can sometimes be the dominant feature, especially in short tubular bones. With healing, the metaphyseal lesions will sclerose, and the periosteal reaction matures as bone thickening. The medial and middle portions of the clavicle are affected, are typically enlarged, and acutely can have either a lytic destructive appearance with periosteal reaction or a sclerotic appearance. Thickening and hyperostosis are features of chronic involvement also.

Bone scanning with 99mTc is useful in the work-up of patients suspected of having CRMO, since the multifocality of the disease can be appreciated. Active lesions, even if clinically asymptomatic, will show radiotracer uptake. Disease activity can also be monitored scintigraphically, since the quiescent phase shows less intense tracer uptake.

On MRI of tubular bones, marrow edema and periosteal reaction, but not adjacent soft-tissue edema (unlike pyogenic osteomyelitis), are seen. Involvement of the clavicle may have associated soft-tissue edema but this edema is well-defined and almost tumoral in appearance, compared with the ill-defined edema of true osteomyelitis. Soft-tissue abscess is also not a feature of CRMO.

Subacute and Chronic Bacterial Osteomyelitis

Brodie's abscess is a manifestation of subacute osteomyelitis, appearing as a geographic area of sclerosis with a lucent center on radiographs and CT. On MRI, it is usually of low signal intensity on T1-weighted sequences and high signal intensity on T2-weighted sequences,

with an enhancing wall of high signal intensity and a center of low signal intensity on contrast-enhanced T1-weighted images (Fig. 6).

Chronic osteomyelitis typically has two appearances [14]. One is the "sclerosing osteomyelitis of Garre", in which there is generalized sclerosis of the medullary canal and bony expansion (Fig. 7). The other appearance

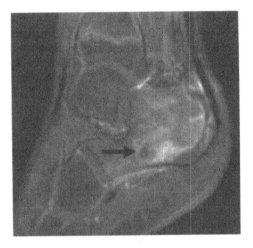

Fig. 6. Brodie's abscess of the calcaneus. Fat-suppressed T1-weighted sequence after intravenous administration of gadolinium contrast shows the low-signal-intensity abscess (*arrow*) with a surrounding high-signal-intensity rim and adjacent enhancing marrow edema

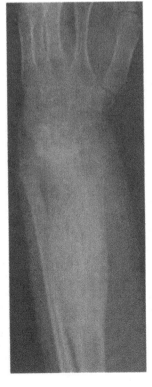

Fig. 7. Chronic sclerosing osteomyelitis of Garre. Oblique radiograph of the distal forearm shows patchy sclerosis and expansion of the distal radius, with involvement of the growth plate and epiphysis

is that of a markedly thickened periosteal reaction, called an "involucrum," that envelops the bone. The involucrum is the bone's way of trying to wall-off the infection. Typically there is a devitalized bony fragment, the "sequestrum," within the center of the medullary canal of the involved bone segment. Since the sequestrum does not have a blood supply, antibiotics cannot reach it and it therefore acts as a safe haven for the offending organism. The sequestrum may not be well-seen on radiographs due to the overlying sclerosis of the involucrum, but can be demonstrated on cross-sectional imaging. An associated feature of this type of chronic osteomyelitis is a sinus track in the cortex, called a "cloaca," which is the body's attempt to expel the sequestrum from the medullary canal. A soft-tissue sinus track extending to the skin is frequently part of this process.

Infection of the Spine

Vertebral osteomyelitis is usually caused by hematogenous spread to the vertebral body, whereas infection of the intervertebral disc ("infectious discitis") is due to osteomyelitis of the adjacent vertebral body that secondarily invades the disc, or to direct contamination of the disc itself during surgical spine procedures or interventional spine procedures such as discography.

Radiographically, the hallmarks of pyogenic infection are loss of disc-space height and destruction of the vertebral endplates, both of which occur early in the course of the disease, usually within the first few weeks of infection (Fig. 8). In contrast, tuberculosis of the spine ("Pott's disease") shows marked osteopenia and bone destruction but with relative sparing of the disc space and endplates until late in the course of the disease, typically over several months. A characteristic late sequela of the vertebral and disc destruction of tuberculous involvement of the thoracic spine is the sharply angled kyphotic "gibbus" deformity. A mimicker of disc-space infection on radiographs is dialysis spondyloarthropathy. People on long-term hemodialysis may have an accumulation of amyloid in the disc space, with resultant narrowing or loss of the disc space and endplate erosion or destruction.

A marrow edema pattern in the adjacent vertebra and endplates is demonstrated on MRI. Typically, there is also high signal intensity within the disc on T2-weighted images and loss of the intranuclear cleft. In addition, both pyogenic and tuberculous spondylitis can have associated paravertebral and epidural abscesses. Tuberculous spondylitis may also demonstrate a subligamentous component, involving either the anterior longitudinal ligament or the posterior longitudinal ligament, through which the infection can spread to adjacent vertebral levels (Fig. 9); the presence of multiple levels of vertebral involvement suggests tuberculosis rather than pyogenic infection, but both fungal infection and sarcoidosis of the spine can also have this multilevel appearance. Fungal infections have a predilection for the posterior elements of the spine and may show preservation of normal disc signal intensity and the intranuclear cleft on T2-weighted images, even with disc involvement [15].

A pitfall in the interpretation of disc-space infection on MRI is severe degenerative disc disease, with disc narrowing, endplate irregularity, and adjacent granulation-type endplate changes [16]. The edema-like pattern in the endplates on either side of the disc can look similar to infection, and the involved regions can show enhancement of

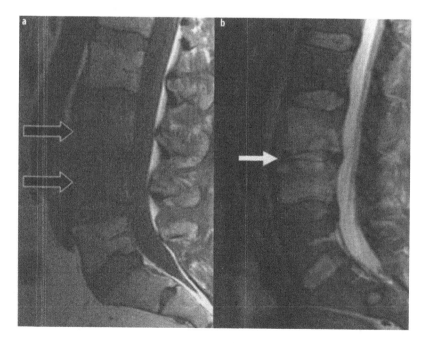

Fig. 8 a, b. Pyogenic disc space infection. **a** Sagittal T1 weighted image shows low-signal-intensity marrow edema in the L3 and L4 vertebrae (*arrows*). **b** Corresponding fat-suppressed T2 weighted sequence shows the high-signal-intensity edema in the vertebrae and narrowing of the intervening disc space (*arrow*)

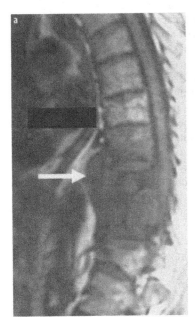
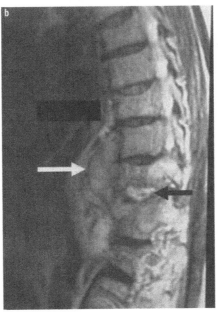

Fig. 9 a, b. Tuberculous osteomyelitis of the spine. Sagittal T1-weighted image (**a**) and sagittal fat suppressed T2-weighted image (**b**) shows involvement of three contiguous lower thoracic vertebrae with an anterior subligamentous abscess (*white arrow*) and preservation of the disc space (*black arrow*)

the vertebral bodies, endplates, and even portions of the disc with intravenous gadolinium administration. CT can be useful for evaluating endplate irregularities in equivocal cases of infection versus degeneration, in order to determine whether the irregularities have sclerotic margins, suggesting chronic degeneration. Gallium-67 using single-photon-emission computed tomography (SPECT) has been demonstrated to be just as sensitive as but slightly more specific than MRI for confirming spinal infection and surrounding soft-tissue involvement [5]. Positron emission tomography (PET) with 18-fluoro-deoxyglucose has been shown to be both more sensitive and specific than MRI for distinguishing endplate changes from infection [17].

The Diabetic Foot

Diabetes is a world-wide malady and has many potential medical complications, one of the most common of which is pedal infection. Clinical assessment of the swollen, red, and hot foot for the presence of osteomyelitis is poor, even in the presence of soft-tissue ulcer, and the radiologist is therefore often asked to participate in the evaluation.

Radiographs should always be performed first because they may provide the diagnosis by showing trabecular or cortical lysis, and because they give an overview of the anatomy and any underlying complicating structural changes, such as occur in diabetic arthropathy; however in many cases more advanced imaging is needed. A meta-analysis of the literature in which weighted averages were determined for various imaging modalities regarding the detection of osteomyelitis in the presence of a soft-tissue ulcer showed that probing for bone or the presence of exposed bone had an average 60% sensitivity and 91%

specificity, radiographs had a weighted average 54% sensitivity and 68% specificity, three-phase bone scan had 81% sensitivity and 28% specificity, labeled-white-cell studies had 74% sensitivity and 68% specificity, and MRI had 90% sensitivity and 79% specificity [18]. MRI also has the advantage of providing the anatomic detail and resolution of bones and soft-tissues needed by the surgeon to perform debridement or limited resections.

The primary sign of osteomyelitis is marrow edema, but evaluation is usually more difficult in the diabetic foot than in the non-diabetic foot because the diabetic foot is often complicated by underlying neuropathic changes. Evaluation of the neuropathic foot must take into account that: (1) normal marrow signal intensity on all pulse sequences excludes osteomyelitis; (2) sclerotic marrow usually excludes an acute or active chronic osteomyelitis; (3) marrow edema of osteomyelitis usually affects the entire bone whereas edema of arthropathy is usually subarticular; and (4) arthropathy usually affects the midfoot, while infection more commonly involves regions of increased pressure such as the toes and heel [19, 20].

Secondary signs of osteomyelitis have also been described in order to increase the accuracy of MRI. For example, cortical destruction is a feature of osteomyelitis but not of reactive marrow edema. A typical finding of cortical destruction is the "ghost sign", which refers to poor definition of the margins of a bone on T1-weighted images which become crisp and look normal after contrast administration [20]. When the ghost sign is present, osteomyelitis should be suspected rather than neuropathic arthropathy. Other secondary signs include cutaneous ulcer, abscess formation, cellulitis, and sinus tract formation [21]. Approximately 90% of pedal osteomyelitis is due to spread from an adjacent cutaneous ulcer, and ulcers tend to occur at points of pressure on the foot, such as under the first and fifth metatarsal heads, at the tips of the toes and around deformed interphalangeal joints, under the calcaneus, and over the malleoli [22]. The most common locations of osteomyelitis parallel these regions of ulcer location, namely the metatarsal heads, phalanges, and calcaneus. Similarly, over 90% of abscesses are associated with ulcers. Soft-tissue infection in the foot does not respect anatomic boundaries and thus can spread from one compartment to another.

Septic Arthritis

Infectious organisms can reach the joint either through direct innoculation, hematogenous spread, or contiguous spread from an adjacent intra-articular site of osteomyelitis. This last mechanism is common in neonates and young children, in whom transphyseal spread of organisms leads to infection of the intracapsular epiphysis [1, 11]. Radiographically, the earliest signs will be generalized soft-tissue swelling and blurring of fat planes about the joint, followed by joint distention due to effusion and synovial thickening. In the septic pediatric hip, the presence of a large joint effusion may laterally displace the femoral head.

Pyogenic arthritis is marked by joint-space narrowing early in the disease due to proteolytic enzymes released by the white-cell exudate, which destroy the articular cartilage. Erosion of bone is concurrent with the cartilage destruction and periarticular osteopenia eventually develops (Fig. 10). In tuberculous arthritis, the main radiographic features are marked periarticular osteopenia with relative preservation of the joint space until late in the disease because the chronic inflammatory exudate of tuberculosis lacks cartilage-destroying proteolytic enzymes (Table 1). "Phemister's" triad refers to the three

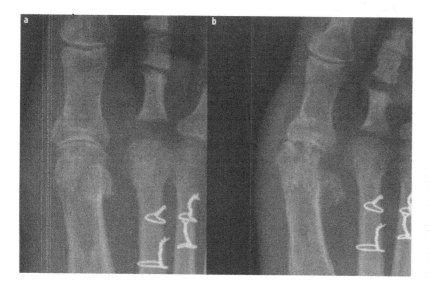

Fig. 10 a, b. Pyogenic septic joint. **a** Initial post-operative AP radiograph of the first toe in a patient who underwent forefoot reconstruction shows soft-tissue swelling and narrowing of the first metatarsophalangeal joint. **b** AP radiograph from the same patient 6 weeks later shows destruction of the first metatarsal head, complete loss of the joint space, and resultant valgus malalignment of the joint

Table 1. Differentiation of acute bacterial and tuberculous infection

	Bacterial	Tuberculous
Bone	Metaphyseal osteolytic lesion with periosteal reaction	1. Metaphyseal osteolytic lesion that can cross the growth plate into the epiphysis. 2. Little periosteal reaction in long bones; "spina ventosa" in short tubular bones
Spine	1. Endplate erosions and loss of disc space early in the disease. 2. Fusion of the vertebrae without deformity late in the disease. 3. Single-level involvement	1. Vertebral body destruction with relative preservation of disc space until late. 2. Subligamentous spread with multilevel involvement. 3. Large paravertebral "cold" abscesses. 4. Gibbus deformity
Joint	Bone erosions and early loss of joint space.	"Phemister's triad": 1. Osteopenia 2. Bone erosions 3. Preservation of the joint space until late in the disease
Abscess	Thick irregular wall with surrounding inflammatory edema	1. Thin smooth wall without surrounding inflammation ("cold") 2. May calcify

typical radiographic features of tuberculous arthritis: marked periarticular osteopenia, relative preservation of the joint space until late in the disease, and small periarticular erosions.

Sonography and MRI are excellent for the evaluation of a suspected septic joint, and both will show changes earlier than radiography. However, the presence of a joint effusion per se does not necessarily indicate a septic joint. This is particularly true for pediatric hips, in which a systemic viral infection can cause a transient but painful reactive sterile synovitis. However, the absence of a joint effusion or synovial thickening in a large joint such as the hip or knee excludes the presence of a septic joint [23, 24]. Septic arthritis in small joints such as in the foot, will have synovial enhancement with infrequent effusions [24].

As noted above, sonography is particularly useful in children since it can be performed quickly and does not require sedation. Sonography demonstrates a joint effusion as an anechoic or a mildly heterogeneous hypoechoic fluid collection. Depending on the acuteness of the process, power Doppler may or may not show hyperemia in the surrounding synovium [25]. A disadvantage of sonography is that it cannot evaluate the underlying bony structures and therefore may miss an early osteomyelitis.

Both the joint and the underlying bony structures are well-evaluated with MRI, although without the use of intravenous contrast it can be difficult to distinguish thickened synovium from joint fluid, since both demonstrate low signal intensity on T1-weighted sequences and high signal intensity on T2-weighted sequences. Intravenous gadolinium contrast administration will demonstrate marked enhancement of the inflamed synovium on a T1-weighted sequence, leaving any joint fluid as low signal intensity. Although there is overlap, pyogenic synovitis tends to be thick and irregular, while tuberculous synovitis tends to be thin and smooth [26]. The distinction between pyogenic arthritis and active rheumatoid arthritis can be difficult, as both may show erosions, marrow edema, and synovial thickening with enhancement.

Potential complications of septic arthritis are growth disturbance if the physis is involved in children, osteonecrosis, degenerative arthritis secondary to incongruity of the joint as a result of articular surface destruction or misshaping of the bone, and auto-fusion of the joint.

Arthroplasty Infection

The first step in the imaging evaluation of a suspected infected prosthesis is plain radiographs. Radiographic findings suggestive of infection include a wide irregular radiolucency around the cement-bone (in the case of cemented components) or metal-bone (in the case of non-cemented components) interface and frank bone destruction. However, a distinction between infectious loosening, mechanical loosening, and loosening due to a non-infectious histiocytic response ("particle disease") often cannot be made on a single radiograph. Usually, previous radiographs are necessary for comparison, with mechan-

ical loosening and a histiocytic response usually taking a slowly progressive course, whereas an acute infection has a more rapid time course and may look more aggressive. However, even this feature is not reliable since infections can be subclinical and smoldering, leading to slowly progressive loosening in an afebrile patient.

Three-phase bone scan can be used but suffers from poor specificity since a cemented femoral component can show increased uptake around the prosthesis for several years after placement, and because a normal non-cemented prosthesis can also show increased radiotracer uptake due to the bony ingrowth that occurs around the prosthesis. Moreover, the presence of new areas of radiotracer uptake compared to prior scans can be caused by both infectious and non-infectious loosening. However, since a normal bone scan is reliable for excluding loosening, it can be used as an initial screening test. Adding a gallium scan to the standard technetium bone scan can improve the diagnostic accuracy for infection: infection is excluded if the gallium scan is normal or has less intense uptake than the corresponding bone scan, and infection is diagnosed when there is uptake of gallium without corresponding Tc uptake or the gallium uptake is more intense than the corresponding Tc uptake.

The combination of labeled white cells and 99mTc-labeled sulfur colloid has excellent results reported, with sensitivity and specificity as high as 100% and 97%, respectively [5]. The imaging feature of infection is radiotracer spatial mismatch in which there is uptake of the labeled white cells with less intense or no uptake of the sulfur colloid. PET scanning also has good to excellent results, with 91% sensitivity and 92% specificity [27], but normal persistent post-surgical uptake around the prosthetic head and neck is a potential pitfall in interpretation [28].

Sonography can be used to evaluate the presence of joint effusion associated with an infected prosthesis. One study suggested that a joint effusion which distends the joint capsule more than 3.2 mm away from the neck of the femur correlates highly with the presence of acute infection, as does the presence of periarticular soft-tissue collections [29]. However, a subsequent investigation found that neither the distension of the anterior capsule nor the echogenicity of the joint fluid or capsule could accurately predict the presence of an effusion [30]. Sonography can also be used to guide aspiration of articular and periarticular fluid.

Artifacts caused by the metal prosthetic components limit the use of MRI, but metal-artifact reduction techniques can decrease dephasing and misregistration, and allow for the assessment of effusion, capsular thickening, osteolysis, and soft-tissue collections. The synovitis of particle disease tends to be thick and of low signal intensity, while that of infection tends to be laminar and of high signal intensity [31, 32].

The gold standard for the evaluation of a clinically suspected infected prosthesis is aspiration, with Gram stain and culture and sensitivity of joint fluid.

References

1. Kothari NA, Pelchovitz DJ, Meyer JS (2001) Imaging of musculoskeletal infections. Radiol Clin North Am 39:653-671
2. Capitanio MA, Kirkpatrick JA (1970) Early roentgen observations in acute osteomyelitis. Am J Roentgenol Radium Ther Nucl Med108:488-496
3. Pineda C, Vargas A, Rodriguez AV (2006) Imaging of osteomyelitis: current concepts. Infect Dis Clin North Am 20:789-825
4. Craig JG, Amin MB, Wu K et al (1997) Osteomyelitis of the diabetic foot: MR imaging-pathologic correlation. Radiology 203:849-855
5. Palestro CJ, Love C, Miller TT (2007) Diagnostic imaging tests and microbial infections. Cell Microbiol 9:2323-2333
6. Fayad LM, Carrino JA, Fishman EK (2007) Musculoskeletal infection: role of CT in the emergency department. Radiographics 27:1723-1736
7. Riebel TW, Nasir R, Nazarenko O (1996) The value of sonography in the detection of osteomyelitis. Pediatr Radiol 26:291-297
8. Chao HC, Lin SJ, Huang YC, Lin TY (1999) Color Doppler ultrasonographic evaluation of osteomyelitis in children. J Ultrasound Med 18:729-734
9. Yao DC, Sartoris DJ (1995) Musculoskeletal tuberculosis. Radiol Clin North Am 33:679-689
10. Soler R, Rodriguez E, Remuinan C, Santos M (2001) MRI of musculoskeletal extraspinal tuberculosis. J Comput Assist Tomogr 25:177-183
11. Schmit P, Glorion C (2004) Osteomyelitis in infants and children. Eur Radiol 14(Suppl 4):L44-L54
12. Demharter J, Bohndorf K, Michl W, Vogt H (1997) Chronic recurrent osteomyelitis: a radiological and clinical investigation of five cases. Skeletel Radiol 26:579-588
13. Jurik AG (2004) Chronic recurrent multifocal osteomyelitis. Semin Musculoskelet Radiol 8:243-53
14. Saigal G, Azouz EM, Abdenour G (2004) Imaging of osteomyelitis with special reference to children. Semin Musculoskelet Radiol 8:255-265
15. Williams RL, Fukui MB, Meltzer CC et al (1999) Fungal spinal osteomyelitis in the immunocompromised patient: MR findings in three cases. AJNR Am J Neuroradiol 20:381-385
16. Mellado JM, Pérez del Palomar L, Camins A et al (2004) MR imaging of spinal infection: atypical features, interpretive pitfalls and potential mimickers. Eur Radiol 14:1980-1989
17. Stumpe KD, Zanetti M, Weishaupt D et al (2002) FDG positron emission tomography for differentiation of degenerative and infectious endplate abnormalities in the lumbar spine detected on MR imaging. AJR Am J Roentgenol 179:1151-1157
18. Dinh MT, Abad CL, Safdar N (2008) Diagnostic accuracy of the physical examination and imaging tests for osteomyelitis underlying diabetic foot ulcers: meta-analysis. Clin Infect Dis 47:519-527
19. Tan PL, Teh J (2007) MRI of the diabetic foot: differentiation of infection from neuropathic change. Br J Radiol 80:939-948
20. Russell JM, Peterson JJ, Bancroft LW (2008) MR imaging of the diabetic foot. Magn Reson Imaging Clin N Am 16:59-70
21. Morrison WB, Schweitzer ME, Batte WG et al (1998) Osteomyelitis of the foot: relative importance of primary and secondary MR imaging signs. Radiology 207:625-632
22. Lederman HP, Morrison WB, Schweitzer ME (2002) MR image of analysis of pedal osteomyelitis: distribution, patterns of spread, and frequency of associated ulceration and septic arthritis. Radiology 223:747-755
23. Zawin JK, Hoffer FA, Rand FF et al (1993) Joint effusion in children with an irritable hip: US diagnosis and aspiration. Radiology 187:459-463
24. Karchevsky M, Schweitzer ME, Morrison WB, Parellada JA (2004) MRI findings of septic arthritis and associated osteomyelitis in adults. AJR Am J Roentgenol 182:119-122
25. Strouse PJ, Di Pietro MA, Adler RS (1998) Pediatric hip effusions: evaluation with power Doppler sonography. Radiology 206:731-735
26. Hong SH, Kim SM, Ahn JM et al (2001) Tuberculous versus pyogenic arthritis: MR imaging evaluation. Radiology 218:848-853
27. Mumme T, Reinartz P, Alfer J et al (2005) Diagnostic values of positron emission tomography versus triple-phase bone scan in hip arthroplasty loosening. Arch Orthop Trauma Surg 125:322-329
28. Zhuang H, Chacko TK, Hickeson M et al (2002) Persistent non-specific FDG uptake on PET imaging following hip arthroplasty. Eur J Nucl Med Mol Imaging 29:1328-1333
29. Van Holsbeeck MT, Eyler WR, Sherman LS et al (1994) Detection of infection in loosened hip prostheses: efficacy of sonography. AJR Am J Roentgenol 163:381-384
30. Weybright PN, Jacobson JA, Murry KH et al (2003) Limited effectiveness of sonography in revealing hip joint effusion: preliminary results in 21 adult patients with native and postoperative hips. AJR Am J Roentgenol 181:215-218
31. Potter HG, Foo LF (2006) Magnetic resonance imaging of joint arthroplasty. Orthop Clin North Am 37:361-373
32. Cahir JG, Toms AP, Marshall TJ et al (2007) CT and MRI of hip arthroplasty. Clin Radiol 62:1163-1171

Compressive and Entrapment Neuropathies of the Upper and Lower Extremities

Javier Beltran[1], Jenny Bencardino[2]

[1] Department of Radiology, Maimonides Medical Center, Brooklyn, NY, USA
[2] Department of Radiology, Hospital for Joint Diseases, New York University, New York, NY, USA

Upper Extremity

Suprascapular nerve syndrome

This condition is produced by the impingement of the suprascapular nerve at the scapular notch or spinoglenoid notch. Proximal entrapment at the scapular notch results in compression of the suprascapular nerve and denervation of both the supraspinatous and infraspinatous muscles. Distal entrapment at the spinoglenoid notch results in compression of the infraspinatous nerve and denervation of the infraspinatous muscle only. Etiologies include paralabral cysts, scapular fractures, hematomas, rotator-cuff tears, overhead activities, soft-tissue and osseous tumors, vascular malformations, thickened transverse scapular or spinoglenoid ligaments, and iatrogenic factors.

Magnetic resonance (MR) findings include denervation edema or fatty atrophy of the affected muscles.

Quadrilateral Space Syndrome

Here, the axillary nerve is compressed in the quadrilateral space. Etiologies include fractures of the proximal humeral head and callus formations, anterior shoulder dislocation resulting in traction and compression, fibrous bands (post-traumatic), soft-tissue and osseous tumors, and paralabral cysts.

MR findings include denervation edema or fatty atrophy of the teres minor and/or deltoid muscle.

Pronator Syndrome

Compression of the median nerve at the level of the pronator teres muscle results in pronators syndrome. Potential sites of entrapment include the space between the superficial (humeral) and deep (ulnar) heads of the pronator teres muscle; at the origin of the flexor digitorum superficialis muscle, where a fibrous arch exists; at the lacertus fibrosus, also known as bicipital aponeurosis; and less commonly, at the supracondylar process of the distal anteromedial humerus (avian spur). Etiologies commonly include elbow trauma, repetitive elbow flexion, supination and pronation of the forearm, and, infrequently, anatomic variants (e.g., accessory bicipital aponeurosis, accessory head of the flexor pollicis longus muscle, palmaris profundus), bicipital bursitis, and soft-tissue masses. Closed reduction of an elbow dislocation can also result in intra-articular entrapment of the median nerve.

The pattern of muscle denervation includes signal abnormalities or atrophy of the pronator teres, flexor carpi radialis, palmaris longus, and flexor digitorum superficialis muscles.

Anterior Interosseous Nerve Syndrome (Kiloh-Nevin Syndrome)

This is caused by compression of the anterior interosseous nerve in the proximal forearm. Etiologies include trauma, cast pressure, bulky tendinous origin of the ulnar head of the pronator teres, soft-tissue masses such as lipoma or ganglion, anomalous or accessory muscles and vessels, and fibrous bands.

MR findings include denervation edema or fatty atrophy of the radial half of the flexor digitorum profundus, flexor pollicis longus, and pronator quadratus.

Cubital Tunnel Syndrome

Compression of the ulnar nerve within the cubital tunnel at the elbow is the cause of cubital tunnel syndrome. Etiologies include "sleep palsy, external compression with pressure from the operating table during surgery, during unconsciousness, in wheelchair-bound patients, in drivers who lean their elbows against hard surfaces, trauma, thickened cubital tunnel retinaculum, anomalous muscles such as anconeus epitrochlearis, tumors including ganglions, lipoma, osteophytes, and osteochondroma [1] (Fig. 1).

MR findings include denervation edema or fatty atrophy of the flexor carpi ulnaris, flexor digitorum profundus, and the ulnar intrinsic muscles of the hand.

Posterior Interosseous Nerve Syndrome (Radial Tunnel Syndrome, Supinator Syndrome)

This results from compression of the posterior interosseous branch of the radial nerve within the radial tunnel. Most commonly, compression of the posterior

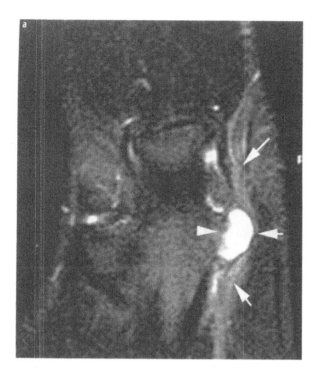

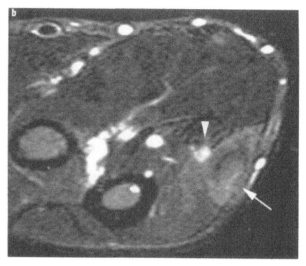

Fig. 1 a, b. Cubital tunnel syndrome. **a** Coronal T1-weighted image demonstrating ganglion cyst (*arrowhead*) within the cubital tunnel, producing compression and displacement of the ulnar nerve (*arrows*). **b** Axial T2-weighted image distal to the elbow joint, demonstrating an enlarged and hyperintense ulnar nerve (*arrowhead*) and early denervation with edema of the flexor carpi ulnaris muscle (*arrow*)

interosseus nerve occurs at the arcade of Frohse (proximal edge of the superficial head of the supinator muscle), but the nerve can also be compressed at its site of exit from the supinator muscle. Other etiologies include abnormal recurrent blood vessels that cross the posterior interosseous nerve (leash of Henry), intermuscular septum between the extensor carpi ulnaris and extensor digitorum minimi, external compression, radial-head fracture and callus formation, hematoma and soft-tissue tumors [2].

MR findings include signs of muscle denervation: abnormal signal intensity or atrophy in the supinator, extensor digitorum, extensor carpi ulnaris, extensor digiti minimi, extensor pollicis longus and brevis, abductor pollicis longus, and extensor indicis, with sparing of the extensor carpi radialis muscle (Fig. 2).

Carpal Tunnel Syndrome

This well-known condition is produced by compression of the median nerve beneath the transverse carpal ligament. Etiologies include anatomic variants, trauma, masses (ganglion cysts, perineural tumors, lipoma, fibrolipomatous hamartoma, gouty tophus), osteophytes from posttraumatic arthritis, synovial thickening due to inflammatory processes and amyloid deposition, acromegaly, edema in hypothyroidism, pregnancy, patients on oral contraceptives, and dynamic changes within the narrow tunnel during repetitive daily activity [3].

MR findings include thenar muscle edema or fatty atrophy; swelling of the median nerve proximal to the

carpal tunnel, resulting in a "pseudoneuroma" and flattening of the nerve within the tunnel (a flattening ratio between the major and minor axis of nerve, determined at the level of the hook of the hamate, >3 is indicative of median nerve pathology). Volar bowing of the flexor retinaculum at the distal carpal tunnel (at the level of the hook of the hamate) is one of the most specific signs.

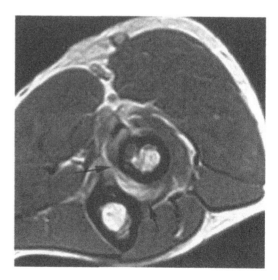

Fig. 2. Late denervation of the supinator muscle. Axial T1-weighted image demonstrating fatty infiltration of the supinator muscle (*arrows*)

Ulnar Tunnel Syndrome (Guyon Canal Syndrome)

This syndrome arises from compression of the ulnar nerve at the ulnar tunnel. Etiologies include trauma, particularly fractures of the hook of the hamate, and soft-tissue tumors, such as ganglion cyst, schwannoma, and lipoma. There is a high prevalence of anomalous muscles and tendons in this region, with common anomalies involving the palmaris longus, abductor digiti minimi, and flexor carpi ulnaris. Ulnar artery aneurysm or thrombosis and "handlebar palsy" have also been described [4].

MR findings include denervation edema or fatty atrophy of the hypothenar muscles (abductor digiti minimi, flexor digiti minimi brevis, and opponens digiti minimi), adductor pollicis, third and fourth lumbricals, and interosseus muscles, depending on the location of lesions.

Superficial Radial Nerve Syndrome (Wartenberg Syndrome, Cheiralgia Paresthetica, Handcuff Neuropathy, or Watch-Strap Nerve Compression)

Entrapment of the sensory branch of the radial nerve results in superficial radial nerve syndrome. Etiologies include trauma (most common), such as watch-strap compression, tight plasters, and postoperative scars; soft-tissue masses, entrapment by fascial bands in the subcutaneous plane as the nerve emerges from a deep location to a superficial one between the brachioradialis and extensor carpi radialis longus tendons, brachioradialis tendon, and extensor carpi ulnaris longus tendon.

MR findings include increased signal intensity of the nerve on T2-weighted and STIR sequences and increased girth of the nerve at and distal to the site of injury due to edema.

Lower Extremity

Piriformis Syndrome

This condition is caused by entrapment of the sciatic nerve at the level of the greater sciatic notch by the piriformis muscle. Etiologies include hypertrophy of the piriformis muscle due to gait disturbances, lumbar lordosis or hip flexion deformities, inflammation of the piriformis muscle secondary to infectious or inflammatory process of the adjacent lower lumbar spine, sacroiliac joint or iliopsoas muscle, spasticity of the piriformis muscles due to cerebral palsy, post-traumatic hematoma or fibrous adhesions of the piriformis muscle, local ischemia and an intramuscular course of the sciatic nerve or peroneal division of the sciatic nerve.

MR findings include increased intraneural T2 signal at the greater sciatic foramen, asymmetry in the size of the piriformis muscle between symptomatic and asymptomatic sides, increased T2 signal in the piriformis muscle, and accessory muscle slips with an intramuscular course of the sciatic nerve.

Iliacus Syndrome

Entrapment of the femoral nerve at the level of the pelvis and groin gives rise to iliacus syndrome. Etiologies include iatrogenic injury from pelvic surgery, hip surgery, hysterectomy, femoral artery catheterization, and arterial bypass procedures; traumatic injury as a result of hip/pelvic fractures, gunshot wounds, and lacerations; enlargement of the iliopsoas muscles secondary to tear, hematoma, or mass; distended iliopsoas bursa; and pseudoaneurysm of the iliac vessels.

MR findings include swelling and/or mass effect from the iliacus or iliopsoas muscle, hematomas, and post-traumatic pseudoaneurysm of the iliac vessels. Denervation edema of the quadriceps femoris muscle may be seen.

Saphenous Neuropathy

This condition may occur within the adductor canal, where its superficial location predisposes it to traumatic contusion or laceration. Etiologies include traumatic contusion or laceration in the adductor canal, iatrogenic injury during knee surgery/arthroscopy, and stretching injury in the setting of posterolateral knee instability.

MR findings include nerve displacement by space-occupying lesions such as parameniscal cysts or ganglia. There is no associated muscle denervation, due to the purely sensory nature of the saphenous nerve.

Obturator Neuropathy

The obturator nerve is formed within the substance of the psoas major muscle by the ventral divisions of the L2, L3, and L4 nerve roots. Etiologies include penetrating/iatrogenic trauma, pelvic and acetabular fractures, post-traumatic hematomas, myositis ossificans, pelvic tumors, and obturator hernia and obturator neuropathy in athletes, with formation of fibrous bands secondary to chronic adductor tendinopathy/osteitis pubis.

MR findings include alterations in the size and signal of the obturator nerve, mass effect from soft-tissue or osseous pelvic tumors, and denervation injury of the medial thigh muscles.

Lateral Femoral Cutaneous Neuropathy (Meralgia Paresthetica)

Entrapment of the lateral femoral cutaneous nerve as it travels under the inguinal ligament or as it pierces the fascia lata is the cause of this neuropathy. Etiologies include avulsion fracture of the anterosuperior iliac spine, pelvic and retroperitoneal tumors, stretching of the nerve due to prolonged leg and trunk hyperextension, leg length discrepancy, iatrogenic factors, prolonged standing, and external compression by belts, weight gain, or tight clothing [5, 6].

MR findings include alteration in size and signal of the entrapped nerve, avulsion injuries of the anterosuperior iliac spine, and mass effect from space-occupying lesions.

Proximal Tibial Neuropathy

This condition may occur within the popliteal fossa as the nerve passes over the popliteus muscles and under the tendinous arch of the soleus muscle. Etiologies include popliteal fossa hematoma, nerve tumors, and Baker's cyst.

MR findings include compression of the tibial nerve in the popliteal fossa, denervation changes in the gastrocnemius and popliteus muscles. Space-occupying lesions in the popliteal fossa can be seen on MR imaging (Fig. 3).

Common Peroneal Neuropathy

The common peroneal nerve is located posteromedial to the biceps femoris muscle in the distal popliteal fossa. At the level of the fibular neck, it gives off three terminal branches: the recurrent articular nerve, the superficial peroneal nerve, and the deep peroneal nerve. Etiologies of *common peroneal neuropathy* include extrinsic compression due to prolonged immobilization, extrinsic compression due to space-occupying lesions, traumatic injury following fibular-head fracture, knee dislocation, or knee surgery, and post-traumatic compartment syndrome.

MR findings include intraneural T2 hyperintensity at the level of the knee joint, space-occupying lesions, and denervation signs involving both the anterior and lateral compartment muscles (Fig. 4).

Anterior Tarsal Tunnel Syndrome

This syndrome is caused by compression of the deep peroneal nerve as it travels deep to the superior and inferior extensor retinacula, or at the level of the talonavicular joint as it travels deep to the extensor hallucis

longus tendon. Distally, the deep peroneal nerve may also be entrapped at the level of the first and second tarsometatarsal joints as it travels in a tight tunnel beneath the extensor hallucis brevis muscle. Etiologies include stretching of the nerve secondary to ankle instability; direct trauma to the dorsum of the foot, hypertrophic extensor hallucis brevis muscle, os intermetatarsum in the proximal first intermetatarsal space, dorsal degenerative spurs at the talonavicular joint, and tight-fitting shoes.

MR findings include denervation atrophy and edema of the anterior compartment muscles.

Superficial Peroneal Neuropathy

The nerve exits through the deep fascia of the lateral leg compartment about 12.5 cm above the tip of the lateral malleolus. Etiologies of superficial peroneal neuropathy include overstretching during inversion and plantar flexion ankle injuries, thickening of the deep fascia of the lateral leg, and lateral compartment muscle hernia/fascial defects.

MR findings include fascial defect or fascial thickening with or without hernia of the peroneal muscle.

Tarsal Tunnel Syndrome

The tarsal tunnel contains the posterior tibial nerve and its branches. Etiologies of tarsal tunnel syndrome include osseous spurs, fracture fragments or tarsal coalition, space-occupying lesions, congenital foot deformities, and systemic diseases (diabetes, peripheral vascular disease) [7, 8].

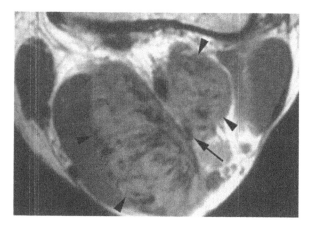

Fig. 3. Proximal tibial neuropathy. Axial T1-weighted image demonstrating fibromatosis in the popliteal fossa (*arrowheads*), producing compression of the tibial nerve (*arrow*)

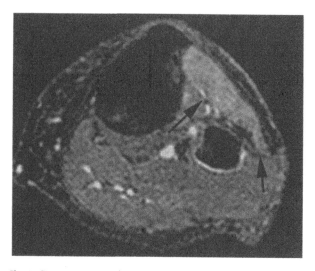

Fig. 4. Common peroneal neuropathy. Axial STIR image demonstrating denervation edema of the muscles of the anterior compartment of the leg (*arrows*), including the tibialis anterior, extensor hallicus longus, extensor digitorum longus, peroneus longus, and peroneus brevis muscles

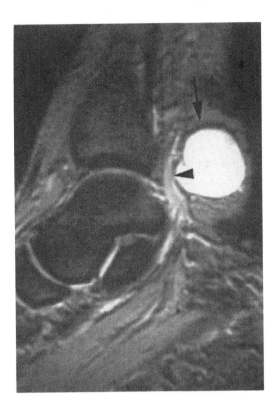

Fig. 5. Tarsal tunnel syndrome. Sagittal gradient-recalled echo (GRE) image demonstrating a large ganglion cyst (*arrow*), producing compression of the posterior tibial nerve (*arrowhead*) at the level of the tarsal tunnel

MR findings include increased size and signal of the tibial nerve and its branches (infrequent), denervation edema of the plantar muscles of the foot, space-occupying lesions, and enhancement of the tarsal tunnel on postgadolinium images (Fig. 5).

Baxter's Neuropathy

This condition may arise secondary to compression of the inferior calcaneal nerve. Etiologies include entrapment by a hypertrophied abductor hallucis muscle, particularly in runners; inferior calcaneal enthesophyte/thickened plantar fascia as the nerve courses anterior to the medial calcaneal tuberosity; stretching secondary to a hypermobile pronated foot: and plantar fasciitis.

MR findings include denervation edema or fatty atrophy of the abductor digiti minimi muscle.

Jogger's Foot

Entrapment of the medial plantar nerve between the abductor hallucis muscle and the anatomic crossover between the flexor digitorum longus and the flexor hallucis longus tendons results in jogger's foot (Henry's knot). Etiologies include heel valgus and excessive pronation while running and a high medial arch [9].

MR findings include muscle denervation edema or atrophy of the abductor hallucis, flexor digitorum brevis, flexor hallucis brevis, and first lumbrical. Space-occupying masses can be found in the fat plane interposed between the abductor hallucis and the flexor digitorum brevis muscles.

Morton's Neuroma

The cause of Morton's neuroma is chronic entrapment of the interdigital nerve under the intermetatarsal ligament. It is more often found at the second and third intermetatarsal spaces.

MR findings include a teardrop-shaped soft-tissue mass emanating from the intermetatarsal space and extending plantarly. The mass typically demonstrates low signal intensity on T1-and T2-weighted images, with variable hyperintensiy on fluid-sensitive sequences. Postcontrast enhancement is often noted.

References

1. Andreisek G, Crook DW, Burg D et al (2006) Peripheral neuropathies of the median, radial, and ulnar nerves: MR imaging features. Radiographics 26(5):1267-1287
2. Bencardino JT, Rosenberg ZS (2006) Entrapment neuropathies of the shoulder and elbow in the athlete. Clin Sports Med 25:465-487
3. Bencardino JT, Rosenberg ZS (2007) Entrapment neuropathies of the upper extremity. In: Stoller DW (ed) Magnetic resonance imaging in orthopaedics and sports medicine, 3rd edn. Lippincott Williams and Wilkins, Baltimore, pp 1933-1976
4. Bordalo-Rodrigues M, Amin P, Rosenberg ZS (2004) MR imaging of common entrapment neuropathies at the wrist. Magn Reson Imaging Clin N Am (12):265-279
5. Erbay H (2002) Meralgia paresthetica in differential diagnosis of low-back pain. Clin J Pain 18:132-135
6. Grothaus MC, Holt M, Mekhail AO et al (2005) Lateral femoral cutaneous nerve: an anatomic study. Clin Orthop Relat Res 437:164-168
7. Delfaut E, Demondion X, Bieganski A et al (2003) Imaging of foot and ankle nerve entrapment syndromes: from well demonstrated to unfamiliar sites. Radiographics 23:613-623
8. Schon LC, Baxter DE (1990) Neuropathies of the foot and ankle in athletes. Clin Sports Med 9:489-509
9. Rask MR (1978) Medial plantar neuropraxia (jogger's foot): report of 3 cases. Clin Orthop Relat Res 134:193-195

Special Aspects of Musculoskeletal Imaging in Children

Diego Jaramillo[1], Paul K. Kleinman[2]

[1] Department of Radiology, The Children's Hospital of Philadelphia, Philadelphia, PA, USA
[2] Department of Radiology, Children's Hospital Boston, Boston, MA, USA

The Changing Skeleton in the Child

In children, the skeleton undergoes multiple changes with age. These age-related transformations determine the distribution of disease, the patterns of injury, and their imaging characteristics. During development, cartilage is converted to bone and hematopoietic marrow to fatty marrow. Most epiphyses and apophyses are cartilaginous at birth and become increasingly ossified [1]. Epiphyseal cartilage has intermediate signal intensity on T1-weighted images and low signal intensity on water-sensitive images. Epiphyseal cartilage is normally hypointense along the body's weight-bearing regions [2]. Within the epiphyseal cartilage there is no capillary network; instead, there are multiple vascular canals which contain the veins and arteries that bring nutrients to the chondrocytes [3]. These can be visible as parallel striations on neonatal sonograms, and Doppler interrogation demonstrates flow within them [4]. Following contrast administration, magnetic resonance imaging (MRI) will show the vascular canals, which become arranged in a radial pattern as the ossification centers develop [5].

The physis, or growth plate, initially a flat disk between the epiphysis and metaphysis, becomes progressively undulated after puberty and ultimately closes [6]. It is of high signal intensity on most MRI sequences and the zone of provisional calcification is uniformly hypointense. With physeal closure, the high signal intensity of cartilage disappears [7]. The interfaces between bone and cartilage are particularly prone to injury [8]. The physis is weakest at the zone of provisional calcification, where endochondral ossification occurs. In infants, physeal injuries are primarily separations of the entire cartilaginous epiphyses [9], whereas in adolescents the fractures through the undulating physis have a complex course [10]. Apophyses tend to be avulsed at the base, where apophyseal cartilage meets the parent bone.

The bony envelope, composed of the periosteum and perichondrium, also changes considerably during childhood. The periosteal attachments are loose and there is a layer of fibrovascular tissue between the bone and the periosteum which is visible on routine MRI. This layer, or "metaphyseal stripe", is of high signal intensity on T2-weighted images, enhances with contrast administration, and disappears during adolescence [11]. The perichondrium is tightly attached to the bone [12]. This helps in fracture remodeling, as the periosteum becomes like the string of a bow – attached to the perichondrium on the physeal side and to the uninjured bone on the other side of the fracture. Tight perichondral attachments limit the spread of subperiosteal collections or tumors. In the classic metaphyseal lesion of infant abuse, the perichondrium retains a rim of juxtaphyseal cortex, seen as a bucket handle or a corner fracture on radiographs [13].

Marrow development follows a predictable pattern, both within each extremity and each individual bone. The marrow, initially entirely hematopoietic, becomes fatty from the periphery (phalanges of the fingers and toes) to the center (proximal humeri and femora) [14]. In each bone, the epiphyses become fatty first, followed by the diaphysis and finally the metaphyses [14]. In the axial skeleton, hematopoietic marrow persists throughout childhood and adolescence. Hematopoietic marrow although predominantly cellular, contains 40% fat and thus on T1-weighted images its signal intensity is higher than that of muscle or marrow infiltrated by disease [15]. Therefore, if on MRI the marrow is of lower signal intensity than adjacent muscle on T1-weighted images or has signal intensity that is close or equal to that of water on water-sensitive sequences, it is likely pathologic [15]. The distribution of marrow also influences the occurrence of disease, as hematopoietic marrow is more highly vascularized and thus prone to blood-borne disease whereas fatty marrow is more prone to osteonecrosis.

The thin, porous bony cortex of the newborn is transformed to dense lamellar bone beginning in the diaphysis; metaphyseal fractures usually occur at the point of transition between the two types of bone [16]. The bones of children often bow rather than break, and fractures, particularly in the radius and ulna, often involve only one cortex [17]. The pelvis of a child is elastic and often breaks in a single place instead of in two places. Fracture healing is faster in younger children.

The ligaments are perhaps the strongest element in the child's skeleton, such that ligamentous injuries are unusual in children under the age of ten. In the knee, the posterior cruciate ligament of the child has a longer horizontal segment and the anterior cruciate ligament (ACL) is more vertical than in the adult [18].

The intrameniscal nutrient vessels are horizontal, bisect the meniscus, originate from the capsular attachment, and do not extend to the articular surface [19]. Meniscal tears are usually vertical in the pediatric population [20].

Normal Age-Related Variants and Related Diseases

Normal variants are often bilateral, but reassuring symmetry is not always present; therefore comparison radiographs are usually not helpful and constitute a source of unnecessary radiation exposure. It is useful to think of variants by site.

Epiphyseal and Apophyseal

Irregularity of the secondary center of ossification of the distal femur is found in approximately two-thirds of boys and 40% of girls [21]. It involves both condyles in 44%, and only the medial condyle in 12%. Accessory centers of ossification are more conspicuous in the posterior femoral condyles, where active ossification is occurring [22]. This active ossification also results in areas of high signal intensity in the epiphyseal cartilage, which at times can look cystic; these are termed "pre-ossification changes".

The tibial tubercle ossifies between 8 and 12 years in girls and 9 and 14 years in boys and is normally irregular. Osgood-Schlatter disease, a chronic avulsive injury to the ossifying tubercle, is characterized on imaging studies by edema in the tubercle, patellar tendon, and adjacent soft tissues; irregularity of the tubercle can be normal and is not sufficient to suspect the disease [23]. The calcaneal apophyseal center ossifies in girls 4-6 years of age and in boys 4-9 years of age, and is uneven, asymmetric, fragmented, and sclerotic. Normal calcaneal sclerosis decreases with disuse of the foot. Sever's disease (calcaneal apophysitis from repetitive trauma [24]) can be diagnosed, just like Osgood-Schlatter disease, by MRI evidence of edema of the marrow of the apophysis.

Physeal

A pseudofracture produced by one end of the physeal disc projecting over the other is easily recognized in the proximal humerus, but can be confused with a lateral condylar fracture in the distal humerus. A normal undulation of the medial distal tibia occurs at the site of normal closure; this is known as Poland's or Kump's bump and is located just above the medial talar hump [7]. The asymmetric closure of the physis accounts for growth arrest after physeal injuries. The irregularity of the physis is also the reason for the complex courses of adolescent fractures of the distal tibia, juvenile Tillaux fracture, and triplane fracture [25].

Metaphyseal

The juxtaphyseal metaphysis of weight-bearing bones can be sclerotic in children between 2 and 6 years of age. The metaphyseal band seen in lead intoxication also affects non-weight-bearing bones such as the fibula [26].

After a period of slowing of growth, there is mineralization of a disc of bone. When the physis migrates away from it, a growth recovery line, the Harris line, is formed [27]. This line, like the rings on a tree, is an indication of prior stress and can be seen in sick neonates as well as in children with leukemia or receiving biphosphonate therapy and in methotrexate osteopathy. Tendinous insertions at metadiaphyseal junctions are prone to repeated minor avulsive injury. The cortex becomes excavated and there can be an appearance of a well-defined lesion on radiographs or on MRI or computed tomography (CT) coronal sections [28]. This is seen most prominently at the insertion of the medial head of the gastrocnemius muscle in the distal medial femoral metaphysis, where it can resemble a neoplasm. In difficult cases, limited CT or MRI can confirm the excavation and the absence of a soft-tissue mass.

The imaging characteristics of the metaphysis are also a reflection of the skeletal history of the child, what Gideon has referred to as the fourth dimension of imaging studies [29]. As the child grows, lesions in the vicinity of the physis are left behind, falsely appearing to migrate towards the diaphysis.

Round Bones

The navicular is the last tarsal bone to ossify. There are normally two ossification centers, but multiple irregular, dense centers can develop and fuse by age 20. Normal irregular ossification should not be confused with aseptic necrosis of the navicular bone (Kohler's disease), which affects older children, is associated with pain, and has characteristic findings of osteonecrosis on MRI, including marrow edema, lack of enhancement, and edema of the surrounding tissues [30].

Accessory ossification centers develop adjacent to the main center of round bones [30]. Some of these are seen in the patella, the tarsal navicular, and the talus. On occasion, these centers can be painful. Scintigraphic evaluation of such "normal variants" can reveal increased uptake; MRI can demonstrate marrow edema and edema of the adjacent soft tissues (Fig. 1).

Advanced Imaging Strategies

Plain radiography is usually the first and often the only diagnostic modality used for evaluation of the skeleton.

Magnetic Resonance Imaging

The modality of choice for evaluating congenital abnormalities of the spine, including vertebral segmentation

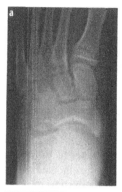
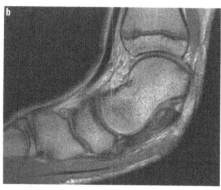
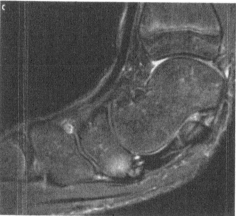
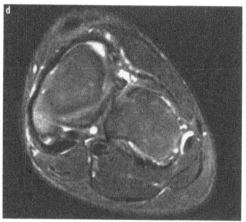

Fig. 1 a-d. 13-year-old with mid foot pain. **a** Frontal radiograph shows a tiny accessory ossicle adjacent to the most proximal aspect of the navicular. **b** Sagittal intermediate weighted image shows the accessory navicular, which has lower signal intensity than the adjacent marrow. **c** Sagittal STIR image shows high signal intensity in the marrow of the navicular and of the accessory ossicle. The tendon of the posterior tibialis is seen to insert in the accessory navicular. There is a bridge of bone joining the accessory navicular to the main bone, which defines it as a developing cornuate variety. **d** Coronal (short axis) T2-weighted imaging shows the insertion of the posterior tibialis tendon into the accessory navicular

defects and significant abnormalities in the location of the conus medullaris (normally at the L2 level, more caudal if the cord is tethered), is MRI [31]. In older children, MRI is optimal for evaluating protrusion or herniation of intervertebral discs, spinal stenosis, and nerve-root compression.

MRI is also the best technique for evaluation of most cases of osteomyelitis, with the exception of infants presenting without localizing signs [30, 32]. Osteomyelitis in children is most often hematogenous and has its primary focus in the metaphysis of long bones, particularly those that grow fast, like the tibia and femur. MRI is crucial in cases of suspected spinal osteomyelitis, as it depicts epidural abscess and extension of the infection into the paraspinal soft tissues. In pelvic osteomyelitis, MRI is useful because the anatomy is complex and involvement of the soft tissues is frequent. Metaphyseal equivalents, bone at the junction with the triradiate cartilage and other synchondroses of the pelvis, are the usual sites of origin and can be easy to miss if they are not specifically sought. Multiple sites are present in nearly 40% of patients and soft-tissue abscesses in 55% [33]. In patients who do not respond after 48 h of antibiotics, MRI can help exclude a subperiosteal or soft-tissue abscess. In osteomyelitis involving the physis, MRI provides adequate mapping of the infection to minimize the

risk of growth arrest during drainage. Gadolinium enhancement is useful to increase the degree of confidence in the diagnosis of an abscess but does not significantly improve the sensitivity or specificity to diagnose osteomyelitis. The use of total-body MRI has facilitated the diagnosis of multifocal disease without localizing signs [34].

A discoid meniscus, one of the most common causes of knee pain in children, is well depicted by MRI, with a reported sensitivity and specificity of 87 and 99%, respectively, if a cut-off width of 15 mm is used [35, 36]. The diagnosis of the incomplete variant of discoid meniscus may more be challenging. For traumatic derangements of the joint, seen mostly in older children and adolescents, MRI can help in the evaluation of meniscal and ligamentous pathologies [20] and in the detection of occult chondral injuries, which are present in nearly one third of patients [37]. ACL tears in the immature patient tend to affect boys more often than girls.

Trauma to cartilaginous structures can also be evaluated by MRI, which can detect epiphyseal separation related to birth trauma or child abuse [9]; extension of a lateral or medial condylar fracture into the unossified epiphysis of the elbow; and chronic stress injury to the physis [38]. Stress injury is most commonly seen as a sports-related phenomenon and the affected physis varies according to the injuring activity: distal radius in gymnasts, proximal humerus and medial epicondyle in baseball players, distal femur in hockey players, and distal tibia in soccer players. MRI shows widening of the physis and areas of premature bridging; if the activity is not discontinued, the physis can close prematurely. In patients with a post-traumatic bony bridge, MRI can define the size and location of the bridge and the percentage of the physis affected by the abnormality. A 3D gradient recalled echo sequence allows axial maximal intensity projections of the physeal cartilage, which permit quantification and mapping of physeal bridging [6].

Juvenile osteochondritis dissecans is diagnosed by a high T2 signal intensity rim, surrounding cysts, high T2 signal intensity cartilage fracture line, and a fluid-filled osteochondral defect [39]. However, these criteria are not as specific for osteochondritis in children as they are in the adult. In children under 10 years of age, it is important to differentiate osteochondritis dissecans from the normal ossification irregularity of the knee, in which the overlying cartilage is intact and there is no evidence of fluid surrounding the lesion.

MRI is also extremely useful for the evaluation of bone ischemia, at three different stages: At presentation, if the radiographs are normal or near normal, it is important to assess whether there is blood flow to the femoral head [40]. In established disease, MRI can define the location of the osteonecrosis, and determine the degree of femoral head involvement, thus predicting the degree of subsequent collapse [41, 42]. MRI can also help in the preoperative evaluation of advanced disease by detecting growth arrest and defining the degree of congruity and containment of the articular surfaces.

Gadolinium-enhanced imaging can detect ischemia related to abduction during treatment for developmental dysplasia of the hip [43, 44]. A global decrease in perfusion is associated with subsequent risk of avascular necrosis of the hip, regardless of the angle of abduction or the age of reduction.

The length of an intramedullary tumor is best depicted on T1-weighted images obtained with a large field-of-view [45, 46]. These images can detect skip lesions while total-body MRI can depict metastatic disease (Fig. 2). It is important to evaluate epiphyseal extension of the tumor, as osteosarcomas involve the epiphysis in 80% of patients. Dynamic gadolinium-enhanced MRI and diffusion-weighted imaging can differentiate between areas of increased activity in tumors and areas of necrosis [46].

Synovial inflammation, as can be seen in juvenile idiopathic arthritis and in seronegative arthritides, is also detected using MRI, and sonography [47, 48]. Active synovial inflammation presents as areas of increased vascularity on Doppler sonography and increased gadolinium enhancement on contrast-enhanced MRI. Synovial proliferation can be well-depicted with both modalities. MRI can also depict early changes in the structure of the cartilage and early cartilaginous erosions.

Cross-sectional Measurements

Glenoid version is the angle between the main axis of the scapula and the glenoid. It is measured in the context of glenoid dysplasia from brachial plexus palsy [49]. Femoral anteversion is determined by obtaining axial slices from the femoral head to the lesser trochanter, and slices through the femoral condyles. A line through the main axis of the femoral neck and another along the posterior surfaces of the distal femoral condyles form the angle of femoral anteversion. The normal angle is 32° at birth and 16° by age 16; it is increased with hip dysplasia and decreased or negative in children at risk for slipped capital femoral epiphysis. Tibial torsion is determined by the angle between a line through the center of the epiphysis (representing the main axis of the proximal tibia) and a line connecting the distal tibial malleoli. Tibial torsion is normally 4° at birth and 14° at 10 years of age; when abnormal, it causes in-or out-toeing [50, 51].

Scintigraphy and PET

Scintigraphy and positron emission tomography (PET) are useful whenever the entire body is to be evaluated, such as for surveillance of metastatic disease (Fig. 2). Metastatic neuroblastoma is best detected using ^{123}I-MIBG, as it accumulates in 90-95% of neuroblastoma metastases [52]. There have not been sufficiently large studies comparing whole-body MRI and ^{18}F-FDG-PET/CT for evaluation of skeletal metastases. Although both techniques have been reported to be of very high sensitivity and specificity, the results of studies so far have not shown a conclusive superiority of one modality over the other. ^{18}F-FDG-PET is useful for diagnosing occult infections such as in patients with fever of unknown origin [53, 54]. Skeletal scintigraphy is also highly sensitive for evaluation of avascular necrosis and early identification of traumatic injuries, such as stress injuries in athletes. In child abuse, skeletal scintigraphy complements the radiographic skeletal survey, particularly when radiographic findings are negative or uncertain. Technetium scintigraphy and fluorine-18 NaF-PET are very sensitive for rib fractures and diaphyseal fractures, but often fail to detect linear skull fractures or certain metaphyseal injuries [55]. It is important to remember that skeletal structures that have not yet ossified have no Tc-99m diphosphonate uptake. For example, a "cold" femoral capital epiphysis during the first 6 months of life does not mean ischemia, and decreased activity in the tarsal navicular below the ages of 2 years in girls and 4 years in boys does not mean Kohler's disease.

Sonography

Sonography is the modality of choice for evaluation of developmental dysplasia of the hip [56, 57]. Sonography is indicated in young infants with an abnormal examination or when there are risk factors, such as a positive family history, breech delivery, oligohydramnios, and three conditions indicating uterine crowding: torticollis, club-

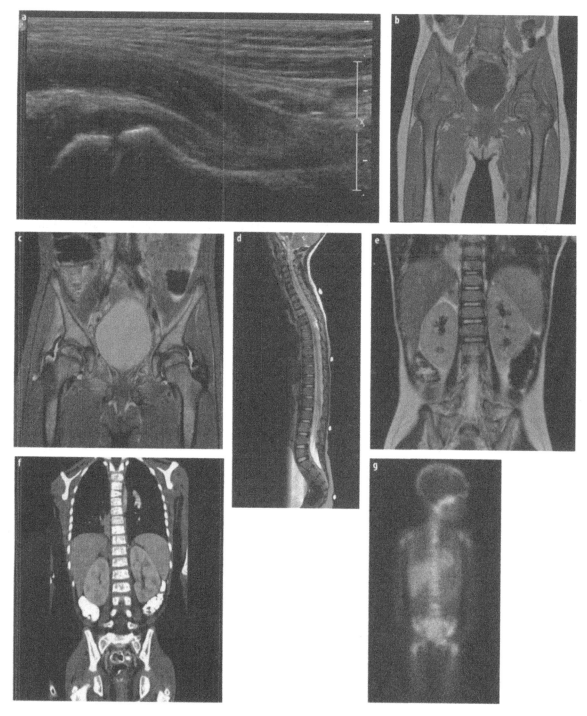

Fig. 2 a-g. 4 year-old boy presenting with left hip pain. Radiographs were difficult to evaluate because the patient was unable to extend the hip. **a** Sagittal ultrasound of the hip shows no evidence of effusion or other abnormality. **b** Coronal T2-weighted image shows that the marrow from the proximal femoral epiphyses (which should be completely fatty by the end of the first year of age) has multiple areas of low signal intensity. Additionally, the marrow of the metaphyses, pelvis, and spine is of very low signal intensity. **c** Coronal STIR images show diffusely increased signal intensity of the marrow and edema of the adjacent musculature, indicative of cellular infiltration. This, together with the findings on theT2-weighted image, suggest leukemia, metastatic neuroblastoma, or some metastatic sarcoma. **d** Sagittal T2-weighted imaging of the entire spine shows diffusely increased signal intensity in the vertebral bodies of T3, T5, and L3, with partial collapse of T5. **e** Coronal T2-weighted image following gadolinium administration shows a right adrenal mass with a central area of decreased enhancement, consistent with a neuroblastoma. **f** Coronal reconstruction of a multidetector CT confirms the right adrenal mass consistent with a neuroblastoma, and the collapse of T5. On bone windows, the texture of multiple bones was inhomogeneous. **g** 223I-MIBG scan shows increased activity throughout the axial skeleton, the proximal humeri, femurs and bony pelvis, consistent with metastatic disease from neuroblastoma

foot, and metatarsus adductus. The study is ideally performed 4-6 weeks after birth, as most of the abnormalities detected in the newborn resolve during this period. In hip dysplasia, sonography demonstrates a shallow, vertical acetabulum, a femoral head covered <50%, a blunted acetabular rim, and, in severe cases, the presence of obstacles to reduction, such as a pulvinar (echogenic fibrofatty tissue within the joint) and an interposed acetabular labrum.

The cartilage of the femoral head and the acetabulum is sonolucent, the bones of the acetabular roof and femoral metaphysis are very echogenic, and the fibrocartilaginous labrum is moderately echogenic. The coronal view, oriented like a frontal radiograph, shows the acetabular morphology. The angle between the iliac wing and the bony acetabulum (the alpha angle) is approximately 60° in the normal newborns. The sonolucent cartilaginous acetabulum is more concave than the bony roof and is in direct contact with the cartilaginous epiphysis. Ossification of the proximal femoral epiphysis, which begins weeks before its radiographic appearance, is protective against avascular necrosis. The transverse motion is best for visualizing articular relationships during the Barlow maneuver. Laxity with a posterior displacement of 6 mm during the Barlow maneuver is seen in infants <2 weeks of age. Immaturity can persist for the first 3 months of life.

Septic arthritis secondary to osteomyelitis usually involves the proximal femur, where the metaphysis is intracapsular. In septic arthritis, sonography can aid in the detection of joint effusion. An effusion is a relatively hypoechoic collection between the capsule and the femoral neck. There is no relationship between the amount or echogenicity of the joint fluid and its likelihood of being infected. On Doppler sonography, increased flow in the capsule is sensitive but not specific for infection [58]. A negative sonogram virtually excludes septic arthritis (Fig. 2). Ultimately, if septic arthritis is suspected and fluid is detected, the hip should be tapped and the fluid analyzed. Kocher defined four criteria for the diagnosis of septic arthritis: reduced range of motion, fever, increased sedimentation rate, and increased white blood cell count. Sonography is only indicated when there is moderate probability of septic arthritis, that is, when two of these criteria are present [59]. A stronger clinical suspicion is an indication for hip drainage, whereas a weaker suspicion only demands observation. Sonography also can assist in providing guidance for the tap. In Legg-Calvé-Perthes disease, sonography can indicate the degree and location of vascular reperfusion [60]. Sonography has been used extensively for the imaging of osteomyelitis, suggested by the presence of fluid in the subperiosteal space and soft tissues or by deep soft-tissue edema and increased perfusion. In the evaluation of tumors, sonography is still the best way to characterize whether the lesion is solid or cystic; for soft-tissue tumors; other findings, such as calcification or tumor vascularity, can also be assessed.

Computed Tomography

In pediatric CT, it is paramount to minimize radiation exposure by optimizing technique and using automatic exposure control and shielding. Exposure factors for pediatric musculoskeletal CT include a kV of 80-100 and a mA of 50-100 [61]. CT is a useful adjunct to plain radiography whenever multiplanar and 3D reconstructions are necessary (Fig. 2). CT is optimal for detection of subtle fractures, such as scaphoid injuries, and suspected elbow injuries. The best images and the least exposure are obtained by imaging the patient prone, with the upper extremity extended over the head and partially flexed at the elbow, and the head moved laterally, such that the elbow is superior to the vertex of the skull and the forearm is angled 45° to the z axis.

In complex fractures, such as Tillaux fractures of the distal tibia, CT can show the number and location of fragments and determine whether the separation between epiphyseal fragments is larger than 2 mm, the threshold beyond which open reduction is necessary. Bony healing in fractures and spondylolysis is also best determined by CT. In a slipped capital femoral epiphysis, CT demonstrates the degree of inferior and posterior displacement of the femoral head and the retroversion of the contralateral femur [62]. In acetabular fractures, 3D reconstructions better demonstrate the relationships between fragments.

In infants with hip dislocation who have undergone reduction and placement of the hips in an abduction cast, CT can be used to assess the position of the femoral heads. Very low exposure factors can be used such that the total ovarian dose is as low as 112 mRad (1.12 mGy) [63]. In adolescents and young adults with undetected hip dysplasia or impingement syndromes, CT demonstrates the configuration and containment of the femoral head, the acetabular architecture, and the development of early degenerative changes in the joint or the acetabular rim. MRI, particularly with volumetric acquisitions and appropriate reformats, is an attractive alternative to CT, entailing no ionizing radiation and providing assessment of the articular cartilage.

Talo-calcaneal coalition is best assessed in the coronal plane, whereas calcaneo-navicular coalitions (which can be diagnosed with oblique radiographs) are best seen in the sagittal plane [64]. Both feet should be studied, as bilateral abnormalities exist in up to 80% of patients and multiple coalitions may occur in 20%. CT images demonstrate a complete osseous fusion if the coalition is bony, or irregularity of the adjacent bones if they are fibrous/cartilaginous. CT is useful to characterize benign osseous lesions, such as normal variants, osteochondromas, and fibrous dysplasia, as the findings can be correlated closely with those of conventional radiographs.

References

1. Rivas R, Shapiro, F (2002) Structural stages in the development of the long bones and epiphyses: A study in the New Zealand white rabbit. J Bone Joint Surg 84-A:85-100

2. Hopkins KL, Li KC, Bergman G (1995) Gadolinium-DTPA-enhanced magnetic resonance imaging of musculoskeletal infectious processes. Skeletal Radiol 24:325-330
3. Jaramillo D, Villegas-Medina OL, Doty DK et al (2004) Age-related vascular changes in the epiphysis, physis, and metaphysis: normal findings on gadolinium-enhanced MRI of piglets. AJR Am J Roentgenol 182:353-360
4. Yousefzadeh DK, Doerger K, Sullivan C (2008) The blood supply of early, late, and nonossifying cartilage: preliminary gray-scale and Doppler assessment and their implications. Pediatr Radiol 38:146-158
5. Barnewolt CE, Shapiro F, Jaramillo D (1997) Normal gadolinium-enhanced MR images of the developing appendicular skeleton: Part I. Cartilaginous epiphysis and physis. AJR Am J Roentgenol 169:183-189
6. Ecklund K, Jaramillo D (2001) Imaging of growth disturbance in children. Radiol Clin North Am 39:823-841
7. Chung T, Jaramillo D (1995) Normal maturing distal tibia and fibula: changes with age at MR imaging. Radiology 194:227-232
8. Shapiro F (2001) Developmental Bone Biology. In: Shapiro F (ed) Pediatric orthopaedic deformities. Academic Press, San Diego, pp 21-53
9. Nimkin K, Kleinman PK, Teeger S et al (1995) Distal humeral physeal injuries in child abuse: MR imaging and ultrasonography findings. Pediatr Radiol 25:562-565
10. Jaramillo D, Kammen BF, Shapiro F (2000) Cartilaginous path of physeal fracture-separations: evaluation with MR imaging – an experimental study with histologic correlation in rabbits. Radiology 215:504-511
11. Laor T, Chun GF, Dardzinski BJ et al (2002) Posterior distal femoral and proximal tibial metaphyseal stripes at MR imaging in children and young adults. Radiology 224:669-674
12. Shapiro F, Holtrop ME, Glimcher MJ (1977) Organization and cellular biology of the perichondrial ossification groove of Ranvier: a morphological study in rabbits. J Bone Joint Surg 59:703-723
13. Kleinman PK, Marks SC Jr (1995) Relationship of the subperiosteal bone collar to metaphyseal lesions in abused infants. J Bone Joint Surg 77:1471-1476
14. Vogler JB, 3rd, Murphy WA (1988) Bone marrow imaging. Radiology 168:679-693
15. Meyer JS, Siegel MJ, Farooqui SO et al (2005) Which MRI sequence of the spine best reveals bone-marrow metastases of neuroblastoma? Pediatr Radiol 35:778-785
16. Ogden J (1991) The uniqueness of growing bones. In: CA Rockwood J, Wilkins K, King R (eds) Fractures in children. JB Lippincott, Philadelphia, pp 50-51
17. Laor T, Jaramillo D, Oestreich AE (1998) Musculoskeletal system. In: Kirks DR, Griscom NT (eds) Practical pediatric imaging: diagnostic radiology of infants and children. Lippincott-Raven, Philadelphia, pp 327-510
18. Kim HK, Laor T, Shire NJ et al (2008) Anterior and posterior cruciate ligaments at different patient ages: MR imaging findings. Radiology 247:826-835
19. Clark CR, Ogden JA (1983) Development of the menisci of the human knee joint. Morphological changes and their potential role in childhood meniscal injury. J Bone Joint Surg [Am] 65:538-547
20. Major NM, Beard LN Jr, Helms CA (2003) Accuracy of MR imaging of the knee in adolescents. AJR Am J Roentgenol 180:17-19
21. Caffey J, Madell SH, Royer C, Morales P (1958) Ossification of the distal femoral epiphysis. J Bone Joint Surg 40-A:647-654
22. Nawata K, Teshima R, Morio Y, Hagino H (1999) Anomalies of ossification in the posterolateral femoral condyle: assessment by MRI. Pediatr Radiol 29:781-784
23. Ogden JA, Southwick WO (1976) Osgood-Schlatter's disease and tibial tuberosity development. Clin Orthop Rel Res 116:180-189
24. Cassas KJ, Cassettari-Wayhs A (2006) Childhood and adolescent sports-related overuse injuries. American family physician 73:1014-1022
25. Brown SD, Kasser JR, Zurakowski D, Jaramillo D (2004) Analysis of 51 tibial triplane fractures using CT with multiplanar reconstruction. AJR Am J Roentgenol 183:1489-1495
26. Blickman JG, Wilkinson RH, Graef JW (1986) The radiologic "lead band" revisited. AJR Am J Roentgenol 146:245-247
27. Ogden J (1990) Injury to the growth mechanisms. In: Ogden J (ed) Skeletal injury in the child. Saunders, Philadelphia, pp 97-174
28. Laor T, Jaramillo D (2009) MR imaging insights into skeletal maturation: what is normal? Radiology 250:28-38
29. Poznanski AK (1978) Annual oration. Diagnostic clues in the growing ends of bone. J Can Assoc Radiol 29:7-21
30. Kan JH, Kleinman PK (2007) Pediatric and adolescent musculoskeletal MRI: a case based approach. Springer, Berlin Heidelberg New York
31. Medina LS, Crone K, Kuntz KM (2001) Newborns with suspected occult spinal dysraphism: a cost-effectiveness analysis of diagnostic strategies. Pediatrics 108:E101
32. Kleinman PK (2002) A regional approach to osteomyelitis of the lower extremities in children. Radiol Clin North Am 40:1033-1059
33. Connolly SA, Connolly LP, Drubach LA et al (2007) MRI for detection of abscess in acute osteomyelitis of the pelvis in children. AJR Am J Roentgenol 189:867-872
34. Darge K, Jaramillo D, Siegel MJ (2008) Whole-body MRI in children: current status and future applications. Eur J Radiol 68:289-298
35. Samoto N, Kozuma M, Tokuhisa T, Kobayashi K (2002) Diagnosis of discoid lateral meniscus of the knee on MR imaging. Magn Reson Imaging 20:59-64
36. Samoto N, Kozuma M, Tokuhisa T, Kobayashi K (2006) Diagnosis of the "large medial meniscus" of the knee on MR imaging. Magn Reson Imaging 24:1157-1165
37. Oeppen RS, Jaramillo D (2003) Sports injuries in the young athlete. Top Magn Reson Imaging 14:199-208
38. Laor T, Wall EJ, Vu LP (2006) Physeal widening in the knee due to stress injury in child athletes. AJR Am J Roentgenol 186:1260-1264
39. Kijowski R, Blankenbaker DG, Shinki K, Fine JP, Graf BK, De Smet AA (2008) Juvenile versus adult osteochondritis dissecans of the knee: appropriate MR imaging criteria for instability. Radiology 248:571-578
40. Lamer S, Dorgeret S, Khairouni A et al (2002) Femoral head vascularisation in Legg-Calvé-Perthes disease: comparison of dynamic gadolinium-enhanced subtraction MRI with bone scintigraphy. Pediatr Radiol 32:580-585
41. de Sanctis N, Rega AN, Rondinella F (2000) Prognostic evaluation of Legg-Calvé-Perthes disease by MRI. Part I: the role of physeal involvement. J Pediatr 20:455-462
42. de Sanctis N, Rondinella F (2000) Prognostic evaluation of Legg-Calvé-Perthes disease by MRI. Part II: pathomorphogenesis and new classification. J Pediatr Orthop 20:463-470
43. Jaramillo D, Villegas-Medina OL, Doty DK et al (1996) Gadolinium-enhanced MR imaging demonstrates abduction-caused hip ischemia and its reversal in piglets. AJR Am J Roentgenol 166:879-887
44. Tiderius C, Jaramillo D, Connolly S et al (2009) Post-closed reduction perfusion magnetic resonance imaging as a predictor of avascular necrosis in developmental hip dysplasia: a preliminary report. J Pediatr Orthop 29:14-20
45. Onikul E, Fletcher BD, Parham DM, Chen G (1996) Accuracy of MR imaging for estimating intraosseous extent of osteosarcoma. AJR Am J Roentgenol 167:1211-1215
46. Reddick WE, Taylor JS, Fletcher BD (1999) Dynamic MR imaging (DEMRI) of microcirculation in bone sarcoma. J Magn Reson Imaging 10:277-285

47. Doria AS, Kiss MH, Lotito AP et al (2001) Juvenile rheumatoid arthritis of the knee: evaluation with contrast-enhanced color Doppler ultrasound. Pediatr Radiol 31:524-531

48. Doria AS, Noseworthy M, Oakden W et al (2006) Dynamic contrast-enhanced MRI quantification of synovium microcirculation in experimental arthritis. AJR Am J Roentgenol 186:1165-1171

49. Waters PM, Smith GR, Jaramillo D (1998) Glenohumeral deformity secondary to brachial plexus birth palsy. J Bone Joint Surg 80:668-677

50. Tomczak RJ, Guenther KP, Rieber A et al (1997) MR imaging measurement of the femoral antetorsional angle as a new technique: comparison with CT in children and adults. AJR Am J Roentgenol 168:791-794

51. Karol LA (1997) Rotational deformities in the lower extremities. Current Opin Pediatr 9:77-80

52. Boubaker A, Bischof Delaloye A (2008) MIBG scintigraphy for the diagnosis and follow-up of children with neuroblastoma. Q J Nucl Med Mol Imaging 52:388-402

53. Bleeker-Rovers CP, Vos FJ, Corstens FH, Oyen WJ (2008) Imaging of infectious diseases using [18F] fluorodeoxyglucose PET. Q J Nucl Med Mol Imaging 52:17-29

54. Bleeker-Rovers CP, Vos FJ, de Kleijn EM et al (2007) A prospective multicenter study on fever of unknown origin: the yield of a structured diagnostic protocol. Medicine 86:26-38

55. Drubach LA, Sapp MV, Laffin S et al (2008) Fluorine-18 NaF PET imaging of child abuse. Pediatr Radiol 38:776-779

56. Rosendahl K, Markestad T, Lie RT (1996) Developmental dysplasia of the hip prevalence based on ultrasound diagnosis. Pediatr Radiol 26:635-639

57. Terjesen T (1998) Ultrasonography for evaluation of hip dysplasia. Methods and policy in neonates, infants, and older children. Acta Orthop Scand 69:653-662

58. Strouse PJ, DiPietro MA, Adler RS (1998) Pediatric hip effusions: evaluation with power Doppler sonography. Radiology 206:731-735

59. Kocher MS, DiCanzio J, Zurakowski D, Micheli LJ (2001) Diagnostic performance of clinical examination and selective magnetic resonance imaging in the evaluation of intraarticular knee disorders in children and adolescents. Am J Sports Med 29:292-296

60. Doria AS, Guarniero R, Molnar LJ et al (2000) Three-dimensional (3D) contrast-enhanced power Doppler imaging in Legg-Calvé-Perthes disease. Pediatr Radiol 30:871-874

61. Chapman VM, Kalra M, Halpern E et al (2005) 16-MDCT of the posttraumatic pediatric elbow: optimum parameters and associated radiation dose. AJR Am J Roentgenol 185:516-521

62. Gekeler J (2007) Radiology of adolescent slipped capital femoral epiphysis: measurement of epiphyseal angles and diagnosis. Operative Orthopadie und Traumatologie 19:329-344

63. Eggli KD, King SH, Boal DK, Quiogue T (1994) Low-dose CT of developmental dysplasia of the hip after reduction: diagnostic accuracy and dosimetry. AJR Am J Roentgenol 163:1441-1443

64. Newman JS, Newberg AH (2000) Congenital tarsal coalition: multimodality evaluation with emphasis on CT and MR imaging. Radiographics 20:321-332; quiz 526-327, 532

Musculoskeletal Ultrasonography

Eugene McNally[1], Stefano Bianchi[2]

[1] Department of Radiology, The Manor Hospital, Headington, Oxford, UK
[2] Institut de Radiologie, Clinique des Grangettes, Geneva, Switzerland

Introduction

Musculoskeletal ultrasound (US) applications continue to show considerable expansion mainly because of technical improvements (development of high-frequency broadband transducers, refined focusing. and sensitive colour and power Doppler technology) and the growing interest of musculoskeletal radiologists. Its low cost, non-invasivity, and possibility to perform the examination directly, e.g., in sport fields, are additional qualities appreciated by the patients. Up to-date, high-level equipment allows the detection of normal anatomic details and identification of a variety of pathologic conditions [1-3]. The possibility to perform a dynamic examination is a specific advantage of US compared to magnetic resonance imaging (MRI) and computed tomography (CT). The introduction of extended-field-of-view technology has allowed the realization of images of larger segments and has facilitated their interpretation by the referring physician. The main disadvantages of US are its limited assessment of internal structures of the joints, bones, and bone marrow.

This chapter presents the basic US aspect of normal and pathologic muscles, tendons, and peripheral nerves, followed by a review of the more common abnormalities of appendicular joints.

Muscles

Ultrasound Anatomy of Muscles

Muscles are composed of muscle fibers and connective tissue, with supporting properties housing vessels and nerves surrounded by loose connective tissue and fat. The muscle fibers insert into intramuscular laminae or tendons (intramuscular fibrous skeleton) that continue with the distal tendon. Ultrasound allows an accurate assessment of the muscles, showing muscle fibers as hypo-anechoic elongated structures while the internal connective tissue (perimysium or fibroadipose septa) appears hyperechoic. In longitudinal sonograms, the perimysium appears as multiples regular hyperechoic lines while in transverse sonograms it has a multiple spotty hyperechoic appearance. The muscle fascia surrounds the muscle belly and presents at US as a regular hyperechoic line encircling the muscle. It s thickness varies among different muscles. At musculotendinous junctions, US depicts the concomitant decrease in the size of the muscle and increase in the size of the tendon. Muscle vessels are easily evaluated with color Doppler technique. A physiological increase in vascularization can be demonstrated during muscle exercise. Dynamic examination is helpful in appreciating muscles changes during contraction. In isometric activation, the muscle shortens and simultaneously enlarges, thus appearing more hypoechoic due to the increase in the size of muscle fibers and relative decrease of the hyperechoic perimysium.

Muscle Diseases

The frequency of muscle trauma has increased due to the rapid expansion in amateur sport activities. US can efficiently locate muscle tears, evaluate their size, differentiate between partial and complete lesions, successfully guide aspiration of hematomas, and allows follow-up and monitoring of healing. Dynamic scans performed during isometric contraction of the affected muscle can help in detecting smaller ruptures. Firm pressure applied through the probe is invaluable in focusing the examination to the point of maximal tenderness, thus shortening the examination time and increasing the possibility to detect subtle injuries that otherwise can go unnoticed. Depending on the site, muscle traumas can be classified as affecting the fascia, muscle, or musculotendinous junction.

Lesions of the Fascia

The most common traumatic lesions of muscle fasciae are herniations. Fascia rupture can involve its central portion or its periosteal attachment. In both cases, US can readily detect and locate the herniations and assess its the diameters [4, 5]. Before starting the US examination it is important to situate clinically the location of the hernia in order to focus the examination and reduce the scanning time. Dynamic scanning obtained with the patient standing, supine, or squatting can increase the pressure inside the muscle compartment, facilitating hernia detection by showing its enlargement through the fascial defect. In smaller lesions, firm pressure with the transducers must be avoided since this can easily reduce the hernia and leads to a false-negative examination. Real-time examination during application of different pressures through the US transducer can improves the assessment of large hernias [4].

Lesion of the Muscles

Traumatic muscles lesions can be due to direct local muscle traumatism (external mechanism) or to maximal powerful contractions performed during simultaneous passive muscle stretching (internal mechanism).

Direct traumatisms are usually observed in contact sports such as rugby or football and mainly involve the quadriceps muscle. The muscle is frequently injured between the knee of a player and the femoral shaft. US shows an ill-defined, hypoechoic, irregular area due to fiber tears, local blood infiltration, and haematoma formation. Post-traumatic muscle calcifications (myositis ossificans) can follow direct muscle trauma and appear as multiple foci of hyperechoic lesions with posterior shadowing. Although, in the proper clinical setting, the US appearance of myositis ossificans is quite typical, standard radiographs are always required to confirm the diagnosis.

Indirect traumatic lesions are mostly located at the myotendinous junctions. Clinical experience and experimental studies [6] have shown that during maximal forceful activation of muscles the first injured site is the musculotendinous junction. Muscles of the lower extremities are more frequently affected. The rectus femoris [7], medial head of the gastrocnemius [8] (Fig. 1) and biceps femoris are involved frequently, since they cross two joints and have a high percentage of muscle type II fibers,

well-suited to rapid forceful activity. Moreover, the possibility of a strain is increased by the fact that these muscles contract in an eccentric manner (i.e., they contract while passively stretched). At US, the retracted muscle fibers show a heterogeneous hypo-hyperechoic appearance due to muscle-fiber rupture and blood infarction. Typically, the fibroadipose septa, which in normal longitudinal images are seen inserting into the distal tendon or aponeurosis, are seen retracted proximally to a variable degree depending on the strength of the trauma. An anechoic fluid collection related to a hematoma is found interposed between the retracted muscle and the tendon in larger lesions. Recently, good results have been reported by US-guided evacuation of the hematoma followed by the application of an elastic bandage, which allows more rapid cicatrization of the tear and an earlier return to sport activities. US can also detect local complications of tears, such as venous thrombosis of the gastrocnemius, which require appropriate treatment.

Non-traumatic muscles disorders are quite uncommon in daily US practice. Muscle tumors are rare. The most common neoplasia is intramuscular lipoma, which appears as a hyperechoic expansible lesion located inside the muscle (intramuscular lipoma) or in the fascial plane among muscles (intermuscular lipomas). The echogenicity of intramuscular lipomas is highly variable. Color Doppler shows absent or weak internal flow signals; these are related to low tumor vascularity. The size of the intramuscular masses cannot be easily assessed by US when the diameters are larger than the size of the probe, although extended field of view technology can be of some help. Moreover, it is sometimes difficult to exactly define the borders of the tumor. For these reasons, MRI with contrast enhancement is almost always required for assessment of muscles masses, particularly in the pre-operative setting.

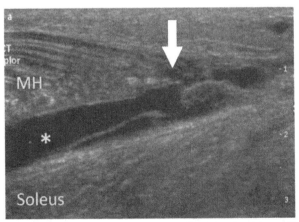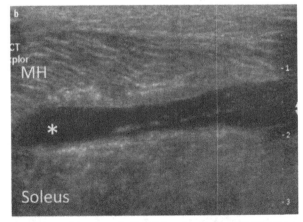

Fig. 1 a, b. Pathologic US appearance of striated muscles. Myotendinous traumatic avulsion. Longitudinal (**a**) and transverse (**b**) US images obtained over the medial aspect of the calf in a patient with tennis leg. (**a**) Note the avulsion of the distal muscle septa of the medial head (*MH*) from the disrupted distal aponeurosis (*arrow*). In both images an anechoic fluid collection (*asterisk*), corresponding to a hematoma, is seen interposed between the medial head and the soleus

Tendons

Ultrasound Anatomy of Tendons

Tendons transmit the forces generated in muscles to bones. They are formed by parallel collagen bundles enfolded by the endotendineum and peritendineum. US allows a detailed assessment of the internal structure of tendons as well as of paratendinous structures. Longitudinal US demonstrates normal tendons as hyperechoic bands of variable thickness characterized by an internal arrangement composed of fine, packed parallel echoes that yield a fibrillar pattern [9]. Such echoes are not related to the collagen bundles but to the interfaces between them and the endotendineum septa [9]. Such echoes are not related to the collagen bundles but to the interfaces between them and the endotendineum septa [9]. Transverse sonograms show tendons as circular or ovoid structures with an internal hyperechoic dotted appearance. It is important to emphasize that the typical US pattern of tendons is evident only when the US beam is perpendicular to them. Any obliquity of the beam results in an artifactual tendon hypoechogenicity, which can simulate a pathologic condition. An accurate technique of examination is therefore essential to avoid diagnostic mistakes.

From the anatomic and biomechanical point of view, tendons can be divided into two main groups. The first group includes tendons that present a straight course and are not prone to friction against other anatomic structures. These tendons are surrounded by paratenon, a loose areolar and adipose tissue envelope adherent to the tendon that facilitates its gliding. At US, the paratenon appears as a hyperechoic tissue in continuity with subcutaneous fat. Tendons of the second group reflect against bones or retinacula and are surrounded by synovial sheaths. The sheath is formed by a visceral layer adherent to the tendon and a parietal layer. Between the two, there is a thin amount of synovial fluid that facilitates frictionless movements, thus preventing tendon damage. The synovial sheath can be appreciated only when the examination is performed with high-resolution equipment and appears as a thin hypoechoic rim surrounding the tendons, related to the physiological amount of normal fluid. The layers of the synovial sheath cannot be visualized in normal conditions.

Tendon Diseases

Tendinosis and Ruptures

Tendinosis is a degenerative disease that results mainly from chronic local microtraumas (Fig. 2). In tendinosis, US shows an enlarged tendon with internal irregularities of the normal internal structure and focal hypoechoic areas [10-11]. Hyperechoic foci with posterior shadowing can be seen in chronic tendinopathy and correspond to tendon calcifications. Histologically, the intratendinous hypoechoic areas correlate with fibromyxoid degeneration while hyperechoic images correlate with calcifications [11].

In partial tear, a localized disruption of some tendon fibers is observed. Since this is almost always associated with changes related to tendinosis, the US distinction between tendon degeneration and small tears is often unfeasible. Nevertheless, high-frequency US can easily differentiate partial from complete tears. This helps the clinician particularly in patients with acute trauma, in which the local edema and pain associated with the injury limit proper physical examination. In full-thickness rupture, a complete disruption of the tendon leads to retraction of the proximal torn edge due to the muscle action. In recent lesions, a hypoechoic hematoma fills the tendon gap whereas in chronic ones granulation tissue can be demonstrated. One of the main applications of US in the evaluation of complete tears is detection of the amount of retraction of the proximal tendon end; this helps in choosing the extent of the surgical incision.

A distinctive type of tendon tears, so-called longitudinal fissurations, can be observed in the ankle tendons. They are particularly evident in the tibialis posterior and peroneal tendons, as a result of repetitive tendons subluxations against the malleoli. US images show tendon splitting as a hypoechoic cleft either partially or completely dividing the tendon into two or more bands. An associated effusion located inside the tendon sheath is usually present and facilitates the recognition of fissures [12].

Inflammatory Conditions

Ultrasound can be used for diagnosing inflammatory conditions affecting tendons of both type 1 and 2. In ten-

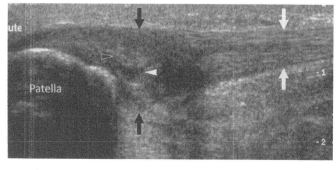

Fig. 2. Pathologic US appearance of tendons. Tendinopathy. Longitudinal US image obtained over the patellar tendon in a patient with "jumper's knee." The distal tendon (*white arrows*) is normal. The affected proximal part (*white arrows*) is swollen and irregular, with hyperechoic (*void arrowhead*) and hypoechoic (black arrowhead) areas indicating degenerative changes

dons of the first group, changes are mainly observed at the level of the peritendon (peritendinitis). Surface irregularities of the outer portion of the tendon appear hypoechoic and do not show a fibrillar appearance. Color Doppler can assess the local inflammatory hyperemia as flow signals into the tendon and in the surrounding tissues. The hallmark of tenosynovitis in tendons of the second group is the presence of an effusion in the tendon sheath. The most common causes of tenosynovitis are trauma, foreign bodies, infection, and arthritis. In post-traumatic tenosynovitis, which can be suspected on the basis of patient history, the fluid collection is usually anechoic. Increased echogenicity of the effusion and the presence of a foreign body within the synovial space can suggest an infective tenosynovitis; however, it must be stressed that a definite diagnosis cannot be made only on the basis of US findings and relies on US-guided fluid aspiration and culture. In tenosynovitis secondary to systemic arthritis, the synovial membrane of the tendon sheath appears hypertrophied and presents at US as hypoechoic villous projections floating inside the effusion. In the most severe cases, the synovial pannus can eventually completely fill the synovial space. Since the hypertrophied synovium can damage the tendons and lead to pathological ruptures, accurate US assessment of tendon borders and echo texture is imperative. In hypertrophic tenosynovitis, color Doppler can help in distinguishing the hypoechoic pannus from effusion, based on the presence or absence of flow signals.

Tendon Dislocation

Dislocation can occur only in tendons of the second group and result from retinacular tears. The most frequent dislocations affect the long head of the biceps tendon, at the shoulder [13], and the peroneal tendons, at the ankle. Due to its tomographic capability, US is well-suited to detect tendon displacement. Transverse images optimally show the relation of the tendons with the osteofibrous tunnels that usually house the tendons. Tears of the retinacula, fibrous bands that hold the tendons in the correct position, can be also detected. Secondary changes, such as tendon sheath effusion due to inflammation of the tendon sheath, are well demonstrated too. Dynamic examination performed during different movements of the arm or foot may detect intermittent subluxation during real-time examination.

Tendon Tumors

Ganglia and the giant cell tumor of the tendon sheath are the most common tendons masses. Ganglia are peritendinous cystic lesions containing mucoid, viscid fluid that usually are found in the hand and foot. They presents at US as multiloculated, well-defined cystic anechoic masses. Rarely, they can grow inside the tendon, thus appearing as hypoechoic internal masses that follow the tendon during dynamic scanning (intratendinous ganglia). Giant

cell tumor of the tendon sheath presents as a painless, slowly growing mass located in close relationship with a tendon. The hand and foot are more commonly affected. US depicts this tumor as a hypoechoic mass with sharp borders located adjacent the tendon. Internal flow signals can be detected at color Doppler. Fibrous and clear cell sarcomas are rare.

Nerves

Ultrasound Anatomy of Nerves

Nerves are formed of nervous fibers grouped in fascicles. The nerve and the fascicles are surrounded by connective tissue, respectively, the epineurium and the perineurium. The US appearance of nerve examined in vitro reflects the nerve's anatomy [14]. Longitudinal sonograms show several hypoechoic parallel linear areas (nerve fascicles) separated by hyperechoic bands (connective tissue), giving the appearance of a fascicular pattern. At transverse scans, the nerve fascicles appear as hypoechoic rounded structures embedded in a hyperechoic background [14, 15] (Fig. 3).

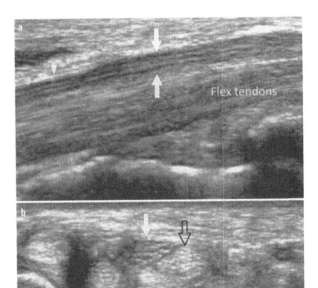

Fig. 3 a, b. Normal US appearance of peripheral nerves. Longitudinal (**a**) and transverse (**b**) US images obtained over the palmar aspect of the wrist. Images show the normal appearance of the median nerve (*white arrows*). Note the internal regular fascicular structure (*white arrowhead*), consisting of parallel hypoechoic nerves fascicles separated by hyperechoic connective tissue. **b** Compare the internal fascicular structure of the nerve with the fibrillar structure of the adjacent flexor digitorum superficialis of the third finger (*void arrow*). *Flex tendons*, Flexor tendons

Most of the peripheral nerves can be identified by US not only on the basis of their appearance but also because of their anatomic location. In doubtful cases, minor movements on dynamic examination performed during muscles activation can help in differentiating peripheral nerves from tendons [16].

Nerve Diseases

Traumatic Lesions

Nerves lesions can result from chronic repetitive microtraumas or a single acute trauma. Recurrent microtraumas are mainly observed in nerves entrapments syndromes, which typically affect nerves that course in unextensible osteofibrous tunnels [17]. US is an effective imaging method to confirm the clinical suspicion of entrapment neuropathy and to plan appropriate treatment since it can depict nerve changes and the cause of the compression. The main nerve findings in chronic entrapments are: localized flattening at the level of compression and proximal bulbous enlargement, hypoechogenicity with loss of fascicular echo texture, and enhanced depiction of flow signals at color Doppler. US can demonstrate different causes of compression [17]. In carpal tunnel syndrome, tenosynovitis of the flexor tendons is seen as an area of hypoechogenicity overlaying the tendons, ganglia as focal anechoic masses without internal flow signals, and accessory muscle as a peculiar muscle architecture and typical behavior at dynamic examination. In cubital tunnel syndrome, elbow osteophytes are depicted as hyperechoic lesions arising from the joint margins.

In nerves injuries secondary to acute traumas, US can appreciate the level of the nerve section as well as the distance between the two nerve ends. This can have practical value in planning operative treatment in patients with multiple traumas at different levels. The defect in the nerve appears as a local discontinuity in nerve fascicles. Partial and complete tears can be differentiated in superficial nerves when a high-resolution probe is deployed. Bulbous neuromas, which present as localized hypoechoic enlargements of the nerve ends, are helpful in detecting the location of the tear.

Nerve Tumors

Most nerve tumors are benign schwannomas and neurofibromas. Schwannomas are encapsulated, well-circumscribed lesions that can be easily treated surgically, while neurofibromas spread within the fascicles and are difficult to remove. The US diagnosis of a nerve tumor is based on the detection of a mass along the course of a nerve in association with clinical signs (Fig. 4). Typically, both tumors present as hypoechoic lesions. A definite differentiation between schwannoma and neurofibroma is difficult to make on the basis of US findings. The value of US in this field is to differentiate compression from extrinsic masses from a nerve tumor. Once a tumor is

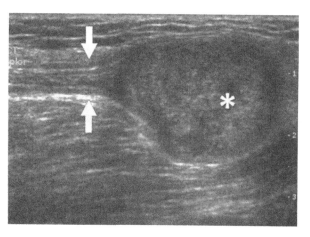

Fig. 4. Pathologic US appearance of peripheral nerves. Schwannoma. Longitudinal US image obtained over the medial aspect of the ankle in a patient with paresthesias of the medial aspect of the foot. The schwannoma (*asterisk*) appears as a well demarcated irregularly hypoechoic mass located along the course of the tibial nerve (*arrows*)

confirmed, US allows its careful location and can accurately measure its longitudinal diameter, which is a crucial factor affecting the choice between end-to-end nerve suture and graft interposition.

Ultrasound of the Shoulder

Ultrasound of the shoulder is one of the most common musculoskeletal applications, second only in our practice to that of the ankle and foot. The typical indication is the assessment and therapy of rotator cuff disease, which consists of supraspinatus tears, tears of the biceps subscapularis and infraspinatus, as well as subacromial subdeltoid bursitis and calcific tendinopathy.

As with musculoskeletal US elsewhere, a thorough knowledge of the anatomy is essential. A key landmark is the bicipital groove, which helps to locate the important anterior structures. These include the biceps tendon, the anterior interval, and the rotator sling; the latter surrounds the proximal biceps tendon, which separates the subscapularis tendon, lying medially, from the supraspinatus tendon, which lies laterally. The majority of rotator cuff pathologies will be localized to this anatomic region. A complete examination also includes examination of the more posteriorly located structures; the infraspinatus tendon, the posterior joint space and labrum, the supraglenoid notch, the subscapularis muscle and, superiorly, the acromioclavicular joint.

The US techniques for joint examination have been well-described. The US committee of the European Society of Skeletal Radiology (ESSR) has made available free to download pdf files illustrating the techniques. The files can be accessed directly from a number of locations including the society's website (www.internationalskeletalsociety.com).

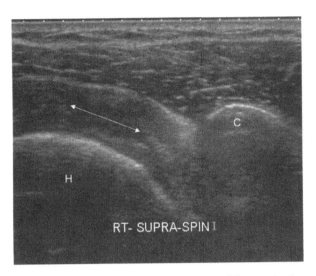

Fig. 5. Axial ultrasound image showing a tear of the anterior free edge of supraspinatus (*arrow*). *H*, Humeral head; *C*, coracoid process

Most supraspinatus tears occur either at the free edge adjacent to the anterior interval (Fig. 5) or in the mid-substance of the supraspinatus tendon. Free edge tears are recognized on axial images by an increase in the gap between the lateral margin of the biceps tendon and the supraspinatus tissue. This gap may be filled with fluid, thickened synovial tissue from adjacent bursitis, or herniation of the overlying deltoid, which collapses into the space created by the tear. A mid-substance tear can also be appreciated on axial images by the presence of a gap between the more anterior and posterior components of the supraspinatus. Once again, the gap may be filled by fluid, bursa, or herniation of the overlying deltoid muscle. Axial images are supplemented by coronal images, which should also include the full extent of the supraspinatus, anterior to posterior. If the tear is filled with fluid, it is usually easy to recognize, whereas a tear that is filled with synovial thickening or deltoid muscle can be more difficult to appreciate. Sonologists should look for an alteration of the normally convex superior configuration of the subacromial subdeltoid bursa. Partial tears are identified by interruptions of the tendon substance, limited to either the joint or the bursal surface. Joint-surface partial tears are more common.

In addition to these primary signs of rotator cuff tear, others have been described that may assist with the diagnosis. Not infrequently, there is bony overgrowth of the foot plate (the bony insertion of the supraspinatus tendon) or increased reflectivity from the articular cartilage surface if the tear overlies cartilage. The presence of fluid in the subacromial subdeltoid bursa, the joint space, or, more importantly, both spaces should be regarded with suspicion as their presence has a high association with rotator cuff tear [18].

Several studies have looked at the accuracy of US in the detection of rotator cuff tears [19]. There is good evidence that the technique is of higher accuracy for full-thickness tears (similar to MRI); rather than partial-thickness tears [20, 21]. However, a deficiency with many of these studies is they do not indicate the size of the rotator cuff tear itself. Large tears should be routinely detected, and accuracies much below 100% indicate poor technique. Small tears are more difficult and careful attention to technique is required to detect them. In this regard, it should be remembered that US is not a static examination; rather, it involves movement of the probe and the patient's arm as well as manipulation of any fluid that may be present in the joint or subacromion subdeltoid bursa, all of which should be used to increase sensitivity.

Pathology in the biceps tendon represents a less common but more important group of injuries. The biceps tendon should be located within its groove in the upper humerus [22], otherwise it is either ruptured or dislocated. Dislocation is in a medial direction, consequently this is the area that should be examined when an empty bicipital groove is found. Care should be taken not to confuse a medially displaced long head of the biceps with the short head of the biceps. The latter can be identified by tracing it proximally to its origin from the coracoid process. If the biceps tendon is dislocated, the next step is to determine whether it lies superficial to the subscapularis tendon, indicating a tear of the rotator interval, or deep to the normal position of subscapularis, indicating an associated tear of that tendon. If the groove is empty and a dislocated biceps is not found, complete rupture is likely. Usually, the retracted tendon end of the torn biceps tendon can be identified low within the groove. Rupture of the biceps is most often a consequence of chronic biceps tendinopathy, which itself is usually caused by chronic attrition against an irregular bony groove. Biceps tendinopathy is recognized by enlargement and loss of reflectivity within the tendon. Occasionally, tendon splits and calcification may be identified. The associated bony changes are easily appreciated. Bony irregularity itself is most frequently caused by chronic rotator cuff disease. Rupture of an otherwise normal tendon is uncommon but may be associated with steroid abuse.

Tears of the subscapularis may occur in isolation but are also more commonly a component of advanced rotator cuff disease [23, 24]. The superior part of the subscapularis should be assessed carefully as tendinopathy and tears often begin in this location.

Calcification is easily identified within any of the rotator cuff tendons [25]; the supraspinatus and subscapularis are the most commonly involved. US is more sensitive than either plain radiography or MRI in the detection of calcification. Various patterns of calcification can be identified, ranging from a few scattered flecks, to an ovoid area of milk of calcium, to a more solid, occasionally ossified conglomerate. The latter are more commonly associated with impingement syndromes and are most often treated initially with subacromial subdeltoid injection. Milk of calcium may be associated with intermittent crystal leak into the subacromial subdeltoid bursa, which causes intense pain simulating septic arthritis. These lesions are best aspirated. US can guide the needle into the calcium collection, which is entered as a single puncture. With sequential injection, aspiration using saline or, preferentially, lidocaine, the milk of calcium can be aspirated.

The most common clinical indication for rotator cuff US is impingement syndrome. In these cases, differentiating patients with or without a rotator cuff tear is the most important imaging goal [26]. In patients who do not have a rotator cuff tear, thickening of the subacromial subdeltoid bursa with or without associated fluid distension can be identified; also, dynamic maneuvers can confirm impingement against the acromium or, more importantly, the coracoacromial ligament. False-negatives and false-positives are associated with this latter finding compared with the more important clinical feature of pain on arm abduction. In patients with confirmed impingement without rotator cuff tear, the subacromial subdeltoid bursa can be injected. In most institutions, this is carried out blindly, often with good results. Following injection, the patient should be re-examined to determine whether there has been improvement in the symptoms. This is called a positive impingement test. In our view, the impingement test should not be regarded as negative without carrying out at least one US-guided procedure. US guidance is straight forward and the injectate, usually a composition of local anesthetic and corticosteroid, can clearly be identified filling the bursa during the procedure.

Other pathologies that can be identified on routine US of the shoulder include tears of the infraspinatus, glenohumeral joint effusions, paralabral cysts, and atrophy of the supraspinatus muscle, which may occur in conjunction with large, chronic rotator cuff tears.

Ultrasound of the Elbow

Ultrasound of the elbow is not one of the more commonly requested US investigations. In adults, its most typical indication is the assessment of epicondylitis [27]. The common flexor and extensor origins can be readily identified on the medial and lateral aspects of the elbow, respectively. The normal common tendon exhibits an echo structure typical of tendons and ligaments elsewhere. The US findings in epicondylopathy include disorganization of the normal echo structure and, frequently, abnormal Doppler signal within the common tendon (Fig. 6). In chronic stages, enthesopathy and calcification occur. US can be used to guide injection or dry-needle therapy in patients whose symptoms are refractive to conservative therapy [28].

The radial and ulnar collateral ligaments can also be assessed with US. The former is important in patients with chronic and refractory disease of the common extensor origin. The ulnar collateral ligament may be injured in isolation, as is commonly associated with throwing sports. US can demonstrate tears of this ligament but medial laxity can be assessed using a valgus stress test [29].

The triceps and biceps tendons are also accessible to US assessment [30]. The triceps is easily examined due to its superficial location although disorders of this ten-

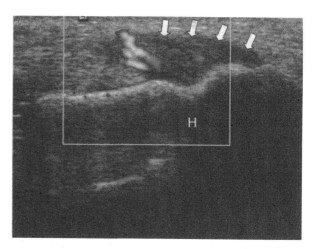

Fig. 6. Long-axis coronal view of the common extensor origin. There is loss of reflectivity (*arrows*) and increased Doppler signal, indicating epicondylitis. *H*, Humerus

don are relatively uncommon. The biceps tendon is more difficult to examine due to its oblique course through the anterior aspect of the joint. The tendon is best seen by displacing the probe medially and angling it laterally with fine manipulation to bring the long axis of the tendon into view. Tilting of the US beam can assist in many cases. The insertion of the biceps is best demonstrated with the forearm in full supranation [31].

US has also been recommended for the assessment of nerve compression syndromes around the elbow. The ulnar nerve is the most frequently examined [32]. Transverse sections can easily demonstrate the nerve within the groove and trace it from proximal to distal, noting any alterations in caliber or compressive lesions throughout its course. Compression is most commonly from adjacent osteophytes. In a proportion of patients the ulnar nerve may either lie outside the groove or be displaceable from it. This is not necessarily associated with symptoms.

The most common cause of median nerve compression is entrapment by the ligament of Struthers, associated with a supracondylar bony process arising from the humerus above the elbow [33]. This results in atrophy of the pronator teres muscle. The detection of muscle atrophy should prompt a search for neural impingement proximal to the elbow joint. Impingement below the elbow joint will not cause pronator muscle atrophy. The common causes are entrapment against the proximal end of the bicipital aponeurosis or by the pronator muscle itself, which leads to anterior interosseous nerve compression.

The radial nerve passes in the posterior arm compartment to the anterior forearm compartment just above the elbow. Entrapment of the radial nerve proximal to the elbow is most commonly associated with fractures of the humerus. Below the elbow, the nerve divides into the posterior interosseous nerve, which passes between the two heads of the supinator. The radial nerve proper continues as a sensory only nerve on the radial aspect of the forearm. Posterior interosseous nerve compression most commonly occurs as the nerve passes between the two heads of the supinator. Edema and atrophy of the extensor muscle groups are a clue. The course and configuration of all three nerves should be examined routinely in patients with nonspecific elbow symptoms. In areas where the nerves pass locations of known impingement, for example, between the supinator and pronator muscle heads, rigorous scrutiny is required.

A number of conditions within the joint are amenable to US diagnosis although, as with many joints elsewhere, a complete review of the articular cartilage surface is not possible. US can readily diagnose effusions and loose bodies. In children, effusion is often the consequence of intra-articular fracture; in such cases, US can be helpful where there is uncertainty regarding the plain film findings. Septic arthritis of the elbow is also not uncommon in children and the US detection of elbow effusion in this clinical context should warrant prompt aspiration for microbiological assessment. One aspect of the articular cartilage that is amenable to US interrogation is the capitellum, although full hyperextension is needed to view its most inferior aspect. The ultrasonologist must be sensitive to subtle changes in curvature as these may indicate an osteochondral lesion. Once detected, stability can be assessed. Unstable lesions are confirmed by demonstrating a step or gap in the articular surface. Grade 4 osteochondral injuries are diagnosed where there has been displacement of the osteochondral fragment, forming a loose body. Loose bodies may be identified in the coronoid or olecranon fossae [34].

Hand and Wrist

Small US probes, utilizing frequencies ranging from 10 to 17 MHz, allow accurate assessment of the superficial tissues of the hand and wrist [35]. The association of standard radiographs with US works well in the evaluation of a large spectrum of disorders, although several conditions cannot be diagnosed by US and require MRI or MRI/CT-arthrography for proper evaluation.

Traumas

Foreign bodies are frequent at the hand and wrist and can be followed by local complications such as infection and granuloma if unrecognized. They appear at US as hyperechoic structures associated with posterior shadowing (bone and vegetable splinters) or comet-tail artifact (glass or metallic fragment). The main utility of US relies on the possibility to detect radiolucent fragments, which are undetectable on standard radiographs. US is excellent in assessing the relationship of the fragment with the adjacent anatomic structures. It also readily detects abscesses, tenosynovitis, or granuloma complicating foreign bodies. US can diagnose rupture of the ulnar collateral ligament of the metacarpophalangeal joint of the thumb and tears of the annular pulleys of the flexor tendons of the fingers. The

dorsal band of the scapholunate ligament can be judged by US but CT- or MRI-arthrography allows a more detailed study of wrist ligaments. All tendons of the hand and wrist are easily evaluated by US, from the myotendinous junction to the bone insertion [35]. Partial tendon ruptures appear as an area of localized swelling and decreased echogenicity inside the tendon. Complete tears are diagnosed when the tendon cannot be appreciated at the level of the injury and the swollen end is detected proximally. Microtraumatic tendon diseases, including De Quervain disease [36] and trigger finger [37], are due to repetitive movements that induce friction at the level of osteofibrous tunnels. US can easily detect tendon swelling, echo texture changes of the retinacula or A1 pulley, as well as synovial sheath effusion. It can also guide a local steroid injection.

Arthritis and Tenosynovitis

Ultrasound allows the diagnosis and follow-up of inflammatory disorders affecting the hand and wrist [38]. At early stages, when osseous erosions are not detected by standard radiographs, it demonstrates para-articular edema and joint and tendon sheath effusions. Later, hypertrophy of the synovial membrane (pannus) producing marginal erosions can be detected. Color Doppler flow studies provide a measurement of the extent of neovascularization within the synovial lining of joints that is not available with other imaging techniques [38] (Fig. 7). Fibrous pan-

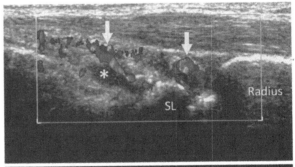

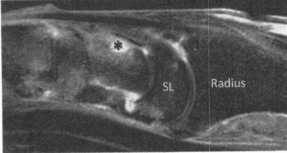

Fig. 7 a, b. Rheumatoid arthritis. Longitudinal color Doppler sonogram obtained over the dorsal aspect of the wrist (**a**), and corresponding T2-weighted fat-saturated MRI image (**b**). US shows the pannus (*asterisk*) as a hypoechoic area containing multiple flow signals (*white arrows*). *SL*, Lunate

nus can be differentiated from active vascular hypertrophy by color Doppler. US aids in guiding a diagnostic joint puncture and allows proper intra-articular injection of steroids.

Entrapment Neuropathies

Entrapment neuropathies of the wrist concern the median nerve at the carpal tunnel [39] and the ulnar nerve at the Guyon tunnel. In both locations, US can show hypoechoic swelling of the involved nerve and loss of its internal fascicular pattern. The cause of the compression (tenosynovitis, ganglia, amyloid deposits.) can be detected by US. In carpal tunnel syndrome, US allows: (1) confirmation of the diagnosis when invasive nerve conduction studies are equivocal or not accepted by the patient; (2) aid in planning surgery by demonstration of anatomic variants, such as a bifid median nerve or presence of median artery, and by detection of expansible masses that cannot be successfully treated by endoscopy.

Soft-Tissues Tumors

Soft-tissue masses are frequently seen in daily clinical practice and can be secondary to a wide variety of causes, including tumors, infection, inflammation, and congenital anomalies [40]. The most common masses of the hand and wrist are ganglia [41] and giant cell tumor of the tendon sheath. Ganglia are depicted as well-demarcated, anechoic masses with regular borders without internal flow signals at color Doppler. In older lesions, internal septa and fibrosis explain the hypoechoic appearance. US-guided aspiration and local steroid injection can be performed in selected cases. A giant cell tumor of the tendon sheath appears at US as a para-articular or paratendinous, 'solid, hypoechoic, well-marginated mass that can present internal signals at color Doppler and cause pressure erosions on the cortical bone of the phalanges. Although the US findings are not specific, the technique is invaluable in the accurate evaluation of tumor size, location, and relationship with surrounding structures as well as in the early diagnosis of local recurrences.

Ultrasound of the Hip

The most common indications in the pediatric population are screening for developmental dysplasia [42, 43] and assessment of the painful hip in the young child [44]. Screening for developmental dysplasia is carried out in all children routinely in a number of European countries, including Austria and Switzerland. In other countries, the UK amongst them, screening of high-risk infants is done in a number of institutions. The risk factors include a breach delivery, family history of developmental dysplasia, congenital anomalies including spinal and foot anomalies, and infants who have a clinical abnormality detected at neonatal screening. The technique is specific and re-

quires the identification of the unossified femoral head firmly seated within the acetabulum. In addition to morphological assessment of femoral head containment, which can be measured using either α- and β-angle measurements or a percentage of femoral head coverage directly, the stability of the femoral head during abduction and dynamic stress is assessed.

An acute painful hip is one of the most common pediatric orthopedic presentations to the emergency department. The majority of cases are due to transient synovitis, which is a self-limiting condition. A small proportion of patients will have septic arthritis, the early detection of which is important is to avoid the devastating complications that can follow a delay in diagnosis. US is used primarily as a tool to detect effusion and guide aspiration. Aspiration is most commonly carried out using a blind technique, following US-guided accurate positioning of the puncture point.

Less common causes of irritable hip include Perthes disease and slipped epiphyses, for which there are specific US findings. In the older child, US can be used to assess snapping tendons including the iliopsoas and iliotibial bands [45]. Painful snapping may be due to a labral tear [46]. US can occasionally demonstrate such tears, particularly if there are associated paralabral cysts but, like its assessment in the menisci and glenoid labrum, the inability to visualize the meniscus in its entirety has significant impact on the negative predictive value.

A number of bursae surround the hip. In younger individuals the iliopsoas initial bursa may be a cause of symptoms. In older individuals gluteus medius tendinopathy and associated trochanteric or subgluteus medius bursal disease is common. Findings in US are variable depending on whether tendon or bursal disease predominates. US-guided therapy is effective. In our experience, the subgluteus medius bursa is more frequently involved than the more commonly known trochanteric bursitis and it is likely that, in the past, many cases of subgluteus medius bursopathy have been called trochanteric bursitis. US can provide more accurate guidance to one, either, or more commonly both of these bursae. This is particularly useful in patients who have failed to respond to an unguided injection.

Within the hip joint itself, US can be used to assess effusion either in the native hip or following hip implantation. Normal values are difficult to define for the anterior joint space size in patients who have undergone hip implantation but 1 cm is often taken as the upper limit of normal. US can also be used to guide aspiration and injection therapy. Post-implantation complications including hematoma, femoral nerve impingement, and iliopsoas bursitis may be detected.

Groin pain is common in sports that involve rapid changes of direction, particularly soccer, American football, and hockey. The differential diagnosis of groin pain includes disorders of the rectus abdominis, the pubic symphysis and its adjacent insertions, the common adductor tendon and adductor insertion, as well as inguinal hernia [47, 48]. Accurate diagnosis of these entities requires a combination of US and high-resolution gadolinium-enhanced MRI. MRI is superior at detecting many of these lesions but is unable to detect herniations that are reduced at the time of examination. Due to its dynamic capability, US is more accurate at identifying inguinal or femoral hernias and in the case of inguinal hernia, detecting whether they are direct or indirect. The inferior epigastric artery is the landmark used to identify the internal ring. Indirect inguinal hernias involve the passage of intra-abdominal fat and, less often, bowel contents through the deep inguinal ring and along the inguinal canal. Direct inguinal hernias are seen as an indentation of the inguinal canal medial to the epigastric artery by the anterior abdominal wall. Not all direct hernias are symptomatic. One additional advantage of US in the assessment of the athlete with groin pain is the ability to link a point of focal tenderness with the anatomic structure associated with it and thus assist in a specific diagnosis and guide injection therapy.

Ultrasound of the Knee

The primary imaging technique for assessing the knee is MRI, as the bone as well as internal and external soft tissues can all be accurately assessed. US is useful when there are focal symptoms related to an extra-articular structure or in the initial evaluation of a soft-tissue mass.

The patellar tendon is the most common structure to be imaged. Patellar tendinosis is an overuse syndrome of adolescence and young adults affecting the proximal tendon adjacent to the inferior pole of the patella. The tendon is focally widened, hypoechoic, and hypervascular on Doppler imaging [49, 50] (Fig. 8). Ultrasound can accurately assess the area of tendinosis and grade the vascular response. Areas of focal degeneration, partial tear, and cyst formation can also be detected. A closely related problem is impingement of the lateral part of the proximal tendon on the lateral femoral condyle. This causes an inflammatory-like mass in the intervening fat which is hypervascular on Doppler. Injection of steroid under US control is helpful in controlling symptoms conditions but

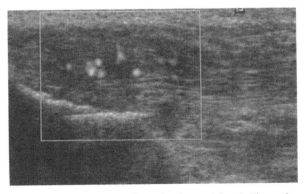

Fig. 8. Proximal patellar tendinopathy (jumper's knee). The tendon is swollen, with a loss of normal reflectivity and increased Doppler signal

should be performed with caution as risk of future tendon rupture is increased.

Although rarely necessary, US can also diagnose Osgood Schlatter's disease [51]. Typically, it presents as a lump of the tibial tubercle in adolescent males athletes. It is essentially a clinical diagnosis and the main purpose of imaging is to reassure the parent and physicians that there is no sinister pathology. US should assess the degree of new bone formation, tendinosis, and its vascular response as well as the presence and extent of deep infrapatellar bursitis.

US is a good first-line investigation for the assessment of periarticular masses and can reliably differentiate solid from cystic lesions [52]. This is an important function, as cystic masses in the majority of patients are benign and can, if clinically indicated, be easily aspirated. A wide variety of cystic masses can be present around the knee. The position of the cyst and its relationship to other structures usually points towards the correct diagnosis. The most common lesions are ganglion, meniscal cyst, and, particularly, synovial cysts. As with other joints, US is a good way to diagnose and aspirate effusions, distinguish simple effusions from synovitis, and, occasionally, detect loose bodies within the joint. The detection of effusion is especially useful in young children and infants with suspected septic arthritis.

Other common applications around the knee include assessment of the extra-articular ligaments, particularly the medial and lateral collateral ligaments and the posterolateral and posteromedial corners.

Important neural structures around the knee include the posterior tibial and the common peroneal nerve [52, 53], which can be compressed as it rounds the neck of the fibula. A ganglion cyst arising from the proximal tibia fibula joint is often implicated. Quadriceps tendon tears can be difficult to assess but a dynamic examination can improve sensitivity.

Ultrasound of the Ankle and Foot

Musculoskeletal diseases of the ankle and foot lend themselves extremely well to US investigation, since clinical examination usually offers only a limited differential diagnosis. Coupled with the superficial position of many of the ligaments and tendons, this has led to the increased use of US as a primary means to assess the ankle and foot. In our practice, these indications now outnumber referrals for other areas of the musculoskeletal system. The approach to differential diagnosis therefore begins with an understanding of the common conditions that leads to symptoms at specific locations.

The principle differential diagnosis of patients presenting with anterior ankle pain are footballer's ankle and tibialis anterior tendinopathy. Footballer's ankle, also called anterior impingement syndrome, is characterised by the presence of a bony spur arising from the anterior aspect of the distal tibia. There may be a corresponding divot on the dorsal aspect of the talus. Between these two, fluid and synovial thickening may be present in the joint. Tendinopathy of the tibialis anterior tendon is much rarer than its posterior counterpart. The normal tendon has a slightly lower reflectivity than other tendons and this must not be taken as pathology. The tendon lies on the anteromedial aspect of the ankle and can be traced to its insertion in the medial cuneiform. Tendinopathy and rupture may occur. Tendinopathy of the anterior tendons, including extensor hallucis and extensor digitorum, are uncommon. The tibiotalar joint can also be appreciated during examination of the anterior ankle. Effusion within the joint can be seen as an echo-poor signal that displaces the anterior fat pad. Increased Doppler flow denotes associated synovitis.

Posterior ankle and heel pain is very much more common. The differential diagnosis focuses primarily on the Achilles tendon and plantar fascia. Consideration should also be given to os trigonum syndrome or posterior impingement and tendinopathy of the flexor hallucis longus.

Chronic Achilles tendinopathy is characterized by focal or diffuse hypoechoic enlargement of the tendon. The most common type involves the proximal two-thirds of the tendon and is termed non-insertional tendinopathy (Fig. 9). This is generally caused by misuse injury often related to abnormal biomechanics of the hindfoot [54]. The ultrasonologist should record the size of the tendon, presence of focal defects, calcification or partial tear, paratenon involvement, and vascularity. When patients complain of pain, there is invariably hypervascularity, which is seen on Doppler [55]. Dry-needling, paratenon injection of local anesthetic and sclerosing therapy are therapeutic options [56]. The second type of Achilles tendinopathy occurs more distally and is called insertional tendinopathy. It may be mechanical in etiology if there is bony enlargement of the posterosuperior corner of the os calcis (Haglund deformity). Insertional Achilles disease may also be associated with enthesopathy elsewhere. US findings include new bone formation, tendinopathy and pre-or retro-Achilles bursitis. The plantar fascia should be examined in all patients complaining of Achilles pain, as plantar fasciitis may be associated with Achilles tendon disease of any type.

The diagnosis of acute complete rupture of the Achilles tendon is usually made clinically. The US report should document the position of the tear, particularly its

relationship with the musculotendinous junction and tendon insertion. In addition, an estimate of the size of the gap should be obtained, both in the resting position and with foot plantar flexion. The majority of tears occur within the tendon itself, between 4 and 6 cm above its insertion (Fig. 10). If the tendon ends are opposed on plantar flexion, then the patient can be treated with a cast. If there is a gap of more than 0.5 cm in plantar flexion, surgery is generally recommended. Tears at the musculotendinous junction are often treated conservatively.

Plantar fasciitis is an important cause of posterior hindfoot pain. In most cases, the symptoms and signs of plantar fasciitis can be differentiated from those of Achilles tendinopathy. However, in some patients, particularly those with insertional Achilles tendon disease, some overlap can occur. The plantar fascia should therefore be examined in all patients presenting with Achilles pain.

There are two components to the plantar fascia in the posterior hindfoot, the central and the lateral bands. A third band, the medial band, arises in the midfoot from the central band. The central band is the most frequently interested. Some authors only describe medial and lateral bands; when such terminology is used, the majority of symptoms are reported as being in the medial band.

The normal US appearance of the plantar fascia is similar to that of ligaments elsewhere. A thin, predominantly echogenic, striated structure is typical of a normal ligament. In patients with plantar fasciitis, there is a loss of this structure accompanied by echo texture with thickening, usually >4.5–5 mm (Fig. 11). Bony irregularity may indicate the formation of spurs. Occasionally, the Doppler

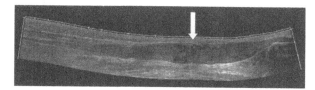

Fig. 10. Similar orientation to Fig. 27. Achilles tendon rupture (*arrow*)

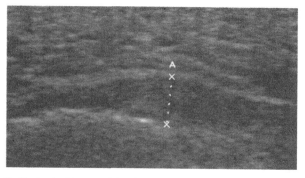

Fig. 11. Sagittal image of the plantar fascia insertion. There is plantar fasciitis with swelling (*between measurement cursors*) and loss of the normal ligament reflectivity

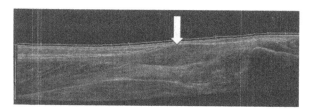

Fig. 9. Long-axis sagittal panoramic image of the Achilles tendon. Note the central fusiform swelling (*arrow*) in a patient with chronic Achilles tendinopathy

signal is also increased but this is not usually a prominent feature. Plantar fasciitis is usually very easy to distinguish from plantar fibroma. These are focal irregular fusiform swellings of the plantar fascia that generally occur more distal to the origin of the ligament. They are frequently multiple and bilateral, a further feature that helps with the differential diagnosis.

Posterior impingement syndrome is a condition related to soft-tissue inflammatory changes around either an os trigonum or a prominent Stieda process. On MRI, signal changes within the os trigonum are characteristic. This is not easy to appreciate on US but occasionally a poor definition of the cortical margin of the bone may be observed. Os trigonum syndrome may be associated with fluid within the flexor hallucis longus tendon sheath, although it must be appreciated that under normal circumstances this sheath may communicate with the tibiotalar joint and consequently even a moderate amount of fluid within the sheath is considered normal. US has an advantage over MRI in differentiating normal fluid from tenosynovitis of the flexor hallucis longus tendon sheath, as increased Doppler blood flow can be detected. The flexor hallucis longus tendon can also be assessed dynamically by gentle movement of the great toe. This is important in detecting sclerosing tenosynovitis, in which there is restricted movement and, occasionally, catching as the tendinopathic tendon becomes constricted in its fibro-osseous tunnel on the dorsal aspect of the os calcis.

Medial ankle pain is common. The medial tendons include the tibialis posterior, flexor digitorum and flexor hallucis longus. By far, the most common tendinopathy detected in the medial side is that of the tibialis posterior. Hypertrophic tendinopathy characterized by enlargement of the tendon and, as a rule, in the tendon sheath must be differentiated from atrophic tendinopathy with loss of tendon caliber [57, 58]. Complete rupture is relatively uncommon but is easy to detect using US.

The ligaments in the medial aspect of the ankle form a complex structure. Broadly, three groups are identified. The deep group comprises two ligaments, the anterior and posterior tibiotalar ligaments. The most common pathology associated with these structures is chronic enthesopathy leading to anteromedial and posteromedial impingement. There is loss of normal reflectivity of the ligament with calcification and increased Doppler signal. The superficial group of ligaments comprise three ligamentous structures named for their origin and insertions. Two of these ligaments run between bony structures, anteriorly the tibionavicular ligament and posteriorly the tibiocalcaneal ligament. The central and most prominent of these three ligaments runs between the tibia and the spring ligament. The third group, the horizontal group, is the spring ligament itself, which has a number of divisions, the principle one being the superficial calcaneal navicular ligament [59]. It can be identified in most patients running deep to the submalleolar portion of the tibialis posterior tendon.

Impingement of the posterior tibial nerve within the tarsal tunnel is a further cause of medial-sided symptoms. The most common cause is a ganglion or synovial cyst arising either from the tibiotalar or the posterior subtalar joints. Cystic lesions causing tarsal tunnel syndrome are easily identified and can be aspirated under US control. These need to be distinguished from neurilemmoma.

Pain on the lateral aspect of the ankle could be due to disorders of the peroneal tendons or the lateral ligament complex. Peroneal tendinopathy is common and most frequently involves the peroneus brevis tendon; it lies anterior to peroneus longus and may become impinged between it and the fibula. A flattened fibula groove or the presence of accessory tendons, such as peroneus quadratus, may predispose to tendinosis. Another common cause is impingement of the peroneal tendons against implanted metalwork. The peroneal tendons should be traced in the axial plane throughout their length from the musculotendinous junction to their insertions. Careful probe control is necessary to avoid an istotrophy during axial imaging particularly as the tendon is traced around the lateral malleolus. It can sometimes be difficult to trace the peroneus longus as it passes under the cuboid bone to insert on the undersurface of the base of the first metatarsal; however, this is an area where impingement within a fibro-osseous tunnel on the under surface of the cuboid can occur. Peroneus brevis should be traced to its insertion at the base of the fifth metatarsal. The peroneal tendons are held in place under the dorsal aspect of the fibula by the peroneal retinaculum. Injuries to this structure may predispose to peroneal subluxation. A dynamic US examination using foot dorsiflexion and internal rotation can assess whether there is abnormal peroneal tendon displacement anterior to the fibula [60].

The main ligaments on the lateral aspect are the tibiofibular ligament, the anterior talofibular ligament, and the calcaneofibular ligament. The anterior pair, the tibiofibular ligament and anterior talofibular ligaments, can easily be identified with careful probe positioning. A history of prior inversion injury is the usual cause of derangement of the anterior talofibular ligament, as it is a rather weak structure and frequently injured. Injury may be associated with the formation of a synovial mass in the anterolateral gutter which can be detected on US. This is termed anterolateral impingement syndrome. The most significant of the lateral ligaments is the calcaneofibular ligament [61]. Its posterior portion can usually be seen lying between the peroneal tendons and the os calcis. The more proximal portion can be difficult to identify but serial dorsal and plantar flexion may bring the full ligament into view. Displacement of the peroneal tendons is also seen in the presence of a competent ligament.

A common indication for US is forefoot pain. If this occurs following acute injury, subtle fractures, post-traumatic synovitis, and injuries to the plantar plate should all be sought. More commonly, the patient complains of chronic pain. The differential diagnosis of metatarsalgia is wide and includes joint disease, Morton's neuroma, and biomechanical disturbances of the metatarsal arch. Less common causes are stress fracture, sesamoiditis, and metatarsal pad bursitis.

Patients with Morton's neuroma frequently complain of pain between the toes, particularly on walking, which is often associated with numbness or tingling in the affected toes. The second/third and the third/fourth interspaces are most commonly affected. Morton's neuroma, a perineural inflammatory lesion, has a variable appearance on US but characteristically is a poorly demarcated, low reflective lesion. A variety of examination techniques have been described but we find that a sagittal orientation of the probe between the metatarsal heads is the most useful. With practice, the normal intermetatarsal space can easily be differentiated from the low-signal neuroma. Many lesions described as Morton's neuroma are likely to be a combination of Morton's neuroma and intermetatarsal bursal disease, but differentiation is not considered particularly significant as the clinical presentation and treatment are similar. As with other areas, US offers advantage over MRI in the investigation of Morton's neuroma since detection can be followed by US-guided therapy.

In younger patients, the differential diagnosis of forefoot pain is extended to include stress fractures, tendon injuries, and injuries to the plantar plate [62]. Stress fractures can be detected by the presence of edema or irregularity of the bony surface, especially of the metatarsal necks. Stress fractures should be considered in patients with pain on exertion. A history of hyperextension injury and pain at the first metatarsal phalangeal joint should prompt a careful examination of the plantar plate, a fibro cartilaginous structure that lies on the plantar aspect of the joint [62]. Other causes of pain in this area include sesamoiditis, which can be diagnosed using US by detecting focal tenderness over the sesamoid associated with poor demarcation of the cortical surface of the bones.

References

1. McNally E (2004) Practical Musculoskeletal Ultrasound. Elsevier, London
2. Bianchi S, Martinoli C (2007) Ultrasound of the musculoskeletal system. Springer-Verlag, Berlin Heidelberg New York
3. Jacobson JA, van Holsbeeck MT (1998) Musculoskeletal ultrasonography. Orth Clin North Am 29:135-167
4. Bianchi S, Abdelwahab IF, Mazzola CG et al (1995) Sonographic examination of muscle herniation. J Ultrasound Med 14:357-360
5. Beggs I (2003) Sonography of muscle hernias. AJR Am J Roentgenol 18:395-399
6. Garrett WE Jr (1996) Muscle strain injuries. Am J Sports Med 24:S2-S8
7. Bianchi S, Martinoli C, Waser NP et al (2002) Central aponeurosis tears of the rectus femoris: sonographic findings. Skeletal Radiol 31:581-586
8. Bianchi S, Martinoli C, Abdelwahab IF et al (1998) Sonographic evaluation of tears of the gastrocnemius medial head ("Tennis leg"). J Ultrasound Med 17:157-162
9. Martinoli C, Derchi LE, Pastorino C et al (1993) Analysis of echotexture of tendons with US. Radiology 186:839-843
10. Kalebo P, Allenmark C, Peterson L et al (1992) Diagnostic value of ultrasonography in partial ruptures of the Achilles tendon. Am J Sports Med 20:378-381
11. Khan KM, Bonar F, Desmond PM et al (1996) Patellar tendinosis (jumpers knee): findings at histopathologic examination, US and MR imaging. Radiology 200:821-827
12. Diaz GC, van Holsbeeck M, Jacobson JA (1998) Longitudinal split of the peroneus longus and peroneus brevis tendons with disruption of the superior peroneal retinaculum. J Ultrasound Med 17:525-529
13. Prato N, Derchi LE, Martinoli C (1996) Sonographic diagnosis of biceps tendon dislocation. Clin Radiol 51:737-739
14. Silvestri E, Martinoli C, Derchi LE et al (1995) Echotexture of peripheral nerves: correlation between US and histologic findings and criteria to differentiate tendons. Radiology 197:291-296
15. Martinoli C, Bianchi S, Derchi LE (1999) Tendon and nerve sonography. Radiol Clin North Am 37:691-711
16. Bianchi S (2008) Ultrasound of the peripheral nerves. Joint Bone Spine 75(6):643-649
17. Martinoli C, Bianchi S, Gandolfo N et al (2000) US of nerve entrapments in osteofibrous tunnels of the upper and lower limbs Radiographics. 20:S199-S213
18. Arslan G, Apaydin A, Kabaalioglu A (1999) Sonographically detected subacromial/subdeltoid bursal effusion and biceps tendon sheath fluid: reliable signs of rotator cuff tear? J Clin Ultrasound 27:335-340
19. Wiener S, Seitz W (1993) Sonography of the shoulder in patients with tears of the rotator cuff: accuracy and value for selecting surgical options. AJR Am J Roentgenol 160(1):103-107
20. Farin PU, Kaukanen E, Jaroma H et al (1996) Site and size of rotator-cuff tear: findings at ultrasound, double-contrast arthrography, and computed tomography arthrography with surgical correlation. Invest Radiol 31(7):387
21. Brenneke SL, Morgan CJ (1992) Evaluation of ultrasonography as a diagnostic technique in the assessment of rotator cuff tendon tears. Am J Sports Med 20(3):287
22. Thain LM, Adler RS (1999) Sonography of the rotator cuff and biceps tendon: technique, normal anatomy, and pathology. J Clin Ultrasound 27(8):446-458
23. Grainger AJ, Tirman PF, Elliott JM et al (2000) MR anatomy of the subcoracoid bursa and the association of subcoracoid effusion with tears of the anterior rotator cuff and the rotator interval. AJR Am J Roentgenol 174(5):1377-1380
24. Chiou HJ, Chou YH, Wu JJ et al (1999) Alternative and effective treatment of shoulder ganglion cyst: ultrasonographically guided aspiration. J Ultrasound Med 18(8):531-535
25. Farin P (1995) Sonographic findings of rotator cuff calcifications. J Ultrasound Med 14(1):7-14
26. McNally E, Rees J (2007) Imaging in shoulder disorders. Skeletal Radiol 36(11):1013-1016
27. Miller TT, Shapiro MA, Schultz E, Kalish PE (2002) Comparison of sonography and MRI for diagnosing epicondylitis. J Clin Ultrasound 30(4):193-202
28. Connell DA, Ali KE, Ahmad M et al (2006) Ultrasound-guided autologous blood injection for tennis elbow. Skeletal Radiol 35(6):371-377
29. De Smet AA, Winter TC, Best TM, Bernhardt DT (2002) Dynamic sonography with valgus stress to assess elbow ulnar collateral ligament injury in baseball pitchers. Skeletal Radiol 31(11):671-676
30. Weiss C, Mittelmeier M, Gruber G (2000) Do we need MR images for diagnosing tendon ruptures of the distal biceps brachii? The value of ultrasonographic imaging. Ultraschall Med 21(6):284-286
31. Bird S (2006) A new method for ultrasound evaluation of the distal biceps brachii tendon. Ultrasound Med Biol 32(5S):294-294
32. Jacobson JA, Jebson PJL, Jeffers AW et al (2001) Ulnar nerve dislocation and snapping triceps syndrome: diagnosis with

dynamic sonography: report of three cases 1. Radiology 220(3):601-605

33. Gessini L, Jandolo B, Pietrangeli A (1983) Entrapment neuropathies of the median nerve at and above the elbow. Surg Neurol 19(2):112-116

34. Miller JH, Beggs I (2001) Detection of intraarticular bodies of the elbow with saline arthrosonography. Clin Radiol 56(3):231-234

35. Bianchi S, Martinoli C, Abdelwahab IF (1999) High-frequency ultrasound examination of the wrist and hand. Skeletal Radiol 28:121-129

36. Giovagnorio F, Andreoli C, De Cicco ML (1997) Ultrasonographic evaluation of de Quervain's disease. J Ultrasound Med 16:685-689

37. Serafini G, Derchi LE, Quadri P et al (1996) High resolution sonography of the flexor tendons in trigger fingers. J Ultrasound Med 15:213-219

38. McNally EG (2008) Ultrasound of the small joints of the hands and feet: current status Skeletal Radiol 37:99-113

39. Buchberger W, Judmaier W, Birbamer G et al (1992) Carpal tunnel syndrome diagnosis with high-resolution sonography. AJR Am J Roentgenol 159:793-798

40. Bianchi S, Della Santa D, Glauser T et al (2008) Sonography of masses of the wrist and Hand. AJR Am J Roentgenol 191:1767-1775

41. Bianchi S, Abdelwahab IF, Zwass A et al (1993) Sonographic findings in examination of digital ganglia: retrospective study. Clin Radiol 48:45-47

42. Harcke H, Grissom L (1990) Performing dynamic sonography of the infant hip. AJR Am J Roentgenol 155(4):837-844

43. Grissom LE, Harcke HT (1999) Ultrasonography and developmental dysplasia of the infant hip. Curr Opin Pediatr 11(1):66-69

44. Berman L, Fink A, Wilson D, McNally E (1995) Technical note: identifying and aspirating hip effusions. Br J Radiol 68(807):306

45. Bianchi S, Martinoli C, Keller A et al (2002) Giant iliopsoas bursitis: sonographic findings with magnetic resonance correlations. J Clin Ultrasound 30(7):437-441

46. Choi YS, Lee SM, Song BY (2002) Dynamic sonography of external snapping hip syndrome. J Ultrasound Med 21(7):753-758

47. Robinson P, Hensor E, Lansdown MJ et al (2006) Inguino-femoral hernia: accuracy of sonography in patients with indeterminate clinical features. AJR Am J Roentgenol 187(5):1168-1178

48. Alam A, Nice C, Uberoi R (2005) The accuracy of ultrasound in the diagnosis of clinically occult groin hernias in adults. Eur Radiol 15(12):2457-2461

49. Cook JL, Khan KM, Kiss ZS et al (2001) Asymptomatic hypoechoic regions on patellar tendon ultrasound: a 4-year clinical and ultrasound followup of 46 tendons. Scand J Med Sci Sports 11(6):321-327

50. Terslev L, Qvistgaard E, Torp Pedersen S et al (2001) Ultrasound and power Doppler findings in jumper's knee: preliminary observations. Eur J Ultrasound 13(3):183-189

51. Blankstein A, Cohen I, Heim M et al (2001) Ultrasonography as a diagnostic modality in Osgood-Schlatter disease. A clinical study and review of the literature. Arch Orthop Trauma Surg 121(9):536-539

52. McCarthy CL, McNally EG (2004) The MRI appearance of cystic lesions around the knee. Skeletal Radiol 33(4):187-209

53. Aulisa L, Tamburrelli F, Padua R et al (1998) Intraneural cyst of the peroneal nerve. Childs Nerv Syst 14(4-5):222-225

54. Maffulli N (1987) Ultrasound diagnosis of Achilles tendon pathology in runners. Br J Sports Med 21(4):158-162

55. Richards PJ, Dheer AK, McCall IM (2001) Achilles tendon (TA) size and power Doppler ultrasound (PD) changes compared to MRI: a preliminary observational study. Clin Radiol 56(10):843-850

56. Ohberg L, Alfredson H (2002) Ultrasound guided sclerosis of neovessels in painful chronic Achilles tendinosis: pilot study of a new treatment. Br J Sports Med 36(3):173

57. Premkumar A, Perry MB, Dwyer AJ et al (2002) Sonography and MR imaging of posterior tibial tendinopathy. AJR Am J Roentgenol 178(1):223-232

58. Miller S, Van Holsbeeck M, Boruta P et al (1996) Ultrasound in the diagnosis of posterior tibial tendon pathology. Foot & Ankle Int 17(9):555-558

59. Mansour R, Teh J, Sharp RJ, Ostlere S (2008) Ultrasound assessment of the spring ligament complex. Eur Radiol 18(11):2670-2675

60. Neustadter J, Raikin SM, Nazarian LN (2004) Dynamic sonographic evaluation of peroneal tendon subluxation. AJR Am J Roentgenol 183(4):985-988

61. Milz P (1996) 13 MHz high-frequency sonography of the lateral ankle joint ligaments and the tibiofibular syndesmosis in anatomic specimens. J Ultrasound Med 15(4):277-284

62. Gregg J, Silberstein M, Schneider T, Marks P (2006) Sonographic and MRI evaluation of the plantar plate: a prospective study. Eur Radiol 16(12):2661-2669

MR Imaging of Articular Cartilage

Lawrence M. White[1], Michael Recht[2]

[1] Department of Medical Imaging, University of Toronto, Toronto, Canada
[2] Department of Radiology, NYU Langone Medical Center, New York, NY, USA

Introduction

Articular cartilage is a highly specialized tissue with a complex ultrastructure and unique biomechanical properties providing for load distribution and a low-friction weight-bearing surface essential for normal pain-free movement of synovial joints.

Magnetic resonance imaging (MRI) is well-established as an accurate non-invasive means of assessing articular cartilage, enabling accurate evaluation of cartilage morphology and volume, and providing insight into its constituent biochemical composition [1-12]. Critical user-dependent image acquisition factors that need to be considered in the accurate MRI evaluation of cartilage include acquisition pulse sequences, image spatial resolution, and overall image signal-to-noise ratio.

Although multiple existing and developing MRI pulse sequences have been evaluated in the assessment of articular cartilage, two classes of pulse sequence acquisitions have been most widely used in this regard; Intermediate-weighted or T2-weighted fast spin echo (FSE) techniques, and three-dimensional (3D) spoiled gradient echo (SPGR) or fast low-angle shot (FLASH) sequences.

Fat suppressed 3D SPGR and FLASH acquisitions provide high-resolution contiguous thin-slice images with high contrast between bright cartilage and dark fluid, bone, fat, and muscle. With 3D SPGR imaging, cartilage abnormalities are seen as morphologic abnormalities of cartilage contour. Fat-saturated 3D SPGR imaging has been shown to be more accurate than standard spin-echo MRI in the detection of cartilage defects in the knee, with sensitivities as high as 93% [6-8]. However, such sequences may be limited in their assessment of internal cartilage pathology and small intrasubstance fissures or defects [13]. Additional potential limitations of SPGR and FLASH acquisitions include their relatively long acquisition times compared to those of FSE imaging sequences and their relative susceptibility to intravoxel dephasing artifacts, which may be important image-quality considerations in the setting of postoperative surgical debris or hardware in patients with prior arthroscopic surgery or prior cartilage repair procedures.

Intermediate and T2-weighted FSE acquisitions can provide high-resolution, high-contrast imaging of articular cartilage in a relatively short acquisition time. FSE imaging acquisitions additionally benefit from inherent magnetization transfer effects within normal cartilage, potentially increasing the relative conspicuity of cartilage abnormalities, with both intermediate and T2-weighted FSE acquisitions providing excellent depiction of surface morphology as well as intrinsic signal changes potentially reflective of intrasubstance pathology. Similar to results obtained in investigations of SPGR imaging, FSE imaging has been shown to have sensitivities as high as 94% in the detection of arthroscopically documented cartilage disease [5]. Of clinical importance, FSE imaging techniques have additionally been shown to be valuable pulse sequences in the diagnostic evaluation of other intra-articular structures, including menisci, ligaments, and subchondral bone.

A series of promising 3D isotropic imaging techniques have recently been developed for clinical imaging. Such imaging sequences provide for the potential acquisition of high-resolution 3D isotropic data, with the flexibility to format data in arbitrary slice thicknesses and imaging planes. Investigational studies of such sequences [14-16] have shown them capable of obtaining high signal-to-noise imaging suitable for cartilage imaging, with initial clinical studies illustrating diagnostic performance comparable to that of conventional standard imaging acquisitions [14].

Magnetic resonance imaging at 3T has the potential advantages of imaging with relatively increased image signal-to-noise ratios or higher spatial resolution at similar imaging acquisition times, compared to 1T or 1.5T imaging (albeit with somewhat increased sensitivity to postoperative metal-related artifacts). In contrast, imaging at low field strength (< 0.5T) should generally be avoided in the evaluation of articular cartilage and has been shown to have substantial limitations in visualization of cartilage pathology compared to imaging at 1.5T [17, 18].

Clinical MR Imaging: Cartilage Lesions

Degenerative Cartilage Disease

Degenerative cartilage disease, or osteoarthritis, is the most common form of arthritis, with symptomatic disease affecting 6-10% of all adults over 30 years of age and illustrating a steep increase in prevalence with increasing age [19]. Early degenerative disease may be seen on MRI as early alterations in cartilage contour morphology (fibrillation, surface irregularity); changes in cartilage thickness, including cartilage thinning or cartilage thickening, which may be an early feature predating cartilage volume loss; or intrachondral alterations in signal intensity, potentially related to premorphologic intra-substance collagen degeneration and increased free water content. Advanced degenerative chondral lesions are typically manifest on MRI as multiple areas of cartilage thinning of varying depth and size, usually seen on opposing surfaces of an articulation. Cartilage defects, when present, typically illustrate obtuse margins and may be associated with corresponding subchondral regions of increased T2-weighted signal, reflective of subchondral edema/cysts, and/or low signal intensity, reflective of subchondral fibrosis or trabecular sclerosis. Other associated MRI findings of degenerative cartilage disease include central and marginal articular osteophytes, joint effusion, and synovitis, as well as subchondral marrow reactive changes such as subchondral cysts and subchondral edema.

Traumatic Cartilage Disease

Traumatic articular cartilage injuries are well-recognized sequelae of acute or repetitive impact or twisting injuries to a joint. The incidence and prevalence of traumatic cartilage injuries has not been fully delineated and is somewhat difficult to gauge clinically. However, surgical studies have highlighted that cartilage lesions are common, with an incidence ranging of 63-66% in patients undergoing arthroscopic surgery [20, 21].

Traumatic injuries may manifest themselves as: cartilage matrix and cellular injury, with a morphologically intact, articular cartilage surface cover; mechanical disruption of articular cartilage, in the form of partial- or full-thickness cartilage fissures, flap tears, and segmental cartilage defects; or osteochondral injuries, involving both articular cartilage and underlying subchondral bone. Associated signal alterations in the subchondral marrow, including bone bruising/edema, or subchondral fracture, may be helpful signs in delineating areas of overlying cartilage injury. Traumatic cartilage fragments may remain in situ, become partially detached, or become loose and displace into the joint space. As a result, recognition of a traumatic chondral defect should prompt careful inspection of the joint for a displaced intra-articular chondral body.

Cartilage Repair

Increased awareness of the prevalence and significance of articular cartilage lesions coupled with the limited natural capacity of cartilage for effective intrinsic repair has contributed to growing interest in surgical techniques for the treatment of articular cartilage lesions. Such operative techniques have advanced considerably over the past decade, paralleling advances in biologic science and incorporating the results of experimental models of cartilage regeneration and repair. In general, surgical treatment options for repair of cartilage lesions currently include marrow stimulation, osteochondral transplantation, and chondrocyte transplantation techniques. The most commonly used techniques are those of local marrow stimulation, but these typically lead to the formation of fibrous repair tissue rather than hyaline cartilage. Accordingly, there has been great interest and increased use of autologous transplantation techniques because of their potential for providing hyaline or "hyaline-like" repair tissue and the promise of better functional results. Success rates for these surgical options vary depending on defect location, size, and depth, the status of underlying subchondral bone and adjacent surrounding cartilage, joint stability, biomechanical joint alignment, and clinical factors, including patient age, weight, and general health status.

MRI is well recognized as a valuable technique in the postoperative evaluation of cartilage repair procedures [13, 22-25]. In addition to a routine assessment of joint anatomy, a complete MRI evaluation of cartilage repair procedures should include specific assessment of: (a) repair tissue, i.e., defect fill, surface morphology, and MR signal characteristics; (b) adjacent cartilage and bone, i.e., repair-tissue integration into native cartilage and subchondral bone, and the MR signal characteristics of subchondral bone, and (c) the articulation, i.e., joint effusion, synovitis, adhesions, and loose bodies.

Functional/Quantitative Parametric Magnetic Resonance Imaging: Cartilage

In addition to conventional imaging, a great deal of investigational interest has been focused on the evaluation and validation of additional MRI strategies as potential surrogate markers of biomechanical and biochemical ultrastructural composition, both within normal healthy cartilage and degenerative and traumatic cartilage disease. Among these MRI techniques are T2 mapping and delayed gadolinium contrast-enhanced magnetic resonance imaging of cartilage (dGEMRIC).

Quantitative T2 mapping and qualitative assessments of the spatial variation of T2 have been correlated to type II collagen matrix organization within normal hyaline articular cartilage [11-13]. The dGEMRIC imaging technique, which displays the distribution of negatively charged gadolinium-based MRI contrast material (gadopentetate dimeglumine) within cartilage, has been validated as an accurate surrogate marker of cartilage tissue glycosaminoglycan (GAG) concentration [10]. These techniques have been investigated as potential markers of early (premorphologic) cartilage disease and as tools to characterize the histologic and biochemical composition and temporal maturation of repair tissue following cartilage repair procedures.

References

1. Disler DG, McCauley TR, Kelman CG et al (1996) Fat-suppressed three-dimensional spoiled gradient-echo MR imaging of hyaline cartilage defects in the knee: comparison with standard MR imaging and arthroscopy. AJR Am J Roentgenol 167:127-132
2. Yao L, Gentili A, Thomas J (1996) Incidental magnetization transfer contrast in fast spin-echo imaging of cartilage. J Magn Reson Imaging 1:180-184
3. Potter HG, Linklater JM, Allen AA et al (1998) MR imaging of articular cartilage in the knee: a prospective evaluation utilizing fast spin-echo imaging. J Bone Joint Surg Am 80:1276-1284
4. Broderick LS, Turner DA, Renfrew DL et al (1994) Severity of articular cartilage abnormality in patients with osteoarthritis: evaluation with fast spin-echo MR vs. arthroscopy. AJR Am J Roentgenol 162:99-103
5. Bredella MA, Tirman PFJ, Peterfy CG et al (1999) Accuracy of T2-weighted fast spin-echo MR imaging with fat saturation in detecting cartilage defects in the knee: comparison with arthroscopy in 130 patients. AJR Am J Roentgenol 172:1073-1080
6. Recht MP, Piraino DW, Paletta GA et al (1996) Accuracy of fat-suppressed three-dimensional spoiled gradient-echo FLASH MR imaging in the detection of patellofemoral articular cartilage abnormalities. Radiology 198:209-212
7. Disler DG, McCauley TR, Wirth CR, Fuchs MD (1995) Detection of knee hyaline articular cartilage defects using fat suppressed three dimensional spoiled gradient-echo MR imaging: comparison with standard MR imaging and correlation with arthroscopy. AJR Am J Roentgenol 165:377-382
8. Konig H, Sauter R, Deimling M, Vogt M (1987) Cartilage disorders: comparison of spin-echo, CHESS, and FLASH sequence MR images. Radiology 164:753-758
9. Chandnani VP, Ho C, Chu P et al (1991) Knee hyaline cartilage evaluated with MR imaging: a cadaveric study involving multiple imaging sequences and intraarticular injection of gadolinium and saline solution. Radiology 178:557-561
10. Bashir A, Gray M, Boutin RD, Burstein D (1997) Glycosaminoglycan in articular cartilage: in vivo assessment with delayed Gd(DTPA)2-enhanced MR imaging. Radiology 205:551-558
11. Rubenstein JD, Kim JK, Morava-Protzner I et al (1993) Effects of collagen orientation on MR imaging characteristics of bovine articular cartilage. Radiology 188:219-226
12. Nieminen MT, Rieppo J, Toyras J et al (2001) T2 relaxation reveals spatial collagen architecture in articular cartilage: a comparative quantitative MRI and polarized light microscopy study. Magn Reson Med 46:487-493
13. Link TM, Stahl R, Woertler K (2007) Cartilage imaging: motivation, techniques, current and future significance. Eur Radiol 17:1135-1146
14. Duc SR, Pfirrmann CWA, Schmid MR et al (2007) Articular cartilage defects detected with 3D Water excitiation true FISP: prospective comparison with sequences commonly used for knee imaging. Radiology 245:216-223
15. Gold GE, Busse RF, Beehler C et al (2007) Isotropic MRI of the knee with 3D fast spin echo extended echo train acquisition (XETA): initial experience. AJR Am J Roentgenol 188:1287-1293
16. Kijowski R, Lu A, Block W, Grist T (2006) Evaluation of the articular cartilage of he knee joint with vastly undersampled isotropic projection reconstruction steady-state free precession imaging. J Mag Reson Imaging 24:168-175
17. Kladny B, Bluckert K, Swoboda B et al (1995) Comparison of low-field (0.2 Tesla) and high-field (1.5 Tesla) magnetic resonance imaging of the knee joint. Arch Orthop Trauma Surg 114:281-286
18. Vahlensieck M, Schneiber O (2003) Performance of an open low-field MR unit in routine examination of knee lesions and comparison with high field systems. Orthopade 32:175-178 [German]
19. Felson DT, Lawrence RC, Dieppe PA et al (2000) Osteoarthritis: new insights. Part 1: the disease and its risk factors. Ann intern Med 133(8):635-646
20. Curl WW, Krome J, Gordon ES et al (1997) Cartilage injuries: a review of 31,516 knee arthroscopies. Arthroscopy 13:456-460
21. Aroen A, Loken S, Hei S et al (2004) Articular cartilage lesions in 993 consecutive knee arthroscopies. Am J Sports Med 32:211-215
22. Alparslan L, Winalski CS, Boutin RD, Minas T (2001) Postoperative magnetic resonance imaging of articular cartilage. Semin Musculoskel Radiol 5:345-363
23. Brown WE, Potter HG, Marx RG et al (2004) Magnetic resonance imaging appearance of cartilage repair in the knee. Clin Orthop 422:214-223
24. Polster J, Recht M (2005) Postoperative MR evaluation of chondral repair in the knee. Eur J Radiol 54:206-213
25. Recht M, White LM, Winalski CS et al (2003) MR imaging of cartilage repair procedures. Skeletal Radiol 32:185-200

NUCLEAR MEDICINE SATELLITE COURSE
"DIAMOND"

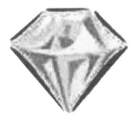

Radionuclide Imaging of Musculoskeletal Infections

Katrin D.M. Stumpe

Nuclear Medicine, Department of Medical Radiology, University Hospital, Zurich, Switzerland

Introduction

Conventional nuclear medicine offers a variety of different methods for the diagnosis of musculoskeletal infections, including three-phase bone scintigraphy, gallium imaging, and labeled leukocyte imaging with indium-111 (^{111}In)-oxine or Tc-99-hexamethyl-propyleneamine oxime (HMPAO) and labeled antibodies against leukocyte surface antigens (antigranulocyte antibodies). However, most of the conventional radionuclide imaging techniques are of low specificity in the detection of low-grade and chronic infections, especially in the axial skeleton due to high physiological uptake in normal bone marrow of the spine.

Fluorine-18 (F-18) fluorodeoxyglucose-positron emission tomography (FDG-PET) represents a promising imaging technique and has shown some advantages compared to conventional radionuclide imaging methods. FDG-PET has the highest diagnostic accuracy for confirming or excluding chronic osteomyelitis [1]. As physiologic FDG uptake in the hematopoietic marrow is relatively low, FDG-PET is successfully performed in patients with infections in the axial skeleton. Similarly, 18-F fluoride PET has shown favorable imaging performance and clinical usefulness compared with bone scintigraphy, which supports the use of 18-F fluoride as a routine bone-imaging radionuclide.

Acute and Chronic Osteomyelitis

Three-phase bone scintigraphy is the radionuclide imaging technique of choice for diagnosing osseous infections, particularly when the involved bone has not been altered by prior trauma, surgery, or infection [2].

To enhance the specificity of bone scintigraphy in patients with underlying bone conditions, gallium-67 imaging is usually performed in conjunction with bone scintigraphy (sequential bone/gallium imaging). The overall accuracy of this approach lies between 65 and 80% [3].

[111]In-labeled leukocytes and antigranulocyte antibodies are neither sensitive nor specific for infection in the axial skeleton [4-6]. The latter imaging methods have appropriate diagnostic accuracy in the peripheral skeleton; however, differentiation between soft-tissue and bone infection is often impossible due to the limited spatial resolution. ^{111}In-labeled leukocyte imaging is the radionuclide technique of choice for diagnosing so-called complicating osteomyelitis, which often must be evaluated in conjunction with 99mTc-sulfur-colloid marrow imaging [7]. This combined technique is often used in patients with prosthetic joints, diabetic foot ulcers, or neuropathic joints. The overall accuracy of combined leukocyte/marrow imaging is approximately 90% [8-11]. The presentation of patients with prosthetic joints or a diabetic foot is complex and discussed later in this chapter.

FDG-PET has advantages over other imaging modalities in the assessment of acute and chronic infections. In contrast to PET, most of the conventional radionuclide studies suffer from a relatively poor spatial resolution and have a low specificity in detecting infections in the axial skeleton.

Our own group evaluated 45 FDG-PET scans in 39 patients with suspected infectious lesions [12]. Eighteen out of 45 PET scans were done in patients in whom acute or subacute osteomyelitis was suspected, with sensitivities of 100% and specificities of 83-99% were described for FDG-PET [12]. In contrast to acute osteomyelitis, low-grade and chronic infections are more difficult to diagnose with the current imaging modalities. In this setting, PET is useful because FDG is avidly taken up by activated macrophages, which predominate in the chronic phase of infection [13, 14]. Guhlmann et al. [15] showed a sensitivity and specificity for FDG-PET of 100 and 92%, respectively, in the assessment of chronic osteomyeltitis in the peripheral ($n = 21$) and axial ($n = 10$) skeleton. These results were confirmed in other studies [16, 17]. Furthermore, a negative FDG-PET scan was shown to virtually rule out osteomyelitis [18,19].

FDG-PET also represents a promising imaging technique in the diagnosis of implant-associated infections in trauma patients [19, 20]. FDG-PET images are not substantially affected by metallic implants inserted for fracture fixation, in contrast to PET imaging of prosthetic-joint devices (Figs. 1, 2). This is most likely due to the more slender materials (e.g., titanium) and different meth-

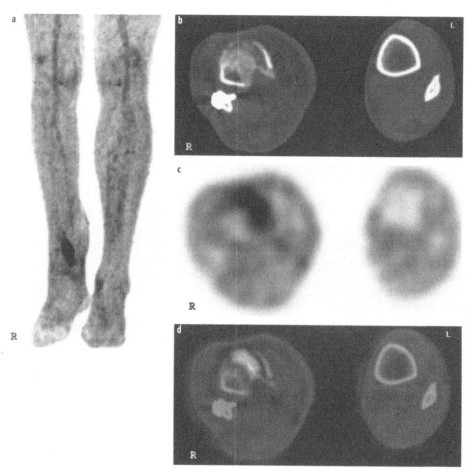

Fig. 1 a-d. A 53-year old man one year after a grade 2 open right pilon tibial fracture. Maximum-intensity-projection (MIP) (**a**) and axial PET image (**c**) show focal increased FDG uptake in the right distal tibia. Axial CT scan (**b**) demonstrates a bony defect of the right tibia posteriorly and an increased density within the right tibia representing spongiosa plastic. A metallic implant is present in the right fibula. Axial co-registered PET/CT (**d**) shows increased FDG uptake in the right distal tibia, representing osteomyelitis. Determination of the exact localization and extension of the infectious foci were only possible with PET/CT. (With permission from [46])

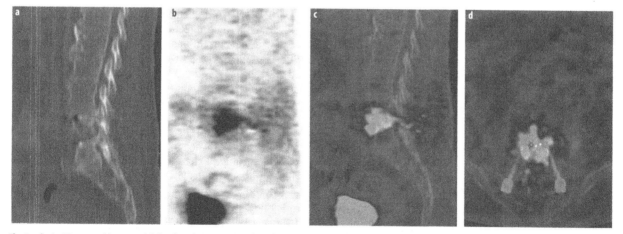

Fig. 2 a-d. A 68-year old man with back pain seven months after the insertion of lumbar spinal hardware. Sagittal CT (**a**) shows osteopenia but no signs of loosening of the pedicle screws at vertebral bodies L4 and L5. Sagittal PET (**b**) and sagittal PET/CT scan (**c**) demonstrate highly increased FDG uptake in the vertebral bodies (L4 and L5) and in the area of the pedicle screws, representing spondylitis. On axial PET/CT scan (**d**), additional increased FDG accumulation in the soft tissues adjacent to L4 and 5 as well as in the soft tissues dorsally is seen. (With permission from [46])

ods (e.g., external fixation) used in trauma patients. FDG-PET has a sensitivity of nearly 100% and a specificity of 88-93% in the diagnosis of chronic musculoskeletal infections, including patients with and without metallic implants or prosthetic replacements [15, 19, 21, 22].

Hartmann et al. recently evaluated the diagnostic value of FDG-PET/CT in trauma patients with suspected chronic osteomyelitis and reported promising results [20], with sensitivity, specificity, and accuracy for FDG-PET/CT ($n = 33$) being 94, 87, and 91% for the whole group; 88, 100, and 90% for disease involving the axial skeleton; and 100, 85, and 91% for disease of the peripheral skeleton, respectively.

Osteomyelitis in the Diabetic Foot

Differentiation between diabetic osteoarthropathy (neuropathic or Charcot joint) and osteomyelitis remains challenging even with the advent of new diagnostic techniques [23]. For pedal osteomyelitis, the most useful radionuclide study is ^{111}In-labeled leukocyte imaging, which has an accuracy of about 80% [24].

Newman et al. [25] prospectively investigated 35 diabetic patients with pedal ulcers and found that ^{111}In-labeled leukocyte scintigraphy was more sensitive (89 vs. 69%) and more specific (69 vs. 39%) than bone scintigraphy for diagnosing pedal osteomyelitis.

FDG-PET is affected by the level of circulating glucose and insulin. Elevated glucose levels decrease FDG uptake because FDG and glucose compete for the same transporters. However, according to a study by Keidar et al., FDG-PET was highly accurate in the detection of clinical suspected osteomyelitis of the foot. PET yielded a false positive result in only one of 18 sites, misdiagnosing osteoarthropathy of the third metatarsal bone as osteomyelitis [26]. Our group was not able to confirm these results [27].

Schwegler et al. [27] compared FDG-PET with 99mTc-labeled antigranulocyte antibody scintigraphy and MRI in diabetic patients with chronic foot ulcers without clinical suspicion for osteomyelitis. FDG-PET and 99mTc-labeled antigranulocyte antibody scintigraphy showed poor sensitivity, detecting only two of seven patients with osteomyelitis of the forefoot. MRI was positive in six of these seven patients. These results support the superiority of MRI over FDG-PET and 99mTc-labeled antigranulocyte antibody scintigraphy and it may also be the preferred imaging modality in patients with nonhealing diabetic foot ulcers.

Disc-Space Infection

Contrast-enhanced MRI is the imaging method of choice in patients with suspected disc space infection. However, differentiation between substantial degenerative (so-called Modic abnormalities) and infectious endplate abnormalities can be difficult. In this setting, three-phase bone scintigraphy is of limited value. Modic et al. [28] reported a sensitivity and specificity of 90 and 78% for bone scintigraphy, and 96 and 92% for MRI, respectively. Before the introduction of PET scanners, bone-gallium scintigraphy was the preferred radionuclide technique for diagnosing spinal osteomyelitis. Love et al. [7] showed that gallium-67 single-photon emission computed tomography (SPECT) was comparable to sequential bone/gallium scintigraphy, yielding a sensitivity of 91% and specificity of 77%. However, FDG-PET is superior in detecting infections of the spine, with higher sensitivities and specificities than obtained with gallium-67-citrate imaging [29-31]. In addition, FDG-PET is useful for excluding disc-space infection in those patients with severe degenerative disc disease of the lumbar spine, in whom the MRI results are often equivocal [29]. FDG-PET did not show FDG uptake in any patient with degenerative disc disease, whereas uptake was found in all patients with endplate abnormalities of infectious origin. The sensitivity and specificity of MRI in detecting disc-space infection were 50 and 96%, while for FDG-PET the corresponding values were 100 and 100%. However, FDG-PET cannot differentiate between bacterial and sterile inflammation (e.g., inflammatory disc disease in patients with ankylosing spondylitis) and biopsy is still necessary [32, 33].

Prosthetic-Joint Infection

Although bone scintigraphy is sensitive for detecting complications of prosthetic surgery, it cannot reliably distinguish aseptic loosening from infection [34]. Sequential bone/gallium imaging is one radionuclide imaging test to diagnose prosthetic-joint infection. But, in contrast to bone scintigraphy alone, it did not result in a major improvement for differentiating infection from other causes of prosthetic failure.

Combined ^{111}In-labeled leukocyte/99mTc-sulfur-colloid marrow imaging remains the gold standard in patients with hip and knee prostheses. Sensitivities and specificities are reportedly 86-100% and 89-94%, respectively [10, 11]. In contrast to patients with metallic implants, PET may not be as useful in the diagnosis of infection in patients with failed total-joint arthroplasties because of the remarkably similar histopathological morphology in patients with septic and aseptic prosthetic loosening [11, 35]. The reason for the increased FDG uptake around the prosthesis in aseptic loosening is an inflammatory reaction to one or more of the prosthetic components. This reaction may, in turn, cause aseptic loosening.

Image interpretation in patients with prosthetic devices can be affected by artifacts induced by attenuation correction. Therefore, examination of non-attenuation-corrected scans is necessary, as these images show less prominent reconstruction artifacts [36].

Initial studies of patients suspected of having total joint infection showed promising results [17, 37, 38]. Zhuang et al. reported sensitivities of 90% and specificities of 89% in the diagnosis of infected lower-limb prostheses [37]. Chacko et al. reported accuracies for FDG-PET of 96% for total hip replacements, 81% for total knee replacements, and 100% for other orthopedic devices [17].

Love et al. [11] investigated 59 patients (40 hip and 19 knee) with FDG-PET using a coincidence detection system and combined ^{111}In-labeled leukocyte and 99mTc-sulfur-colloid marrow imaging. The accuracy of FDG-PET for diagnosing infection of the failed prosthetic joint in this series was low, between 47 and 71% depending on the different criteria used by the authors to evaluate the images. This is in contrast to the high accuracy of 95% obtained for combined ^{111}In-labeled leukocyte and 99mTc-sulfur.colloid marrow imaging.

Data from our group [35] in a study of patients with total hip replacement had an accuracy of 69%, comparable to the results of Love et al. [11]. FDG-PET was unable to differentiate between aseptic loosening and infection.

In another study performed by our group, FDG uptake was examined in 28 patients with painful total knee arthroplasty, with uptake found to be related to the location of soft-tissue pain [39]. Increased FDG uptake was found in the synovial membrane in all patients except one patient independent of the clinical diagnosis (Fig. 3). FDG uptake in the synovial membrane was already described by Manthey et al., who suggested that it contributed to the

false-positive findings in patients with suspected infected prostheses [40]. In agreement with the results of other studies, our data [39] indicate that periprosthetic uptake is not only associated with infection [11, 38, 40, 41].

Very recently, Chryssikos et al. [42] prospectively investigated 113 patients with 127 painful hip prostheses. The authors reported that FDG PET findings were suggestive of infection if increased uptake was observed at the stem-prosthesis interface. Sensitivity, specificity, and accuracy were 85, 93, and 91%, respectively. However, due to the different study results among various groups, more prospective data are needed to define the value of FDG-PET in patients with prosthetic joints.

18-F Fluoride

18-F fluoride PET imaging is a promising imaging technique in musculoskeletal diseases. This method has provided excellent results in the evaluation of back pain in children and adolescents in whom osseous abnormalities were seen on CT imaging [43, 44]. In addition, 18-F fluoride PET has been used to predict bone viability after trauma or reconstructive surgery [45]. It is more accurate than planar scintigraphy or SPECT with 99mTc-labeled diphosphonates for localizing and characterizing benign and malignant bone disorders.

References

1. Termaat MF, Raijmakers PG, Scholten HJ et al (2005) The accuracy of diagnostic imaging for the assessment of chronic osteomyelitis: a systematic review and meta-analysis. J Bone Joint Surg Am 87:2464-2471
2. Schauwecker DS (1992) The scintigraphic diagnosis of osteomyelitis. AJR Am J Roentgenol 158:9-18
3. Meyers SP, Wiener SN (1991) Diagnosis of hematogenous pyogenic vertebral osteomyelitis by magnetic resonance imaging. Arch Intern Med 151:683-687
4. Chung JK, Yeo J, Lee DS et al (1996) Bone marrow scintigraphy using technetium-99m-antigranulocyte antibody in hematologic disorders. J Nucl Med 37:978-982
5. Jacobson AF, Gilles CP, Cerqueira MD (1992) Photopenic defects in marrow-containing skeleton on indium-111 leucocyte scintigraphy: prevalence at sites suspected of osteomyelitis and as an incidental finding. Eur J Nucl Med 19:858-864
6. Gratz S, Braun HG, Behr TM et al (1997) Photopenia in chronic vertebral osteomyelitis with technetium-99m-antigranulocyte antibody (BW 250/183). J Nucl Med 38:211-216
7. Palestro CJ, Torres MA (1997) Radionuclide imaging in orthopedic infections. Semin Nucl Med 27:334-345
8. Mulamba L, Ferrant A, Leners N et al (1983) Indium-111 leucocyte scanning in the evaluation of painful hip arthroplasty. Acta Orthop Scand 54:695-697
9. Palestro CJ, Kim CK, Swyer AJ et al (1990) Total-hip arthroplasty: periprosthetic indium-111-labeled leukocyte activity and complementary technetium-99m-sulfur colloid imaging in suspected infection. J Nucl Med 31:1950-1955
10. Palestro CJ, Roumanas P, Swyer AJ et al (1992) Diagnosis of musculoskeletal infection using combined In-111 labeled leukocyte and Tc-99m SC marrow imaging. Clin Nucl Med 17:269-273

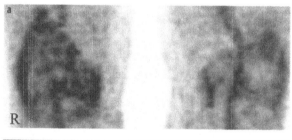
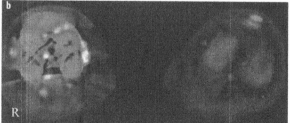

Fig. 3 a, b. A 79-year-old man who underwent right-knee replacement and subsequently experienced pain. MIP PET (**a**) and axial PET/CT (**b**) show strongly increased FDG uptake in the synovial membrane of the right knee, including the suprapatellar recess. FDG uptake is also seen in the contralateral left joint, at the site of painful osteoarthritis. The diagnosis was made through rotational CT, demonstrating severe femoral malrotation of the prosthesis. (With permission from [46])

Metabolic Bone Disease

Paul J. Ryan

Department of Nuclear Medicine, Medway Maritime Hospital, Gillingham, UK

Introduction

Metabolic bone disease encompasses a number of disorders that typically show involvement of the entire skeleton. They are mostly associated with increased bone turnover and increased uptake of radiolabeled diphosphonate. The increased uptake produces heightened contrast on bone scan between bone and soft tissues, deceptively giving the appearance of excellent image quality. In more severe cases, there may be characteristic patterns of abnormality, including one or more of the following metabolic features [1]:

1. Increased tracer uptake in the long bones
2. Increased tracer uptake in the axial skeleton
3. Increased uptake in the periarticular areas
4. Faint or almost absent kidney images
5. Prominent calvaria and mandible
6. Beading of the costochondral junctions
7. "Tie" sternum

In mild cases, the bone scan may often appear normal and detection of disease suffers from the difficulty of subjective interpretation. Thus, the bone scan is rarely used for the detection of metabolic bone disease on its own, although it can be used in a complementary role. It should be recognized that the sensitivity of the bone scan for focal metabolic bone disease, such as Paget's disease, and the focal complications of metabolic bone disease, such as fracture and pseudofracture, is very good. This is where the major applications of bone scintigraphy are found in clinical practice.

Primary Hyperparathyroidism

The bone scan in hyperparathyroidism may show slight generalized increased activity with high bone to soft tissue ratios but rarely the obvious metabolic features. As most cases are mild and asymptomatic, the high generalized uptake is not a consistent diagnostic finding. In one study the bone scans of only four out of 20 patients showed increased uptake [2]. In clinical practice, the suggestion of hyperparathyroidism on bone scan is most likely to occur as part of the investigation of hypercal-

cemia. It is important to be aware that high uptake can persist for up to a year following parathyroidectomy. In addition, calcification of the lungs and stomach can occur in severe hyperparathyroidism and is detectable on bone scan. This rapidly resolves following successful treatment. Ectopic calcification is not, however, a diagnostic feature and can be found in malignancy. In advanced primary hyperparathyroidism, brown tumors may occur. These can be single or multiple and confusion is possible with skeletal metastases, since these will also be visualized as focal defects on bone scan.

Osteomalacia

The bone scan in osteomalacia will show the classical features of metabolic bone disease although in the early stages will be normal [3]. The reason for the increased uptake in osteomalacia, a condition in which there is a mineralization defect, is uncertain. Suggested explanations are that there is so much osteoid present that even though mineralization is occurring more slowly the total mineralizing area is increased. Alternatively, there may be increased diffusion of tracer in an extremely large osteoid pool. However, the increased uptake is most likely to be due to secondary hyperparathyroidism since the clinical impression is that the bone scan appearances in osteomalacia reflect the degree of hyperparathyroidism present. Focal abnormalities due to pseudofractures may also be seen and the bone scan provides a sensitive means of their detection, particularly in the ribs, where they may be missed by conventional radiology. The detection of pseudofractures is probably the most useful application of the bone scan in osteomalacia. On occasion, the bone scan can be useful for diagnosis when other investigations have proved to be equivocal.

Renal Osteodystrophy

The most common appearance of bone scan images in renal osteodystrophy is of generalized increased tracer uptake throughout the skeleton, as in other metabolic bone

11. Love C, Marwin SE, Tomas MB et al (2004) Diagnosing infection in the failed joint replacement: a comparison of coincidence detection 18F-FDG and 111In-labeled leukocyte/99mTc-sulfur colloid marrow imaging. J Nucl Med 45:1864-1871

12. Stumpe KD, Dazzi H, Schaffner A, von Schulthess GK (2000) Infection imaging using whole-body FDG-PET. Eur J Nucl Med 27:822-832

13. Babior BM (1984) The respiratory burst of phagocytes. J Clin Invest 73:599-601

14. Kaim AH, Weber B, Kurrer MO et al (2002) Autoradiographic quantification of 18F-FDG uptake in experimental soft-tissue abscesses in rats. Radiology 223:446-451

15. Guhlmann A, Brecht-Krauss D, Suger G et al (1998) Chronic osteomyelitis: detection with FDG PET and correlation with histopathologic findings. Radiology 206:749-754

16. Zhuang H, Duarte PS, Pourdehand M et al (2000) Exclusion of chronic osteomyelitis with F-18 fluorodeoxyglucose positron emission tomographic imaging. Clin Nucl Med 25:281-284

17. Chacko TK, Zhuang H, Nakhoda KZ et al (2003) Applications of fluorodeoxyglucose positron emission tomography in the diagnosis of infection. Nucl Med Commun 24:615-624

18. Guhlmann A, Brecht-Krauss D, Suger G et al (1998) Fluorine-18-FDG PET and technetium-99m antigranulocyte antibody scintigraphy in chronic osteomyelitis. J Nucl Med 39:2145-2152

19. de Winter F, van de Wiele C, Vogelaers D et al (2001) Fluorine-18 fluorodeoxyglucose-position emission tomography: a highly accurate imaging modality for the diagnosis of chronic musculoskeletal infections. J Bone Joint Surg Am 83-A:651-660

20. Hartmann A, Eid K, Dora C et al (2006) Diagnostic value of (18)F-FDG PET/CT in trauma patients with suspected chronic osteomyelitis. Eur J Nucl Med Mol Imaging 34:704-714

21. Schiesser M, Stumpe KD, Trentz O et al (2003) Detection of metallic implant-associated infections with FDG PET in patients with trauma: correlation with microbiologic results. Radiology 226:391-398

22. De Winter F, Gemmel F, Van De Wiele C et al (2003) 18-Fluorine fluorodeoxyglucose positron emission tomography for the diagnosis of infection in the postoperative spine. Spine 28:1314-1319

23. Chatha DS, Cunningham PM, Schweitzer ME (2005) MR imaging of the diabetic foot: diagnostic challenges. Radiol Clin North Am 43:747-759, ix

24. Palestro CJ, Tomas MB (2000) Scintigraphic evaluation of the diabetic foot. In: Freeman LM (ed) Nuclear Medicine Annual: Lippincott Williams & Wilkins, Philadelphia, pp 143-172

25. Newman LG, Waller J, Palestro CJ et al (1991) Unsuspected osteomyelitis in diabetic foot ulcers. Diagnosis and monitoring by leukocyte scanning with indium in 111 oxyquinoline. Jama 266:1246-1251

26. Keidar Z, Militianu D, Melamed E et al (2005) The diabetic foot: initial experience with 18F-FDG PET/CT. J Nucl Med 46:444-449

27. Schwegler B, Stumpe KD, Weishaupt D et al (2008) Unsuspected osteomyelitis is frequent in persistent diabetic foot ulcer and better diagnosed by MRI than by 18F-FDG PET or 99mTc-MOAB. J Intern Med 263:99-106

28. Modic MT, Feiglin DH, Piraino DW et al (1985) Vertebral osteomyelitis: assessment using MR. Radiology 157:157-166

29. Stumpe KD, Zanetti M, Weishaupt D et al (2002) FDG positron emission tomography for differentiation of degenerative and infectious endplate abnormalities in the lumbar spine detected on MR imaging. AJR Am J Roentgenol 179:1151-1157

30. Schmitz A, Risse JH, Grunwald F et al (2001) Fluorine-18 fluorodeoxyglucose positron emission tomography findings in spondylodiscitis: preliminary results. Eur Spine J 10:534-539

31. Gratz S, Dorner J, Fischer U et al (2002) 18F-FDG hybrid PET in patients with suspected spondylitis. Eur J Nucl Med Mol Imaging 29:516-524

32. Wendling D, Blagosklonov O, Streit G et al (2005) FDG-PET/CT scan of inflammatory spondylodiscitis lesions in ankylosing spondylitis, and short term evolution during antitumour necrosis factor treatment. Ann Rheum Dis 64:1663-1665

33. Chew FS, Kline MJ (2001) Diagnostic yield of CT-guided percutaneous aspiration procedures in suspected spontaneous infectious diskitis. Radiology 218:211-214

34. Levitsky KA, Hozack WJ, Balderston RA et al (1991) Evaluation of the painful prosthetic joint. Relative value of bone scan, sedimentation rate, and joint aspiration. J Arthroplasty 6:237-244

35. Stumpe KD, Notzli HP, Zanetti M et al (2004) FDG PET for differentiation of infection and aseptic loosening in total hip replacements: comparison with conventional radiography and three-phase bone scintigraphy. Radiology 231:333-341

36. Goerres GW, Ziegler SI, Burger C et al (2003) Artifacts at PET and PET/CT caused by metallic hip prosthetic material. Radiology 226:577-584

37. Zhuang H, Duarte PS, Pourdehnad M et al (2001) The promising role of 18F-FDG PET in detecting infected lower limb prosthesis implants. J Nucl Med 42:44-48

38. Reinartz P, Mumme T, Hermanns B et al (2005) Radionuclide imaging of the painful hip arthroplasty: positron-emission tomography versus triple-phase bone scanning. J Bone Joint Surg Br 87:465-470

39. Stumpe KD, Romero J, Ziegler O et al (2006) The value of FDG-PET in patients with painful total knee arthroplasty. Eur J Nucl Med Mol Imaging 33:1218-1225

40. Manthey N, Reinhard P, Moog F et al (2002) The use of [18F]fluorodeoxyglucose positron emission tomography to differentiate between synovitis, loosening and infection of hip and knee prostheses. Nucl Med Commun 23:645-653

41. Love C, Tomas MB, Marwin SE et al (2001) Role of nuclear medicine in diagnosis of the infected joint replacement. Radiographics 21:1229-1238

42. Chryssikos T, Parvizi J, Ghanem E et al (2008) FDG-PET imaging can diagnose periprosthetic infection of the hip. Clin Orthop Relat Res 466:1338-1342

43. Ovadia D, Metser U, Lievshitz G et al (2007) Back pain in adolescents: assessment with integrated 18F-fluoride positron-emission tomography-computed tomography. J Pediatr Orthop 27:90-93

44. Lim R, Fahey FH, Drubach LA et al (2007) Early experience with fluorine-18 sodium fluoride bone PET in young patients with back pain. J Pediatr Orthop 27:277-282

45. Forrest N, Welch A, Murray AD et al (2006) Femoral head viability after Birmingham resurfacing hip arthroplasty: assessment with use of [18F] fluoride positron emission tomography. J Bone Joint Surg Am 88 Suppl 3:84-89

46. Stumpe KD (2007) PET and PET/CT Imaging in infection and inflammation. In: Wahl RL (ed) Categorical course in diagnostic radiology: clinical PET and PET/CT imaging syllabus. The Radiological Society of North America, pp 185-201

disorders with some or all of the typical metabolic features. The severest and most striking scan appearances found in metabolic bone disease are seen in the more extreme cases of renal osteodystrophy. The 24-h whole-body retention is increased and bone to soft tissue ratios are elevated. On occasion, ectopic calcification can be visualized on bone scintigraphy, for example in the lungs, stomach, or kidneys. Aluminum toxicity rarely occurs nowadays but when present produces poor bone scan images with heightened background due to inhibition of tracer uptake in bone. Aluminum is deposited at the calcification front and blocks mineralization. In clinical practice, there is little indication for bone scanning to detect metabolic bone disease in renal osteodystrophy but it is important to be aware of the possible appearances. Obviously, if a metabolic bone scan appearance is detected this would require further evaluation.

Osteoporosis

The bone scan is mainly used for the diagnosis and age determination of fractures, particularly collapsed vertebrae. It can also detect co-existent disease and exclude alternative diagnoses. Other roles include the detection of unsuspected fractures and fracture complications, such as osteomyelitis and non-union. The bone scan is also useful for the diagnosis of regional osteoporotic syndromes, such as transient osteoporosis of the hip, regional migratory osteoporosis, and algodystrophy. It has a potentially useful role in the evaluation of new therapies since the detection of new vertebral fractures is recognized as the most appropriate endpoint for osteoporosis prevention studies.

Although not usually used for diagnosis, the bone scan can demonstrate features that are suggestive, such as relatively low uptake of tracer into the skeleton, which gives a "washed out" appearance and poor vertebral definition (reduced bone to soft tissue ratios) [4]. There may be loss of vertebral height due to a marked kyphosis, and closeness of the rib cage to the pelvis can be seen in patients with multiple vertebral fractures. These features may alert the physician to the presence of osteoporosis if it had not previously been suspected. It is also not uncommon for fractures (e.g., vertebrae or ribs) to be first detected on bone scan, which then leads to a diagnosis of osteoporosis.

Spinal Osteoporosis

Vertebral fractures are associated with a characteristic intense linear pattern of increased tracer uptake corresponding to the site of fracture. This activity then fades over a period of 6-18 months, such that the intensity of uptake helps in the assessment of the age of the fracture [5]. In the clinical situation of a patient presenting with acute back pain and vertebral fracture detected on X-ray, the bone scan can assist in the evaluation as to whether pain is attributable to a recent fracture. A normal scan excludes a recent fracture and in this situation another cause of pain should be sought. In the patient with more chronic back pain and multiple collapsed vertebrae, the bone scan is useful to help detect whether a new fracture has occurred. This can often be difficult on X-ray, where good reproducible views can be difficult to obtain. The development of further back pain in this context is almost impossible to evaluate without a bone scan. The bone scan can also suggest other causes of vertebral collapse, such as metastases, infection, or Paget's disease. When compared with X-ray results, a positive bone scan nearly always implies a significant vertebral fracture if the vertebral height is more than 3 SD below the mean [6].

The advent of new interventional treatments for osteoporosis, such as vertebroplasty and kyphoplasty, has enlarged the role of the bone scan in the assessment of vertebral fracture. Both techniques work best in the acute or sub-acute setting and are less effective at pain relief if performed >6 months after the fracture has occurred. The bone scan can help determine whether any vertebrae may be suitable for such treatments and in the context of multiple fractures determine which are most amenable to treatment. In clinical practice, such patients will also be investigated with magnetic resonance imaging (MRI) to determine whether there are contraindications to intervention and also to assess the age of the fracture. The bone scan and MRI scan are complementary, as the MRI features of an acute fracture settle much faster than those of the bone scan. Another use of the bone scan is to detect new fractures in a patient with multiple fractures, to help in the selection of patients for parathyroid hormone anabolic therapy. These treatments are expensive and often restricted to those who have continued to sustain fractures despite conventional therapy with bisphposphonates. Demonstration of disease progression by the development of new fractures can enable a patient to become eligible for treatment.

SPECT

The addition of single photon emission computed tomography (SPECT) has improved the diagnostic ability of the bone scan, with further enhancement recently achieved by the advent of hybrid SPECT/CT scanners. SPECT enables separate evaluation of the different parts of the vertebra, such as the body, pedicle, facet joint, pars inter articularis, and lamina and spinous process. In the diagnosis of acute vertebral fracture, localization of activity to the vertebral body and associated with the collapsed vertebra, as seen on SPECT/CT, helps to establish the diagnosis. Patients with multiple fractures and chronic back pain can be difficult to assess in clinical practice. In many cases, there is increased activity in the facet joints above or below the involved vertebra or in the lower lumbar spine at L4/L5 and L5/S1 [7]. The detected facet arthropathy can then be used to select local treatment if necessary.

Fractures

Patients with vertebral fractures commonly have fractures at other sites. An important role of the bone scan is the early detection of suspected fractures in patients with normal or equivocal X-ray findings. Previously unrecognized fractures of the pelvis are commonly found on bone scan in the sacrum where a vertebral fracture was suspected, or the pubic rami where a hip fracture was suspected. In the sacrum, the positive identification of a fracture can be important not only for secure diagnosis but also because such fractures are suitable for cement fixation by sacroplasty, a technique similar to vertebroplasty. Unsuspected fractures of the ribs, femoral neck, humerus, scapulae, radius, and ribs may first be detected only on the bone scan. The classical appearance is a linear increased uptake during the blood-flow, blood-pool, and static images, which is very different from the findings in skeletal metastases. Ribs fractures are, however, typically focal; if multiple, they are distributed in a linear pattern. Complications of fracture, such as avascular necrosis and complex regional pain syndrome, can also be detected.

Paget's Disease

Paget's disease of bone is a common disorder, particularly in the UK and in northern European countries and areas populated by descendents from there. A prevalence of 5% has been estimated for UK patients over 60 years of age. In the great majority of affected individuals the condition is asymptomatic and may only be discovered incidentally, following the detection of an elevated serum alkaline phosphatase, or as an incidental finding on X-ray or isotope bone scan. In the past, Paget's disease was regarded as an untreatable disorder and was to a large degree neglected. However, in recent years, with the advent of powerful antiresorptive agents, effective therapies are now available and the condition is regarded as treatable

Bone Scan Appearances

The bone scan appearances in Paget's disease are usually characteristic with the predominant feature, being strikingly increased uptake distributed throughout most or all of the affected bone [8]. The only common exception to this is osteoporosis circumscripta (lytic disease involving the skull), in which tracer uptake may only be intense at the margin of the lesion. Paget's disease, in contrast to other skeletal pathologies, tends to preserve or enhance the normal anatomy. The appearance of individual lesions may be quite dramatic and pagetic bone appears to be picked out, as the borders between normal and abnormal bone are clearly delineated. In affected vertebrae, the transverse spinous processes will frequently be involved; this may be an important feature in the differential diag-

nosis. The vertebral appearance of Paget's disease has been described as a "Mickey Mouse" sign, with uptake having an inverted triangular pattern. Other case reports have described the "black beard" sign of monostotic disease of the mandible and the "short pants" sign of spinal, pelvic, and upper femoral disease. Expansion and distortion of the involved bones can often be recognized. In the appendicular skeleton, lesions are bound by the articular surface and progress into the shaft. The advancing lesion may be seen to have a sharp V-shaped edge, which corresponds to the lytic flame-shaped resorption front seen on radiographs.

The typical findings of Paget's disease are easily recognizable. When polyostotic disease is present, there is seldom any doubt as to the diagnosis. Indeed it is usually possible to distinguish Paget's disease from metastatic disease when they co exist. However, both are common conditions and inevitably some diagnostic difficulty arises, particularly when scan appearances are atypical. Furthermore, metastases do occur in pagetic bone, but despite its high vascularity this occurs perhaps less often than one would expect. A frequent situation that arises is that of a patient with a known primary tumor who has a bone scan performed to screen for skeletal metastases, with Paget's disease found incidentally. Where any uncertainty exists, individual sites of involvement must be carefully evaluated and X-rayed. Rarely, when the bone scan appearances are atypical, a CT scan or biopsy is performed. Lesions in the spine are usually the most problematic, particularly when vertebral collapse or degenerative disease is present. SPECT can be useful to assess spinal disease when uptake is seen throughout the vertebra including the transverse processes. SPECT can be also useful to evaluate cranial disease. Following therapy for Paget's disease, particularly with the more powerful bisphosphonates, the uniform uptake on bone scan may change to a more focal distribution and this may be particularly true as re-activation occurs [9]. Confusion could occur with metastases if the findings are not recognized as reflecting the response to treatment.

Compared to X-rays, the bone scan is more sensitive and it has the advantage of being easily able to assess the entire skeleton. Very rarely, a lesion will be seen on X-ray but not on the bone scan – a finding usually attributed to burnt out disease. Although the bone scan is usually effective at detecting fractures, these may be less well identified in pagetic bone because of the high background uptake. Also, osteosaracomas may not be identified although reduced uptake is generally found in this tumor.

In evaluating the response to therapy, the bone scan is useful about 3-6 months following the start of treatment. Biochemical findings will respond more quickly but do not allow for the assessment of individual bones. In some patients, alkaline phosphatase levels are not markedly elevated before therapy, particularly in those with monostotic disease, in which case the bone scan becomes an even more valuable tool for following the patient. Pagetic lesions show variable response to therapy even amongst lesions in the same patient. In general, less active lesions are more likely to respond completely. The change in bone scan activity is a good predictor of the need for further therapy. The use of ^{18}FDG PET has been investigated in Paget's disease and uptake can sometimes be seen in Pagetic lesions but in the majority there is no uptake [10].

References

1. Fogelman I, Citrin DL, Turner JG et al (1979) Semiquantitative interpretation of the bone scan in metabolic bone disease. Eur J Nucl Med 4:287-289
2. Weighmann T, Rosenthall L, Kaye M (1977) Technetium 99m pyrophosphate bone scan in hyperparathyroidism. J Nucl Med 18:231
3. Fogelman I, McKillop JH, Bessant RG et al (1978) The role of bone scanning in osteomalacia. J Nucl Med 19:245-248
4. Sy WM (1981) Osteoporosis. In: Sy WM (ed) Gamma images in benign and metabolic bone disease. CRC, Boca Ralton, FL, pp 223-239
5. Fogelman I, Carr D (1988) A comparison between bone scanning and radiology in the evaluation of patients with metabolic bone disease. Clin Radiol 31:321-326
6. Ryan PJ, Fogelman I (1994) Osteoporotic vertebral fractures. Comparison with radiography and bone scintigraphy. Radiology 190:669-672
7. Ryan PJ, Evans PA, Gibson T, Fogelman I (1992) Osteoporosis and chronic low back pain. A study with single photon emission computed bone scintigraphy. J Bone Miner Res 7:1455-1459
8. Serafini AN (1976) Paget's disease of bone. Semin Nucl Med 6:47-58
9. Ryan PJ, Gibson T, Fogelman I (1992) Bone scintigraphy following pamidronate therapy for Paget's Disease of Bone. J Nucl Med 33:1589-1593
10. Cook GJR, Maisey M, Fogelman I (1999) Fluorine 18 FDG PET in Paget's disease of Bone. J Nucl Med 43:259-268

Radionuclide Imaging and Therapy of Inflammatory Joint Lesions

Torsten Kuwert

Department of Nuclear Medicine, Friedrich-Alexander University of Erlangen-Nürnberg, Erlangen, Germany

Radionuclide Imaging

The spectrum of inflammatory disorders of the joints includes degenerative osteoarthritis (OA) and autoimmune diseases such as rheumatoid arthritis (RA) and psoriatic arthritis (PA). Further diseases to be considered in this context are metabolic disorders such as gout or chronic inflammatory processes such as pigmented villonodular synovialitis (PVNS). Bacterial infections of the joints and, in particular, of joint prostheses are another example of diseases producing inflammatory joint lesions. Furthermore, the differential to be considered in pain of the joints includes also non-inflammatory diseases such as occult fractures or tumors growing near or in the joints.

More than 50% of subjects older than 60 years suffer from OA. The disease is caused by degeneration of the cartilage of the joint, leading in its worst case to its complete destruction. The radiological hallmarks of OA are joint space narrowing, osteophytes, and subchondral cysts, also called geodes. OA may affect any joint of the body, being most frequently in the spine, hip, knee, and hands. In the hands, the term "Heberden's polyarthrosis" has been coined to denote the isolated involvement of the distal interphalangeal joints. The isolated involvement of the proximal interphalangeal joints is called Bouchard's polyarthrosis. Degeneration of the intervertebral disks leads to narrowing of the intervertebral space and osteochondrosis. Further sequelae are facet arthritis and pseudospondylolisthesis, which is defined as a misalignment of the vertebral bodies. OA may be inactive or active; in the latter case synovialitis also occurs, leading to joint effusions and pain.

Autoimmune joint diseases are characterized by the production of antibodies directed against various body proteins. All autoimmune joint diseases may lead to joint destruction as endpoint if not treated properly.

Rheumatoid arthritis (RA) is the most common of these disorders. It is more frequent in women than in men and has a peak incidence at 40 years of age, but may also affect children. In its early stages, it is characterized by synovialitis, joint effusion, and marrow edema in the articulating bones. Typical further radiological signs of RA are subchondral erosions. Symmetrical involvement of the proximal interphalangeal joints and the carpus is typical of RA, but also the large joints may be affected.

Serologically, RA is characterized by the so-called rheumatoid factors, which are autoantibodies against immunoglobulins. A large group of inflammatory joint diseases lack these autoantibodies and are subsumed under the heading of seronegative spondylarthropathies. This group includes psoriatic arthritis, ankylosing spondylitis, and the various forms of reactive arthritis. In these disorders, involvement of the spine and the sacroiliac joints is frequently seen.

Psoriatic arthritis is found in approximately 10% of subjects suffering from psoriasis. Its pattern is asymmetrical; an involvement of all joints in one finger or toe is occasionally seen and pathognomonic. Enthesiopathies are another hallmark of this disease.

Ankylosing spondylitis (AS) typically leads to inflammation of various elements of the spine, such as the facets' joints or the disks. In extreme cases, the spine will completely lose its flexibility and thoracic kyphosis develops.

Reactive arthritis is a sequela of infection with various pathogens, including yersiniae, chlamydiae, and borreliae. However, it is not caused by direct infection of the joints involved, but by ill-characterized immunological phenomena such as cross-reactivity of synovial and bacterial antigens. Reactive arthritis is frequently self-limiting and has no characteristic patterns of joint involvement. Reiter's disease belongs to this group and is characterized by the triad of arthritis, urethritis, and conjunctivitis. Rheumatic arthritis occurring after tonsillar angina caused by streptococci is a further well-known member of this category and may occur together with cutaneous manifestations such as erythema nodosum, endocarditis, or – even more rarely – a hyperkinetic disorder called Sydenham's chorea.

Infectious arthritis involves in most cases one joint only and is usually caused by direct bacterial infection of the joint. It can be diagnosed by the demonstration of massive granulocytic infiltration of the joint fluid and is treated by antibiotics. A diagnostic dilemma is the infection of a joint prosthesis since the use of magnetic resonance imaging (MRI) as well as X-ray computed tomography (CT) is limited by artifacts arising from the metal implants.

Gout and chondrocalcinosis are characterized by the deposition of crystalline substances in various joint tissues, leading to an inflammatory reaction in the joint. If not treated properly, this has deleterious effects on the joint involved.

PVNS is a very rare benign disorder of the synovial tissue, occurring in adults between the ages of 20 and 50 years (for further literature, see [1]). It exists in three subtypes, a focal and a diffuse form restricted to the joint as well as a form extending to the tendon sheath, also termed "giant cell tumor of the tendon sheath". The diffuse form restricted to the joint resembles the chronic synovitis of RA.

The above-mentioned diseases lead to pain in the joints involved. Pathologically, the soft-tissue structures of the affected joints may be chronically or acutely inflamed; this is particularly true of the synovia, but also adjacent structures such as the tendons and ligaments may be involved in that process. Joint inflammation leads to joint remodeling. Bone tissue may hypertrophy locally, as in the case of osteophytes, encountered in OA, or of syndesmophytes in AS. However, it may also undergo resorption and destruction, as in the case of subarticular osteoporosis or periarticular erosions in RA.

Imaging capitalizes on the visualization of various aspects of the pathogenesis of joint disease (for further literature, see [2] and [3]):As a first step, planar radiography is usually performed, providing information on any disturbances of bone integrity, such as erosions, subchondral cysts, or osteophytes. On these images, the width of the joint space may also be assessed, allowing the diagnosis of effusions or joint space narrowing, both of which are typical for OA.

Ultrasound of the joints is valuable to assess the related soft-tissue structures such as tendons or the synovia. This technique enables also the detection of joint effusions or of a Baker's cyst of the knee.

CT is only rarely used in the workup of inflammatory joint disease but can be of benefit when trauma has occurred. It is, however, used to complement single-photon emission computed tomography (SPECT, see below) in a "one-stop shop" procedure, since hybrid cameras combining the two modalities have now been installed in several institutions.

MRI certainly is the gold standard of imaging joint inflammations since it allows the visualization of soft-tissue and osseous lesions. T1-weighted sequences are valuable as they depict the anatomy with high resolution and allow the detection of, among others, erosions, subchondral cysts, osteomyelitis, edema, and avascular necrosis. T2-weighted sequences may, in particular, permit the detection of inflammatory processes, joint effusions, and bone marrow edema, which is an early indicator of pathology.

Three-phase bone scintigraphy (BS) performed after injection of Tc-99m-labeled polyphosphonates has two advantages: (1) its high sensitivity, especially in the early stages of the rheumatoid disorders and of OA, and (2) assessment of the whole skeleton. BS may therefore be used to rule out inflammatory disease in a patient presenting with pain in or discomfort of the joints. A further indication is the determination of inflammatory activity in OA, e.g., in facets' arthritis or osteochondrosis. Furthermore, it may help in differentiating the various disorders, by demonstrating typical patterns of joint involvement. BS suffers from some limitation in specificity. The recent introduction of SPECT/CT hybrid scanners may help overcome this problem [4-6] (Fig. 1).

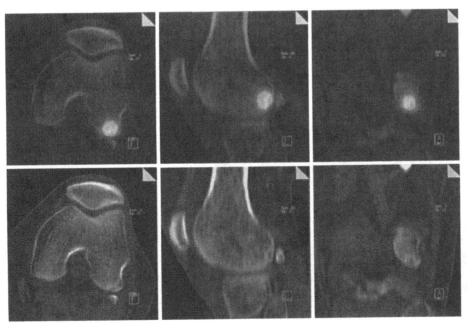

Fig. 1. The upper row shows fusion images between skeletal SPECT obtained after injection of Tc-99-labeled polyphosphonate and CT of a painful knee. Increased bone metabolism projects to a circumscribed region where an accessory bone, the so-called fabella, articulates with the femur. The lower row shows the corresponding CT images, the right image is a magnified view, featuring subcortical sclerosis and a subchondral cyst in the femur as signs of osteoarthritis

Scintigraphy performed after either injection of leuko-cytes labeled with In-11-oxim (IOX) or Tc-99m-hexam-ethylaminooxim (HMPAO) as well as after injection of Tc-99m-antigranulocyte antibodies (GAB) has been proven to be a highly specific method for localizing acute bacterial infection. Recent work has proven that also these types of scintigraphy benefit from SPECT/CT hybrid imaging (for further references see [6] and [7]) (Fig. 2).

Since labeling leukocytes with IOX or HMPAO is time-consuming, GAB-scintigraphy has replaced scintig-raphy with radioactively labeled leukocytes in most insti-tutions. Its drawbacks are mainly due to the pattern of normal distribution of GAB, which concentrates also in bone marrow. Consecutively, the diagnosis of infection localized in the stem skeleton is confronted with some difficulty with this method. Its specificity is also reduced in the diabetic foot, due to the occurrence of bone mar-row islands accumulating GAB.

F-18-deoxyglucose (FDG) accumulates also in inflam-matory cells. This reduces the specificity of positron emission tomography (PET) with this tracer in oncology, but serves as the basis for its use in diagnosing inflam-mation. FDG is taken up not only by granulocytes but al-so by macrophages [8]. Therefore, also chronic inflam-matory processes concentrate this tracer and are thus amenable to diagnosis by FDG-PET. This is of the case in rheumatoid arthritis and activated OA. Since FDG does not usually accumulate in bone marrow, it may also be used to search for inflammatory sites in the stem skele-ton. Some evidence has demonstrated a higher accuracy of FDG-PET compared to GAB-scintigraphy in diagnos-ing bacterial infection of joint prostheses (for literature, see [9]), although studies comparing FDG-PET/CT to GAB-SPECT/CT are still missing.

F-18-fluoride concentrates in bone as a function of bone metabolism, in analogy to the TC-99-labeled polyphosphonates (for further literature, see [10]). F-18-fluoride-PET has been shown to be more accurate than skeletal scintigraphy in staging cancer patients. Its use in orthopedics and rheumatology has as yet not been stud-ied systematically. It may be of use when the metabolic activity of comparatively small parts of the skeleton have to be investigated (Fig. 3).

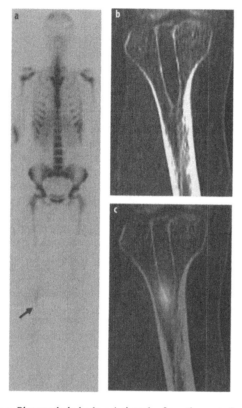

Fig. 2 a-c. Planar whole-body scintigraphy from the ventral aspect (**a**) shows accumulation of Tc-99m-antigranulocyte antibodies in the region of the right knee (*arrow*). The CT of that region (**b**) dis-closes a cavity in the femur as a remnant of a knee prosthesis. The fusion image (**c**) allows exact localization of the inflammatory process with relation to this cavity

Therapy

For most inflammatory joint diseases, systemic anti-in-flammatory medication is administered. In some cases, the disease may progress, in which case local therapy of the joints involved becomes a necessity. The latter may

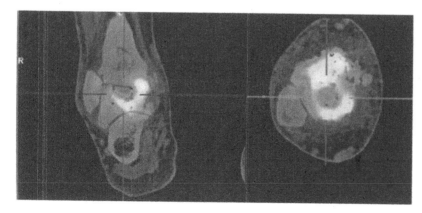

Fig. 3. F-18-fluoride PET image of the foot in axial (*left*) and transaxial (*right*) orientations and fused to the corresponding CT images. Consecutive to post-traumatic osteoarthritis, fluoride uptake is increased in the talus and adjacent structures. The cross marks an avi-tal fragment of the talus, one not accumulat-ing the tracer

consist of intra-articular injection of anti-inflammatory agents such as cortisone or of surgical therapy.

Radiosynoviorthesis (RSO) involves the intra-articular injection of radionuclides emitting β-radiation such that the dose is delivered at a high rate at a short distance (for a review, see [11]). The target organ is the synovium, which is the connective tissue lining the joint cavity. The radionuclides used are bound to colloids, which are rapidly phagocytized by the macrophages of the inflamed synovium. Because the particles are sufficiently large to prevent leakage from the joint, the levels of radiation delivered to the rest of the body are negligible. Rarely, the radiopharmaceutical is injected para-articularly or leaks for other reasons into neighboring tissue. In this case, radionecrosis may ensue.

RSO may be indicated in therapy-refractory synovialitis of any cause. Synovialitis can be demonstrated by the accumulation of Tc-99m-labeled polyphosphonates in the so-called pool phase of three-phase bone scintigraphy. Absolute contraindications are pregnancy, breast feeding, a ruptured Baker's cyst, local skin infection, and massive hemarthrosis. Bone destruction and significant cartilage loss are relative contraindications. The interval between RSO and previous joint puncture should be at least two weeks, that between RSO and joint surgery at least six.

RSO may alleviate pain and reduce joint effusion. Extensive evidence has been published on its success rates, which vary between 40 and 90%, depending on the underlying disease, its severity, and the joint treated.

References

1. Kat S, Kutz R, Elbracht T et al (2000) Radiosynovectomy in pigmented villonodular synovitis. Nuklearmedizin 39:209-213
2. Backhaus M, Sandrock D, Schmidt WA (2002) Bildgebende Verfahren in der Rheumatologie. Dtsch Med Wochenschr 127:1897-1903 [German]
3. Backhaus M, Burmester GR, Sandrock D et al (2002) Prospective two year follow up study comparing novel and conventional imaging procedures in patients with arthritic finger joints. Ann Rheum Dis 61:895-904
4. Even-Sapir E, Flusser G, Lerman H et al (2007) SPECT/Multislice Low-Dose CT: a clinically relevant constituent in the imaging algorithm of nononcologic patients referred for bone scintigraphy. J Nucl Med 48:319-324
5. Schillaci O (2005) Hybrid SPECT/CT: a new era for SPECT imaging? Eur J Nucl Med Mol Imaging 32:521-524
6. Mariani G, Flotats A, Israel O et al (2008) Clinical applications of SPECT/CT: new hybrid nuclear medicine imaging system. IAEA, Vienna
7. Bar-Shalom R, Yefremov N, Guralnik L et al (2008) SPECT/CT in 99mTc-HMPAO-labeled leukocyte scintigraphy for diagnosis of infection. J Nucl Med 47:587-594
8. Deichen J Th, Prante O, Gack M et al (2003) Uptake of F-18-deoxyglucose in human monocyte-macrophages in vitro. Eur J Nucl Med Mol Imaging 30:267-273
9. Strobel K, Stumpe KDM (2007) PET/CT in musculoskeletal infection. Sem Musculoskeletal Radiol 11:353-364
10. Even-Sapir E, Metser U, Flusser G et al (2004) Assessment of malignant skeletal disease: initial experience with 18F-fluoride PET/CT and comparison between 18F-fluoride PET and 18F-fluoride PET/CT. J Nucl Med 45(2):272-278
11. Schneider P, Farahati J, Reiners C (2005) Radiosynovectomy in rheumatology, orthopedics, and hemophilia. J Nucl Med 46:48S-54S

Radionuclide Imaging of Bone Metastases

Einat Even-Sapir Weizer

Department of Nuclear Medicine, Tel Aviv Sourasky Medical Center, Sackler School of Medicine, Tel Aviv University, Tel Aviv, Israel

Introduction

Skeletal imaging of oncologic patients is aimed at identifying early bone involvement, to determine the extent of the disease, and to monitor the response to therapy [1]. Detection of malignant bone involvement is either direct, by visualization of tumoral infiltration, or indirect, by detecting the reaction of bone to the presence of malignant cells. The vast majority of bone metastases initiate as bone marrow micrometastases. As the lesion enlarges within the marrow, the surrounding bone undergoes osteoclastic (resorptive) and osteoblastic (depositional) activity. Based on the balance between these two processes, metastasis can be lytic, sclerotic (blastic), or mixed [2, 3]. In nuclear medicine, ^{18}F-fluordeoxyglucose (^{18}F-FDG), a PET tracer, directly accumulates in tumor cells and may therefore identify malignant bone involvement even at early stages, when confined to the marrow, before cortical bone reaction has occurred, while increased accumulation of ^{99m}Tc-MDP-methylene diphosphonate (the tracer used for bone scintigraphy) or 18F-fluoride, a bone-seeking PET tracer, depends on the presence of secondary reactive osteoblastic changes [3, 4].

Scintigraphic lesions often require further correlation with contemporaneous CT. Hybrid techniques, such as SPECT-CT and PET-CT, recently introduced in clinical practice, provide better anatomic localization of scintigraphic findings and may improve the diagnostic accuracy of SPECT and PET in detecting malignant bone involvement [4].

Imaging Using Single-Photon-Emitting Tracers and Gamma Cameras

^{99m}Tc-MDP is the most commonly used bone tracer for the detection of bone metastases with gamma cameras. The compound, an analogue of pyrophosphate, is chemisorbed onto bone surface and its uptake depends on local blood flow and osteoblastic activity. The focal accumulation of ^{99m}Tc-MDP in bone metastases is due to the increased osteoblastic reaction that commonly accompanies bone metastases [3]. Based on these characteristics, bone scintigraphy (BS) with ^{99m}Tc-MDP is highly sensitive for detection of the osteoblastic-type metastases predominating in oncologic diseases such as prostate cancer. In the past, virtually all patients with newly diagnosed prostate, breast, or lung cancer underwent a baseline ^{99m}Tc-MDP BS and then annual follow-up studies. This "automatic" referral for BS was abandoned such that currently BS is indicated only in patients who are at high-risk for bone metastases or have a clinical suspicion of malignant bone involvement [5]. At present, the use of ^{18}F-FDG-PET whole-body imaging (discussed below) in the routine imaging algorithm of various human malignancies may obviate the need to perform a separate BS. The latter remains, however, the primary imaging modality in oncologic diseases for which FDG PET is not the routine, mainly prostate cancer [6].

The BS procedure initiated as two-dimensional (planar) data. Later, with the introduction of SPECT, in which reconstructed data are provided in three planes: transaxial, coronal, and sagittal, it became apparent that the latter technology improves the diagnostic accuracy of BS in the detection of bone pathology. It was reported that SPECT detects 20-50% more lesions than planar BS and allows for a straightforward comparison with other tomography-based techniques, such as CT and MRI. The better localization of lesions by SPECT has been reported to improve the specificity of BS, mainly for lesions located at the vertebral column [7]. The use of SPECT has been limited, at least until recently, to a relatively localized skeletal region. However, with the introduction of novel software algorithms that yield rapid multi-field SPECT views when combined with BS, it will likely become a full tomographic procedure [8].

^{99m}Tc-MDP BS has a few albeit major limitations. It is insensitive for the detection of early bone marrow involvement and lytic metastases. It cannot accurately separate active malignant disease from repair processes, as the latter are also associated with high bone turnover. Therefore, the procedure is of a limited value for monitoring the response to therapy. The accumulation of ^{99m}Tc-MDP is not specific for malignancy and may be detected in other bone conditions associated with high bone turnover, including trauma, osteomyelitis, osteoporosis, metabolic bone disease, and degenerative changes. The detection of a solitary or only a few bone lesions on BS often indicates the need to further assess these lesions by CT [1]. Hybrid systems composed of gamma camera and CT are now commercially available [9].

Imaging Using Positron-Emitting Tracers and Positron Emission Tomography

Positron emission tomography a whole-body tomographic data. It is characterized by a high-contrast resolution and the ability to absolutely quantify of tracer uptake. The number of PET devices has rapidly grown, with the technique changing from being a research tool to a routine modality in the imaging algorithm of oncologic patients.

Two main PET tracers that are clinically used for the assessment of metastatic skeletal spread: ^{18}F-FDG, the most commonly used tracer in oncologic patients for detection of both soft-tissue and bone tumor sites, and ^{18}F-fluoride, a bone-seeking agent.

[18]F-Fluordeoxyglucose (^{18}F-FDG)

This glucose analog gains entry into cells by glucose membrane transporter proteins, which are overexpressed in many tumor cells. Due to the slow rate of dephosphorylation by these cells, the compound becomes trapped within them. The normal red marrow demonstrates low-intensity [18]FDG uptake. Increased marrow uptake may suggest the presence of early bone marrow malignant involvement prior to an identifiable bone reaction, therefore preceding the detection of early metastases by BS and CT [10] (Fig. 1). Although ^{18}F-FDG-PET reportedly is appropriate for detecting all types of bone metastases, there are data suggesting that ^{18}F-FDG-PET is more sensitive in detecting lytic rather than sclerotic metastases. It is assumed that the avidity of ^{18}F-FDG in lytic metastases reflects their high glycolytic rate and relative hypoxia, while sclerotic metastases are relatively acellular, less aggressive, not prone to hypoxia, and therefore show lower or no ^{18}F-FDG-avidity [10].

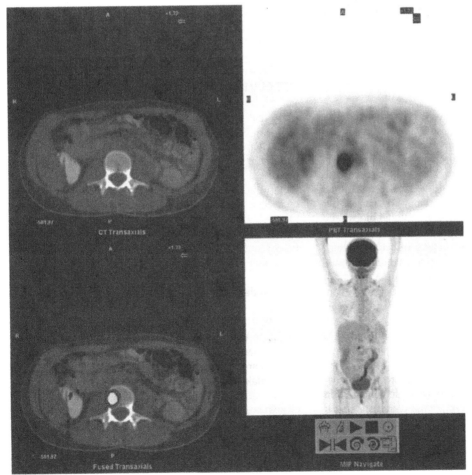

Fig. 1. ^{18}F-FDG PET/CT study in a 34-year-old female patient with breast cancer. The patient was referred to the study due to rising markers, 2 years after removal of the primary tumor, radiotherapy, and while on hormonal therapy. On PET data (*upper right* transaxial image; *bottom right*, an overview maximum-intensity projection image), focal increased uptake is detected. The latter appears to be located, based on the fused image (*bottom left*) at the right aspect of the L3 vertebra. On CT (*upper left*), the bone looks normal with no morphological abnormality. This finding represents an early metastasis confined to the bone marrow prior to any accompanying cortical abnormality

Breast Cancer

^{18}F-FDG-PET was found to be superior to BS in detecting both malignant bone involvement in patients with breast cancer and early marrow-based lesions. The latter are predominately lytic, with only minimal osteoblastic reaction, and are overlooked on BS [11, 12] (Fig. 1). The sensitivity of ^{18}F-FDG-PET in detecting sclerotic metastases is somewhat lower, encouraging some authors to recommend complementary use of BS and ^{18}F-FDG-PET for optimizing the detection of sclerotic and lytic metastases, which may be present in patients with breast cancer. However, the current use of hybrid PET-CT imaging technique simplifies this issue, as sclerotic lesions overlooked by PET can be identified by the CT data of the study.

Lung Cancer

Bone metastases are diagnosed at initial presentation in 3.4-60% of patients with non-small cell lung carcinoma (NSCLC). Up to 40% of lung cancer patients with proven bone metastases are asymptomatic. Before the era of ^{18}F-FDG-PET, the staging algorithm of patients with NSCLC included CT of the thorax through the liver and adrenals, CT and/or MRI of the brain, and BS. Recently, ^{18}F-FDG-PET and PET-CT were reported valuable in assessing the presence of soft-tissue and bone spread in patients with NSCLC, obviating the need to perform a separate BS [13].

Lymphoma

^{18}F-FDG-PET has become a routine imaging modality for staging and monitoring the response to therapy in patients with lymphoma. Lymphoma involvement is commonly marrow-based. It appears that in some of the patients in whom positive PET findings were considered false-positive due to negative bone marrow biopsy, the PET results turned out to be true-positive when repeat biopsy was carried out using the positive PET site to guide the optimal biopsy site [14]. In the interpretation of a baseline ^{18}F-FDG-PET study prior to therapy, the finding of a pattern of heterogeneous, patchy marrow with increased activity should raise the suspicion of marrow lymphomatous involvement. A pattern of diffuse uptake, mainly seen in Hodgkin's disease, is more commonly associated with reactive hematopoietic changes or myeloid hyperplasia [15].

Secondary bone involvement may occur in up to 25% of lymphoma patients, while primary bone lymphoma is an uncommon disease. ^{18}F-FDG-PET was found to be more sensitive than BS and CT in the detection of osseous involvement in lymphoma. A valuable contribution of the CT data of PET/CT in lymphoma patients is that it allows the identification of vertebral collapse, the presence of soft-tissue paravertebral masses, epidural masses, or neural foramen invasion, complications, that may accompany vertebral lymphoma [16].

Multilple Myeloma

Since myeloma lesions tend to be predominantly lytic, BS is considered less sensitive than X-ray and CT, overlooking almost half of the abnormal sites of disease identified radiographically. Myelomatous marrow involvement precedes bone destruction and can be identified by MRI and ^{18}F-FDG-PET. The use of ^{18}F-FDG-PET in patients with multiple myeloma is accumulating. In patients with monoclonal gamopathy, a positive ^{18}F-FDG-PET reliably implies active disease, whereas a negative study strongly supports the diagnosis of monoclonal gamopathy of undetermined significance (MGUS) [17]. ^{18}F-FDG-PET is also valuable in identifying unexpected medullary and extra-medullary sites of disease missed by X-ray, CT, or BS [18].

Monitoring Response

Bone may remain morphologically abnormal on CT even when the disease is "burnt out." Radiotracers whose accumulation reflects high bone turnover, i.e., ^{99m}Tc-MDP and ^{18}F-fluoride, are inadequate in the accurate assessment of the therapeutic response, as both viable bone metastasis and repair processes are associated with increased bone turnover and may have similar appearances. A potential advantage of ^{18}F-FDG-PET is in the assessment of the response to therapy given the direct mechanism of ^{18}F-FDG uptake, which is related to tumor cell activity rather than to the osteoblastic reaction. Normalization of ^{18}F-FDG uptake in a bony site associated with increased uptake prior to therapy indicates a favorable response [1]. However, it should be borne in mind that uptake during ^{18}F-FDG-PET may be affected by therapy [19]. If ^{18}F-FDG-PET is performed too soon after chemotherapy (less than 2 weeks apart), it may result in metabolic shutdown of the tumor cells and a false-negative PET study. At different time points after radiotherapy, bone included in the radiation field may show increased, normal, or reduced uptake of ^{18}F-FDG compared to neighboring bone. Similarly, treatment with granulocyte colony-stimulating factors (GCSF) may induce a diffusely increased FDG uptake in the marrow, which can mask malignant infiltration [20, 21].

[18]F-Fluoride

This PET bone-seeking agent has an uptake mechanism similar to that of the single-photon emitting tracer, ^{99m}Tc-MDP. However, the pharmacokinetic characteristics of ^{18}F-fluoride are better than those of ^{99m}Tc-MDP. Moreover, its bone uptake is two-fold higher; it does not bind to protein; and its capillary permeability is higher with fast blood clearance and a better target-to-background ratio. Regional plasma clearance of ^{18}F-Fluoride was reported to be three to ten times higher in bone metastases compared with that in normal bone [3]. ^{18}F-Fluoride-PET is a highly sensitive modality for detection of bone abnormalities [22-24].

Although the mechanism of uptake of ^{18}F-fluoride depends on bone turnover, it is very sensitive in the detection not only of osteoblastic metastases but also of lytic ones, as the latter even when considered "pure lytic", nonetheless have minimal osteoblastic activity but enough for detection by ^{18}F-fluoride-PET. ^{18}F-fluoride is not tumor-specific and accumulates excessively in benign bone lesions. The use of novel hybrid PET-CT systems has significantly improved the limited specificity of ^{18}F-fluoride-PET, as the CT part of the study allows morphologic characterization of the scintigraphic lesion and accurate separation between benign lesions and metastases [25]. In patients with prostate cancer, ^{18}F-fluoride-PET-CT has been found to be superior to planar and SPECT BS and plays a complementary role to ^{18}F-fluorocholine study [8, 26]. Due to its relatively higher cost and the limited availability of the tracer, the technology has not yet become a routine imaging modality for detecting malignant bone involvement.

Functional-Anatomic Hybrid Imaging: SPECT-CT and PET-CT

Scintigraphic lesions often require further validation with a contemporaneous morphologic imaging modality, mainly CT. Novel integrated systems consisting of SPECT or PET (functional) and CT (anatomic) installed in a single gantry have been recently introduced into routine clinical practice. Data of the two modalities are acquired at the same clinical setting so that each lesion is characterized by its tracer uptake (SPECT or PET) and morphologic appearance (CT). The CT part of hybrid imaging may range from low-dose non-diagnostic CT to full-dose multi-slice diagnostic CT with IV contrast injection [9, 27].

The better localization of scintigraphic lesions based on the CT data allows separation between physiological and pathological uptake. In the case of SPECT and PET tracers such as ^{131}iodine, ^{111}In-somatostatin, ^{67}Ga-citrate (SPECT tracer), and ^{18}F-FDG (PET tracer), which may identify soft-tissue and bone tumor sites, the fused data assist in localizing the scintigraphic abnormality to the correct tissue [9].

SPECT-CT and PET-CT have been found to improve the specificity of ^{99m}Tc-MDP, ^{18}F-FDG-PET, and ^{18}F-Fluoride-PET, which, as noted above, may accumulate also in benign bone lesions [25, 28]. The CT part of the PET-CT study was found to be valuable in identifying complications, including epidural involvement and neural foramen invasion, reported to occur in ~10% of vertebral metastases. These complications require early diagnosis and treatment prior to the development of permanent neurological deficits [29]. PET-CT can be used for radiotherapy planning. The CT information thus obtained can be used for the purpose of volume planning, while the PET data allow better delineation of the tumor margins. Ultimately, a more rational approach to radiotherapy planning is an achievable goal by PET-CT [30].

Conclusions

In ^{18}F-FDG-avid tumors, ^{18}F-FDG PET allows the identification of early bone marrow as well as cortical metastases. Successful therapy is evidenced by a decline in the intensity of ^{18}F-FDG uptake. ^{18}F-fluoride-PET is a highly sensitive modality for detecting bone metastases, but it is not yet a routine procedure and is still reserved for selected high-risk patients. ^{99m}Tc-MDP bone scintigraphy has been, for years, the most widely used modality for evaluating the presence of skeletal metastases. While in patients undergoing ^{18}F-FDG PET, it is not indicated, it remains the primary imaging modality for the assessment of malignant bone involvement in diseases, mainly prostate cancer, in which PET imaging is not the routine.

Novel hybrid systems composed of PET or SPECT and CT allow for the acquisition of both modalities at the same clinical setting and the generation of fused functional-anatomical images. These novel techniques have been found to improve the diagnostic accuracy of scintigraphic techniques in detecting malignant bone involvement.

References

1. Hamaoka T, Madewell JE, Podoloff DA et al (2004) Bone imaging in metastatic breast cancer. J Clin Oncol 22:2942-2953
2. Roodman GD (2004) Mechanisms of bone metastasis. N Engl J Med 350:1655-1664
3. Blake GM, Park-Holohan SJ, Cook GJ, Fogelman I (2001) Quantitative studies of bone with the use of 18F-fluoride and 99mTc-methylene diphosphonate. Semin Nucl Med 31:28-49
4. Even-Sapir E (2005) Imaging of malignant bone involvement by morphologic, scintigraphic, and hybrid modalities. J Nucl Med 46:1356-1367
5. Smith TJ, Davidson NE, Schapira DV et al (1998) American Society of Clinical Oncology 1998. Update of recommended breast cancer surveillance guidelines. J Clin Oncol 17:1080-1082
6. Schoder H, Larson SM (2004) Positron emission tomography for prostate, bladder, and renal cancer. Semin Nucl Med 34:274-292
7. Gates GF (1998) SPECT bone scanning of the spine. Semin Nucl Med 28:78-94
8. Even-Sapir E, Metser U, Mishani E et al (2006) The detection of bone metastases in patients with high-risk prostate cancer: 99mTc-MDP planar bone scintigraphy, single-and multi-field-of-view SPECT, 18F-fluoride PET, and 18F-fluoride PET/CT. J Nucl Med 47:287-297
9. Keidar Z, Israel O, Krausz Y (2003) SPECT/CT in tumor imaging: technical aspects and clinical applications. Semin Nucl Med 33:205-218
10. Cook GJ, Houston S, Rubens R et al (1998) Detection of bone metastases in breast cancer by ^{18}FDG PET: differing metabolic activity in osteoblastic and osteolytic lesions. J Clin Oncol 16:3375-3379
11. Abe K, Sasaki M, Kuwabara Y et al (2005) Comparison of ^{18}FDG-PET with ^{99}mTc-HMDP scintigraphy for the detection of bone metastases in patients with breast cancer. Ann Nucl Med 19:573-579
12. Port ER, Yeung H, Gonen M et al (2006) (18)F-2-fluoro-2-de-oxy-d:-glucose positron emission tomography scanning affects surgical management in selected patients with high-risk, operable breast carcinoma. Ann Surg Oncol 13:677-684

13. Cheran SK, Herndon JE, Patz EF (2004) Comparison of whole-body FDG-PET to bone scan for detection of bone metastases in patients with a new diagnosis of lung cancer. Lung Cancer 44:317-325

14. Pakos EE, Fotopoulos AD, Ioannidis JP (2005) ^{18}F-FDG PET for evaluation of bone marrow infiltration in staging of lymphoma: a meta-analysis. J Nucl Med 6:958-963

15. Carr R, Barrington SF, Madan B et al (1998) Detecion of lymphoma in bone marrow by whole-body positron emission tomography. Blood 91:3340-3346

16. Even-Sapir E, Lievshitz G, Perry C et al (2006) Fluorine-18 Fluorodeoxyglucose PET/CT patterns of extranodal involvement in patients with non-Hodgkin Lymphoma and Hodgkin's disease. PET Clinics1:251-263

17. Durie BGM, Waxman AD, D'Agnolo A, Williams CM (2002) Whole-body 18F-FDG PET identifies high-risk myeloma. J Nucl Med 43:1457-1463

18. Schirrmeister H, Bommer M, Buck A et al (2002) Initial results in the assessment of multiple myeloma using F-18 FDG PET. Eur J Nucl Med Mol Imag 29:361-366

19. Israel O, Goldberg A, Nachtigal A et al (2006) FDG-PET and CT patterns of bone metastases and their relationship to previously administered anti-cancer therapy. Eur J Nucl Med Mol Imaging 33:1280-1284

20. Clamp A, Danson S, Nguyen H et al (2004) Assessment of therapeutic response in patients with metastatic bone disease. Lancet Oncol 5:607-616

21. Kazama T, Faria SC, Varavithya V et al (2005) FDG PET in the evaluation of treatment for lymphoma: clinical usefulness and pitfalls. Radiographics 25:191-207

22. Cook GJ, Fogelman I (2001) The role of positron emission tomography in skeletal disease. Semin Nucl Med 31:50-61

23. Schirrmeister H, Kuhn T, Guhlmann A et al (2001) Fluorine-18 2-deoxy-2-fluoro-D-glucose PET in the preoperative staging of breast cancer: comparison with the standard staging procedures. Eur J Nucl Med 28:351-358

24. Even-Sapir E, Mishani E, Flusser G, Metser U (2007) ^{18}F-Fluoride positron emission tomography and positron emission tomography/computed tomography. Semin Nucl Med 37:462-469

25. Even-Sapir E, Metser U, Flusser G et al (2004) Assessment of malignant skeletal disease: initial experience with 18F-fluoride PET/CT and comparison between 18F-fluoride PET and 18F-fluoride PET/CT. J Nucl Med 45:272-278

26. Beheshti M, Vali R, Waldenberger P et al (2008) Detection of bone metastases in patients with prostate cancer by F-18 fluorocholine and F-18 fluoride PET-CT: a comparative study. Eur J Nucl Med Mol Imaging 35:1766-1774

27. Antoch G, Vogt FM, Freudenberg LS et al (2003) Whole-body dual-modality PET/CT and whole-body MRI for tumor staging in oncology. JAMA 290:3199-3206

28. Strobel K, Exner UE, Stumpe KD et al (2008) The additional value of CT images interpretation in the differential diagnosis of benign vs. malignant primary bone lesions with 18F-FDG-PET/CT. Eur J Nucl Med Mol Imag 35:2000-2008

29. Metser U, Lerman H, Blank A et al (2004) Malignant involvment of the spine: assessment by 18F-fluorodeoxyglucose PET/CT. J Nucl Med 45:279-284

30. Ell PJ (2006) The contribution of PET/CT to improved patient management. Br J Radiol 79:32-36

Radionuclide Imaging of Degenerative Joint Diseases

Klaus Strobel

Department of Nuclear Medicine, University Hospital Zurich, Switzerland

Introduction

The incidence of degenerative joint diseases increases with age and therapeutic procedures such as joint replacement are expensive [1]. Conventional bone scintigraphy with Tc99m-phosponates is very sensitive in the diagnosis of osteoarthritis. SPECT, SPECT/CT, and 18F-fluoride PET(/CT) increase the performance of planar bone scintigraphy and provide brilliant images even in complex anatomic regions such as the spine or the foot [2-4]. Differentiation between degenerative joint disease and bone metastases is one of the most important questions in clinical practice. Since uptake in scintigraphy does not always correspond with the symptoms of the patient, exact clinical correlation is crucial.

Degenerative Spine

Degenerative lesions in the spine are very common and are predominantly found in the lower lumbar and cervical regions. Findings such as the "mid-cervical-lateral-focus," are highly suggestive of degenerative disease and should not be misinterpreted as bone metastases in cancer patients (Fig. 1)

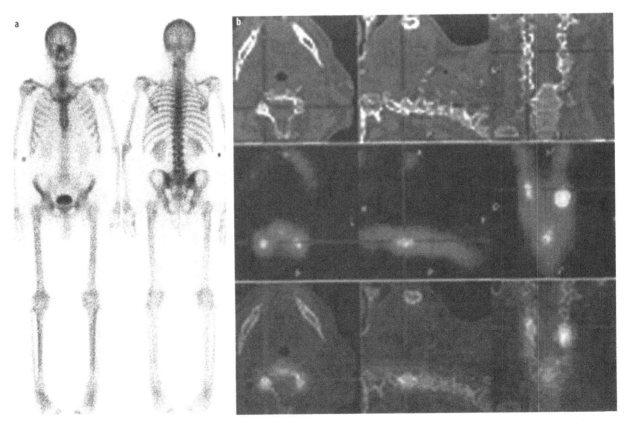

Fig. 1 a, b. Planar (a) and SPECT/CT (b) images of a "mid-cervical-lateral-focus", representing facet joint osteoarthritis

[5]. Bone scintigraphy and SPECT(/CT) can play an important role in identifying patients with lower back pain who profit from facet joint injections [6, 7] (Figs. 2, 3). Another interesting indication is the evaluation of degenerative lesions and complications after spine fusion surgery (Fig. 4). In this population the value of MRI is limited because of metal artifacts; instead, fluoride-PET/CT provides the orthopedic surgeon with important information.

Degenerative Lesions in the Wrist and Hand

Bone scintigraphy is very sensitive in the detection of degenerative lesions in the wrist and finger joints (Fig. 5). The pattern of uptake distribution helps to differentiate osteoarthritis from rheumatologic diseases like rheumatoid arthritis.

Degenerative Knee

The imaging reference standard for the diagnosis of osteoarthritis of the knee is MRI. However, as shown recently in patients with chronic medial knee pain, increased uptake in bone scintigraphy is more sensitive than the bone marrow changes demonstrated in MRI [8, 9]. SPECT imaging of the knee is highly sensitive for the diagnosis of patellofemoral abnormalities [10].

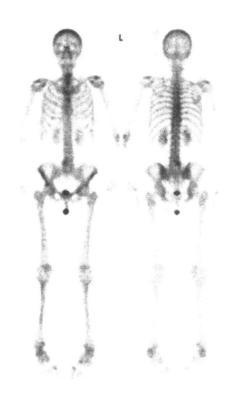

Fig. 2. Planar bone scintigraphy (anterior and posterior view). Atypical degenerative uptake in the lumbar spine caused by spondylosis/osteochondrosis

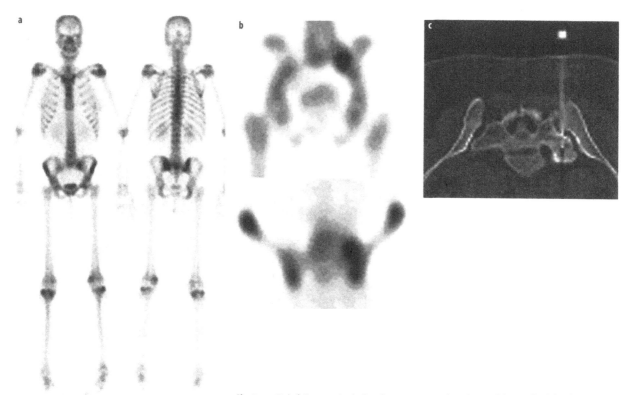

Fig. 3 a-c. Painful enoarticulation in a young patient imaged imaged with planar bone scintigraphy (a), SPECT (b) and treated with CT-guided injection (c)

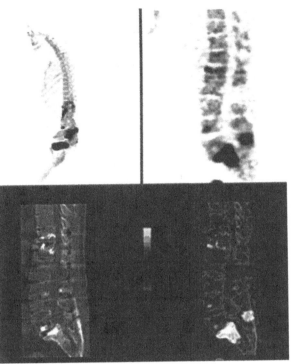

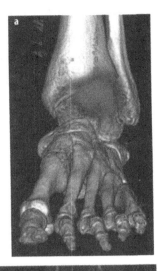

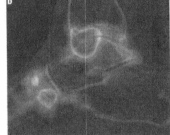

Fig. 4. Fluoride-PET/CT after spine-fusion surgery and vertebro-plasty with insufficiency fractures (Th12, L1, L2), sacral osteomyelitis, and failed fusion L5/S1

Fig. 6 a, b. Osteoarthritis in the upper ankle joint imaged with fluoride -PET/CT (**a**, 3-D reconstruction; **b**, sagittal fused image)

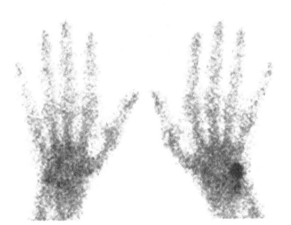

Fig. 5. Pisotriquetral joint osteoarthritis

Degenerative Lesions in the Ankle and Foot

SPECT/CT and fluoride PET/CT are increasingly used in the imaging evaluation of patients with unclear foot pain (Figs. 6, 7). In these situations, these techniques provide important information that supplements the clinical data, by showing lesions with increased bone turnover and the corresponding structural damages. In certain cases, scintigraphy might be more sensitive than MRI.

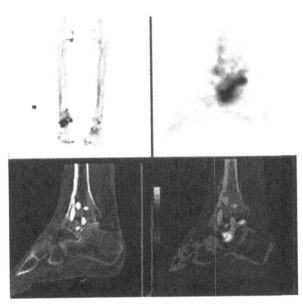

Fig. 7. Osteoarthritis of the subtalar joint after fusion of the upper ankle joint, imaged with fluoride-PET/CT

Degenerative Lesions and FDG-PET/CT

Degenerative lesions can take up FDG to a certain extent, thereby leading to misinterpretations in tumor patients. Often this uptake is markedly lower than the FDG-uptake of metastases. CT helps to increase the specificity (Fig. 8) [11, 12].

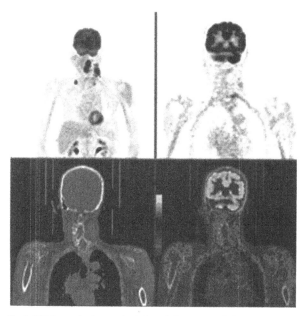

Fig. 8. FDG-uptake in cervical facet-joint osteoarthritis in a patient with tonsilar cancer and bilateral lymph node metastases

References

1. MacLean CH, Knight K, Paulus H et al (1998) Costs attributable to osteoarthritis. J Rheumatol 25:2213-2218
2. Strobel K, Burger C, Seifert B et al (2007) Characterization of focal bone lesions in the axial skeleton: performance of planar bone scintigraphy compared with SPECT and SPECT fused with CT. AJR Am J Roentgenol 188:W467-W474
3. Utsunomiya D, Shiraishi S, Imuta M et al (2006) Added value of SPECT/CT fusion in assessing suspected bone metastasis: comparison with scintigraphy alone and nonfused scintigraphy and CT. Radiology 238:264-271
4. Romer W, Nomayr A, Uder M et al (2006) SPECT-guided CT for evaluating foci of increased bone metabolism classified as indeterminate on SPECT in cancer patients. J Nucl Med 47:1102-1106
5. Kim DW, Kim SC, Krynyckyi BR et al (2005) Focally increased activity in the lateral aspect of the mid cervical spine on bone scintigraphy is almost always benign in nature. Clin Nucl Med 30:593-595
6. Pneumaticos SG, Chatziioannou SN, Hipp JA et al (2006) Low back pain: prediction of short-term outcome of facet joint injection with bone scintigraphy. Radiology 238:693-698
7. Dolan AL, Ryan PJ, Arden NK et al (1996) The value of SPECT scans in identifying back pain likely to benefit from facet joint injection. Br J Rheumatol 35:1269-1273
8. Buck FM, Hoffmann A, Hofer B et al (2008) Chronic medial knee pain without history of prior trauma: correlation of pain at rest and during exercise using bone scintigraphy and MR imaging. Skeletal Radiol Dec 3 [Epub ahead of print]
9. Boegard T, Rudling O, Dahlstrom J et al (1999) Bone scintigraphy in chronic knee pain: comparison with magnetic resonance imaging. Ann Rheum Dis 58:20-26
10. Lorberboym M, Ami DB, Zin D et al (2003) Incremental diagnostic value of 99mTc methylene diphosphonate bone SPECT in patients with patellofemoral pain disorders. Nucl Med Commun 24:403-410
11. Nakamura H, Masuko K, Yudoh K et al (2007) Positron emission tomography with 18F-FDG in osteoarthritic knee. Osteoarthritis Cartilage 15:673-681
12. Rosen RS, Fayad L, Wahl RL (2006) Increased 18F-FDG uptake in degenerative disease of the spine: Characterization with 18F-FDG PET/CT. J Nucl Med 47:1274-1280

Radionuclide Evaluation of Primary Bone and Soft-Tissue Tumors

Chistiane Franzius

MR- and PET/CT-Center Bremen-Mitte, Bremen, Germany

Introduction

This presentation reviews the applications of nuclear medicine imaging techniques in the evaluation of primary bone and soft-tissue malignomas in children, adolescents, and adults. The focus is on three-phase bone scintigraphy, positron emission tomography using ^{18}F-fluoro-deoxy-glucose (FDG-PET), and the combination of PET and computed tomography (PET-CT). These imaging techniques are used for the grading, staging, and response control of tumors as well as for the diagnosis of tumor recurrence.

Tumors

Musculoskeletal tumors are a heterogeneous group, comprising various tumor entities with different biologies, patterns of malignancy, and therapeutic options. The incidence of malignant primary musculoskeletal tumors is very low: 1/100,000 for primary bone tumors and 3/100,000 for primary soft-tissue tumors. Different age patterns are associated with the different tumor entities. Some, such as embryonal rhabdomyosarcomas, osteosarcomas, and Ewing tumors, mainly or exclusively occur in childhood and adolescence whereas others, such as chondrosarcomas and malignant fibrous histiocytomas, are predominantly seen in the elderly. The metastatic spread of sarcomas is mainly hematogenous, reaching the lungs and the bones. However, soft-tissue sarcomas also spread via the lymphatics. The presence or absence of metastases, the tumor histology, and the tumor grade are the main aspects influencing treatment.

Imaging Techniques

Three-Phase Bone Scintigraphy

Primary Bone Tumors and Tumor-Like Lesions

Even in the age of cross-sectional imaging, primary bone tumors were best classified using a conventional X-ray image. With the advent of CT and magnetic resonance imaging (MRI), further information on tumor localization and extension has become available [1]. A bone scan in which tracer uptake is increased in all three phases supports the diagnosis of a primary malignant bone tumor. However, the pattern is not specific, as acute inflammation shows the same tracer-uptake behavior. Additionally, in some benign lesions, e.g., osteoid osteoma or Paget's disease of the bone, tracer uptake is also clearly increased in all three phases. A normal or only marginally increased blood-pool phase and a moderately increased bone phase indicate the benign character of a lesion; but, again, there are exceptions. Nonetheless, in general, the bone scan offers the advantage of whole-body information and consequently allows a statement on the singularity or multifocal occurrence of lesions, with reasonably low radiation exposure.

Subsequent to the chemotherapy of primary bone tumors, bone scintigraphy can be used for therapy control. A decrease in tracer uptake in the blood-pool phase and in the bone phase of more the 30% indicates a good response [2, 3]. However, even in good responders tracer uptake may be increased during chemotherapy due to flare phenomena. Therefore, the therapeutic response should be assessed by bone scintigraphy after the end of chemotherapy.

Osseous Metastases

In both primary osseous and soft-tissue malignomas, bone scintigraphy is a fast and sensitive technique to detect or exclude osseous metastases [4]. The advantage of whole-body information is evident. Bone metastases are usually visualized by bone scan 3-6 months earlier than by X-ray [5]. However, the specificity of skeletal scintigraphy is relatively low, only 60-70%. Therefore, verification or falsification of suspicious lesions is often necessary. While many studies have demonstrated the superiority of MRI over bone scintigraphy in the detection of osseous metastases, especially in the vertebral column [6, 7], whole-body MRI is still too expensive to be used in clinical routine and capacity is still limited. FDG-PET is more sensitive and more specific than bone scan in the detection of osseous metastases, as it offers whole-body tomography with higher spatial resolution than obtained with planar imaging and SPECT [8]. However, the expense and limited availability restrict the widespread use of FDG-PET.

A distinctive feature of osteosarcoma and its metastasis is the production of premature osseous matrix, the point of contact of the radio-labeled phosphonates. Therefore, skeletal scintigraphy is very sensitive in the detection of osseous metastases of osteosarcoma and even soft-tissue metastases are often visible on the bone scan [9, 10]. Because of this characteristic feature, therapy with bone-seeking radiopharmaceuticals can be administered to patients with osteosarcoma. Nevertheless, despite highly efficacious chemotherapy, patients with osteosarcomas still have a poor prognosis if adequate surgical control cannot be obtained. These patients may benefit from therapy with radiolabeled phosphonates, such as Sm-153-EDTMP (samarium-153 ethylenediaminetetramethylene phosphonic acid) [11, 12].

Conventional Scintigraphy and SPECT Using Other Tracers

Several other tracers for conventional scintigraphy and SPECT, such as [67]Gallium, [201]Thallium, Tc-sestamibi, and Tc-tetrofosmin, are used in the diagnosis, grading, and post-chemotherapy evaluation of primary musculoskeletal tumors. However, the impact of these tracers has decreased since the broad clinical introduction of FDG-PET. A detailed review of these applications has been published by Pneumaticos et al. [13].

FDG-PET

Grading

Since the late 1980s, a correlation between FDG uptake by musculoskeletal tumors and the grade of malignancy has been known [14, 15] and confirmed by many authors (reviews in [16, 17]), with the exception of a study by Kole et al. [18]. Most authors reported, not surprisingly, an overlap in the FDG uptake intensity of low-grade malignant tumors and benign processes [19]. Although FDG-PET has the potential to differentiate between high-grade malignant and low-grade malignant/benign processes with high accuracy [17, 20-23], it cannot replace a biopsy. Sarcomas may be very heterogeneous in composition such that assessment of the areas of a lesion with the highest malignancy is essential. A practical problem is that a biopsy of a small portion of the tumor is not always representative of the overall character of the tumor (sampling error). Therefore, the non-invasive grading information obtained by FDG-PET can be the crucial factor for the strategy of biopsy or tumor resection [24].

Prognosis

Several studies have shown that the initial FDG uptake of a primary sarcoma is a prognostic parameter [23, 25-29].

In a retrospective study of 209 patients, multivariate analyses showed that the maximum standardized uptake value (SUV) is a statistically significant, independent predictor of patient survival [25]. Another study demonstrated that the heterogeneity of FDG distribution within the primary sarcoma is a strong predictor of outcome [30].

Staging

A tumor's T-stage classification is based on morphological criteria; accordingly, morphological imaging procedures are superior to functional imaging techniques in this field. In primary bone tumors, lymph node metastases are very rare whereas in primary soft-tissue sarcomas they are a frequent occurrence. To date, there are no studies concerning lymph node detection by FDG-PET in these tumor entities. Some studies demonstrated that, compared with FDG-PET, spiral thoracic CT yields better detection of pulmonary metastases of sarcoma [31-34]. In the detection of osseous metastases of Ewing tumors, FDG-PET is superior to skeletal scintigraphy [35]. A prospective study of pediatric sarcoma patients demonstrated the relevant impact of PET staging information on therapeutic decisions [36]. In myeloma patients, MRI is superior to FDG-PET in the detection of bone marrow involvement as well as lesions of the spine and pelvis. FDG-PET can, however, significantly contribute to an accurate whole-body evaluation in myeloma patients [37-40].

Control of Therapy

In primary osseous sarcoma, patient response to neoadjuvant chemotherapy can be evaluated using FDG-PET [41-48]. In 1999, Schulte and colleagues demonstrated in 27 patients that decreased FDG uptake in osteosarcomas closely correlates with the amount of tumor necrosis induced by polychemotheapy [43]. In the study of Nair and colleagues, tumor necrosis was accurately predicted by FDG-PET in 15/16 patients based on visual assessment alone, and in 14/15 patients by determination of the final tumor/background ratio [42]. In addition, FDG-PET seems to be superior to skeletal scintigraphy in this clinical setting [44]. In 17 patients with primary malignant bone tumors (11 osteosarcomas, 6 Ewing sarcomas), FDG-PET was able to clearly differentiate between good and poor responders by means of the change in the tumor/background ratio between pre-and post-therapeutic scans. According to the results of bone scintigraphy, eight patients with a good response to neoadjuvant chemotherapy were falsely classified as poor responders [44]. In a recent study of 33 patients with osteosarcoma and Ewing tumors, both post-therapeutic SUV and the ratio post-therapeutic SUV/pre-therapeutic SUV correlated with the histopathologic assessment of response and thus potentially could be used as a noninvasive surrogate to predict patient response [41].

In all studies, the standard of reference was the histologically assessed grade of tumor necrosis after resection of the primary tumor. As yet, however, there are no data concerning the early assessment of therapeutic response – for instance, after one or two cycles of chemotherapy. In the future, FDG-PET results might lead to an early change in patient management and, likewise, influence surgery in patients with primary osseous tumors. However, other authors describe that FDG-PET monitoring of the therapeutic response has limited benefits [49, 50].

Diagnosis of Recurrences

The detection of a local relapse is frequently hampered by post-therapeutic changes after surgery, chemotherapy, and/or radiotherapy. Furthermore, prosthesis material may affect the quality of images obtained by CT or MRI. Several studies have shown that FDG-PET has a high sensitivity and specificity in the detection of local recurrences of musculoskeletal tumors [51-53] (review in [16]). Furthermore, within the same examination, FDG-PET can visualize distant recurrences [54].

FDG PET/CT

During the last several years, combined PET-CT scanners have been introduced into the clinical routine. An improvement with respect to the diagnosis of musculoskeletal tumors by combined PET-CT compared to separately acquired PET and CT has yet to be established. In musculoskeletal tumors, CT is mainly used to evaluate the lung, while the primary tumor is more frequently imaged by MRI. However, CT can demonstrate both the soft-tissue component of a tumor and the accompanying osseous destruction. Therefore, PET-CT image fusion in evaluating the primary tumor might be useful to determine the areas of the tumor with the highest malignancy. This, in turn, could guide biopsy or influence the strategy of tumor resection. Furthermore, in a single examination, PET-CT provides morphological and functional information regarding the primary tumor and information about pulmonary and other distant metastases. It has been demonstrated for Ewing tumor patients that PET-CT is significantly more accurate than FDG-PET alone in the detection and localization of lesions and that it improves tumor staging [55].

Non-FDG-PET

There are only single experiments and studies using non-FDG tracer in sarcoma (e.g., [56]). Uptake of the proliferation marker F-18-fluorodeoxythymidine correlated significantly with tumor grade [57].

References

1. Reiser M, Semmler W (2002) Magnetresonanztomographie, 3rd edn. Springer, Berlin, Heidelberg, New York
2. Erlemann R, Sciuk J, Bosse A et al (1990) Response of osteosarcoma and Ewing sarcoma to preoperative chemotherapy: assessment with dynamic and static MR imaging and skeletal scintigraphy. Radiology 175:791-796
3. Knop J, Delling G, Heise U, Winkler K (1990) Scintigraphic evaluation of tumor regression during preoperative chemotherapy of osteosarcoma. Skeletal Radiol 19:165-172
4. Bares R (1999) Leitlinien für die Skelettszintigraphie. Nuklearmedizin 38:251-253
5. O'Mara RE (1988) Bone scanning in osseous metastatic disease. JAMA 229:1915-1917
6. Algra PR, Bloem JL, Tissing H et al (1991) Detection of vertebral metastases: comparison between MR imaging and bone scintigraphy. Radiographics 11:219-232
7. Link M, Sciuk J, Fründt H et al (1995) Wirbelsäulenmetastasen - Wertigkeit diagnostischer Verfahren bei der Erstdiagnose und im Verlauf. Radiologe 35:21-27
8. Grant F, Fahey F, Packard A et al (2008) Skeletal PET with F-18-fluoride: applying new technology to an old tracer. J Nucl Med 49:68-78
9. Petersen M (1990) Radionuclide detection of primary pulmonary osteogenic sarcoma: a case report and review of the literature. J Nucl Med 31:1110-1114
10. Othman S, El-Desouki M (2003) Bone scan appearance in aggressive osteogenic sarcoma with pleural, lung, bone, and soft-tissue metastases. Clin Nucl Med 28:926
11. Franzius C, Bielack S, Sciuk J et al (1999) High-activity Samarium-153-EDTMP therapy in unresectable osteosarcoma. Nuklearmedizin 38:337-340
12. Anderson PM (1998) Sm-153-EDTMP therapy with stem cell support in patients. In: Bruland OS (ed) Towards the eradication of osteosarcoma metastases. The Norwegian Radium Hospital, Oslo, pp 87-88
13. Pneumaticos SG, Chatziioannou SN, Moore WH, Johnson M (2001) The role of radionuclides in primary musculoskeletal tumors beyond the "bone scan". Crit Rev Oncol Hematol 37:217-226
14. Kern KA, Brunetti A, Norton JA et al (1988) Metabolic imaging of human extremity musculoskeletal tumors by PET. J Nucl Med 29:181-186
15. Tateishi U, Yamaguchi U, Seki K et al (2006) Glut-1 expression and enhanced glucose metabolism are associated with tumor grade in bone and soft tissue sarcomas: a prospective evaluation by [F-18]fluorodeoxyglucose positron emission tomography. Eur J Nucl Med Mol Imaging 33:683-691
16. Franzius C, Schulte M, Hillmann A et al (2001) Klinische Wertigkeit der Positronen-Emissions-Tomographie (PET) in der Diagnostik der Knochen- und Weichteiltumore. 3. Konsensuskonferenz 'PET in der Onkologie', Ergebnisse der Arbeitsgruppe Knochen und Weichteiltumore. Chirurg 72:1071-1077
17. Bastiaannet E, Groen H, Jager PL et al (2004) The value of FDG-PET in the detection, grading and response to the therapie of soft tissue and bone sarcomas) a systematic review and meta-analysis. Cancer Treat Rev 30:83-101
18. Kole AC, Nieweg OE, Hoekstra HJ et al (1998) Fluorine-18-fluorodeoxyglucose assessment of glucose metabolism in bone tumors. J Nucl Med 39:810-815
19. Hamada K, Tomita Y, Qiu Y et al (2008) F-18-FDG-PET of musculoskeletal tumors: a correlation with the expression of glucose transporter 1 and hexokinase II. Ann Nucl Med 22:699-705
20. Schulte M, Brecht-Krauss D, Heymer B et al (1999) Fluorodeoxyglucose positron emission tomography of soft tissue tumors: is a non-invasive determination of biological activity possible? Eur J Nucl Med 26:599-605
21. Schulte M, Brecht-Krauss D, Heymer B et al (2000) Grading of tumors and tumorlike lesions of bone: evaluation by 2-(fluorine-18)-fluoro-2deoxy-D-glucose positron emission tomography. J Nucl Med 41:1695-1701
22. Eary JF, Conrad EU, Bruckner JD et al (1998) Quantitative (F-18) fluorodeoxyglucose positron emission tomography in pretreatment and grading of sarcoma. Clin Cancer Res 4:1215-1220

23. Brenner W, Conrad EU, Eary JF (2004) FDG PET imaging for grading and prediction of outcome in chondrosarkoma patients. Eur J Nucl Med Mol Imaging 31:189-195

24. Hain S, O'Doherty M, Bingham J et al (2003) Can FDG-PET be used to successfully direct preoperative biopsy of soft tissue tumours? Nucl Med Commun 24:1139-1143

25. Eary JF, O'Sullivan F, Powitan Y et al (2002) Sarcoma tumor FDG uptake measurement by PET and patient outcome: a retrospective analysis. Eur J Nucl Med Mol Imaging 29:1149-1154

26. Franzius C, Bielack S, Flege S et al (2002) Prognostic significance of F-18-FDG and Tc-99m-methylene diphosphonate uptake in primary osteosarcoma. J Nucl Med 43:1012-1017

27. Brenner W, Eary J, Hwang W et al (2006) Risk assessment in liposarcoma patients based on FDG PET imaging. Eur J Nucl Med Mol Imaging

28. Hawkins DS, Schuetze SM, Butrynski JE et al (2005) [F-18] Fluorodeoxyglucose positron emission tomography predicts outcome for Ewing sarcoma family of tumors. J Clin Oncol 23:8828-8834

29. Schuetze S, Rubin B, Vernon C et al (2005) Use of positron emission tomography in localized extremity soft tissue sarcoma treated with neoadjuvant chemotherapy. Cancer 103:339-348

30. Eary J, O'Sullivan F, O'Sullivan J, Conrad E (2008) Spatial heterogeneity in sarcoma F-18-FDG uptake as a predictor of patient outcome. J Nucl Med 49:1973-1979

31. Franzius C, Daldrup-Link HE, Sciuk J et al (2001) FDG-PET for detection of pulmonary metastases from malignant primary bone tumors: comparison with spiral CT. Ann Oncol 12:479-486

32. Lucas JD, O'Doherty MJ, Wong JCH et al (1998) Evaluation of fluorodeoxyglucose positron emission tomography in the management of soft-tissue sarcoma. J Bone Joint Surg (Br) 80-B:441-447

33. Gyoerke T, Zajic T, Lange A et al (2006) Impact of FDG PET for staging of Ewing sarcomas and primitive neuroectodermal tumours. Nucl Med Commun 27:17-24

34. Iagaru A, Chawia S, Menendez L, Conti P (2006) F-18-FDG PET and PET/CT for detection of pulmonary metastases from musculoskeletal sarcomas. Nucl Med Commun 27:795-802

35. Franzius C, Sciuk J, Daldrup-Link HE et al (2000) FDG-PET for detection of osseous metastases from malignant primary bone tumors: comparison with bone scintigraphy. Eur J Nucl Med 27:1305-1311

36. Voelker T, Denecke T, Steffen I et al (2007) Positron emission tomography for staging of pediatric sarcoma patients: results of a prospective multicenter trial. J Clin Oncol 25:5435-5441

37. Zamagni E, Nanni C, Patriarca F et al (2007) A prospective comparison of F-18-fluorodeoxyglucose positron emission tomography-computed tompgraphy, magnetic resonance imaging and whole-body planar radiographs in the assessment of bone disease in newly diagnosed multiple myeloma. Haematologica 92:50-55

38. Fonti R, Salvatore B, Quarantelli M et al (2008) F-18-FDG PET/CT, Tc-99m-MIBI, and MRI in evaluation of patients with multiple myeloma. J Nucl Med 49:195-(200

39. Hur J, Yoon C, Ryu Y et al (2008) Comparative study of fluorodeoxyglucose positron emission tomography and magnetic resonance imaging for the detection of spinal bone marrow infiltration in untreated patients with multiple myeloma. Acta Radiol 49:427-435

40. Nanni C, Rubello D, Zamagni E et al (2008) F-18-FDG PET/CT in myeloma with presumed solitary plasmocytoma of bone. In Vivo 22:513-517

41. Hawkins DS, Rajendran JG, Conrad EU et al (2002) Evaluation of chemotherapy response in pediatric bone sarcomas by [F-18]-fluorodeoxy-d-glucose positron emission tomography. Cancer 94:3277-3284

42. Nair N, Ali G, Green AA et al (2000) Response of osteosarcoma to chemotherapy. Evaluation with F-18 FDG-PET scans. Clin Positron Imaging 3:79-83

43. Schulte M, Brecht-Krauss D, Werner M et al (1999) Evaluation of neoadjuvant therapy response of osteogenic sarcoma using FDG-PET. J Nucl Med 40:1637-1643

44. Franzius C, Sciuk J, Brinkschmidt C et al (2000) Evaluation of chemotherapy response in primary bone tumors with F-18-FDG-PET compared with histologically assessed tumor necrosis. Clin Nucl Med 25:874-881

45. Evilevitch V, Weber W, Tap W et al (2008) Reduction of glucose metabolic activity is more accurate than change in size at predicting histopathologic response to neoadjuvant therapy in high-grade soft-tissue sarcomas. Clin Cancer Res 14:715-720

46. Benz M, Allen-Auerbach M, Eilber F et al (2008) Combined assessment of metabolic and volumetric changes for assessment of tumor response in patients with soft-tissue sarcoma. J Nucl Med 49:1579-1584

47. Benz M, Evilevitch V, Allen-Auerbach M et al (2008) Treatment monitoring by F-18-FDG PET/CT in patients with sarcomas: interobserver variability of quantitative parameters in treatment-induced changes in histopathologically responding and nonresponding tumors. J Nucl Med 49:1038-1049

48. Ye Z, Zhu J, Tian M, Zhang H et al (2008) Response of osteogenic sarcoma to neoadjuvant therapy: evaluated ba F-18-FDG PET. Ann Nucl Med 22:475-480

49. Huang T, Liu R, Chen T et al (2006) Comparison between F-18-FDG positron emission tomography and histology for the assessment of tumor necrosis rates in primary osteosarcoma. J Chin Med Assoc 69:372-376

50. Iagaru A, Masamed R, Chawla S et al (2008) F-18 FDG PET and PET/CT evalation of response to chemotherapy in bone and soft-tissue sarcomas. Clin Nucl Med33:8-13

51. Franzius C, Daldrup-Link HE, Wagner-Bohn A et al (2002) FDG PET for detection of recurrences from malignant primary bone tumors: Comparison with conventional imaging. Ann Oncol 13:157-160

52. Bredella MA, Caputo GR, Steinbach LS (2002) Value of FDG positron emission tomography in conjunction with MR imaging for evaluating therapy response in patients with muscusceletal sarcomas. Am J Roentgenol 179:1145-1150

53. Johnson GR, Zhuang H, Khan J et al (2003) Roles of positron emission tomography with fluorine-18 deoxyglucose in the detection of local recurrent and distant metastatic sarcoma. Clin Nucl Med 28:815-820

54. Arush M, Israel O, Postovsky S et al (2007) Positron emission tomography/computed tomography with (18) fluoro-deoxyglucose in the detection of local recurrence and distant metastases in pediatric sarcoma. Pediatr Blood Cancer 24: epub ahead of print

55. Gerth H, Juergens K, Dirksen U et al (2007) Significant benefit of multimodal imaging: PET/CT compared with PET alone in staging and follow-up of patients with Ewing sarcoma. J Nucl Med 48:1932-1939

56. Tang G, Wang M, Tang X et al (2003) Synthesis and evaluation of O-(3-[18F]fluoropropyl) -L-tyrosine as an oncologic PET tracer. Nucl Med Biol 30:733-739

57. Buck A, Herrmann K, Bueschenfelde C et al (2008) Imaging bone and soft tissue tumors with the proliferation marker [F18]fluorodesoxythymidine. Clin Cancer Res 14:2970-2977

Radionuclide Imaging of Musculoskeletal Disorders in Children

Ariane Boubaker

Service de Medicine Nucleaire, Centre Hospitalier Universitaire Vaudois, Lausanne, Switzerland

Introduction

Bone scintigraphy (BS) with ^{99m}Tc-labeled diphosphonates (^{99m}Tc-DPD) is the second most common nuclear medicine procedure performed in children and adolescents after renography. Common indications are suspicion of infections/inflammations, trauma, and tumors. BS is a simple and non-invasive procedure and does not need special preparation [1-3]. Cooperation of the child and parents can be easily obtained by a trained staff. A dedicated examination room and the use of distraction techniques (videos, music, and books) will work efficiently for patient immobilization during the acquisition. A proper time schedule with late acquisition performed after feeding and during the normal daytime sleeping period will allow infants and children to be examined without sedation. Local anesthetic cream should be applied at least 45 min before injection and the child should be encouraged to drink, especially between contrast injection and late imaging, to increase spontaneous voiding and lower radiation burden. A high-quality examination is mandatory and can be obtained by having the child lie directly on the collimator of the camera. Three-phase (vascular, blood pool, and late) imaging is routinely used to assess infection/inflammation, trauma, and primary bone tumors, with delayed imaging only being generally performed to assess bone metastases. As a rule, the patient's whole body must be examined in anterior and posterior projections 2-4 h after injection, and high-count static views are preferred to a whole-body scan in children younger than 5 years. For late images, low-energy high- or ultra-high-resolution collimators should be used, with static views of 50-100 kcounts for the hands, feet, and knees, and 300-500 kcounts for the axial skeleton. For the evaluation of back pain or lesions of the axial skeleton, single photon emission computed tomography (SPECT) or SPECT/CT is mandatory, whereas the use of a pinhole collimator is preferred for imaging the extremities [1, 2, 4]. BS has a high sensitivity for the early detection of bone lesions and changes in osseous metabolism, such that a negative examination generally rules out significant pathology. When bone metastases are diagnosed on BS, other tracers, such as ^{123}I-metaiodobenzylguanidine (MIBG) or ^{111}In-octreotide, can be used to stage the disease and to provide

more specific information for follow-up during and after treatment (Fig. 1). More recently, ^{18}F-fluoro-2-deoxy-D-glucose (^{18}F-FDG) PET or PETCT has been introduced in pediatric nuclear medicine and is already recognized as a useful diagnostic procedure in lymphoma patients. This approach will probably be useful in primary bone tumors and soft-tissue sarcoma, both for staging and follow-up during and after treatment, but up to now there are few published studies in small groups of patients. Another issue is the lack of specificity of ^{18}F-FDG in the differentiation of benign from malignant bone lesions.

Inflammations and Infections

Acute hematogenous infections of the osteoarticular system are common in children, occurring at a rate of 5.5-13/100,000 children, being more frequent below the age of 5 years [5, 6]. The differential diagnosis of a child presenting with limb pain and fever includes transient synovitis, cellulitis, acute osteomyelitis, and osteoarthritis. The usual scintigraphic patterns of these disorders are described in Table 1. Over the last 20 years, the pathogens identified in culture by conventional means or polymerase chain reaction (PCR) has evolved and *Kingella Kingae* has replaced *Haemophilus influenzae* since the introduction of vaccination, but the most common pathogen identified in acute hematogenous osteomyelitis (AHO) and septic arthritis remains *Staphylococcus aureus* (54-89% of cases) [6-8]. It should be emphasized that a pathogen can be identified in only 26-38% of blood cultures. Bone biopsy is rarely performed and imaging remains the modality of choice for the diagnosis of osteoarticular infection [9, 10]. It is essential to have access to the clinical history of the child, because the duration of symptoms, introduction of antibiotic therapy before performing the bone scan, bone biopsy, or joint aspiration will change the osteoblastic reaction and influence the result of the study. Imaging too early (<24 h) after the onset of the symptoms may lead to a false-negative bone scan, caused by the edema of the involved bony area. Another pitfall encountered when performing a bone scan early after the onset of symptoms is the increased joint pressure due to arthritis.

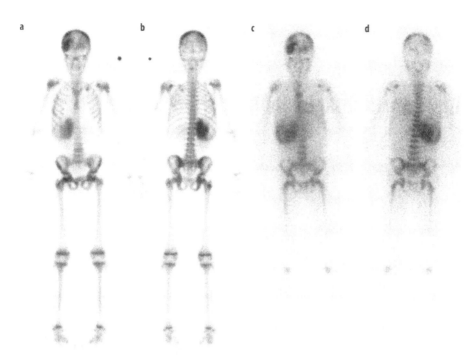

Fig. 1 a-d. A 12-year old boy presenting with fever and pain in the right hip over a period of a few days. A three-phase bone scintigraphy was performed to search for possible acute hematogenous osteomyelitis. Whole-body scan performed in anterior (**a**) and posterior (**b**) projections demonstrated multiple foci of increased uptake of Tc-99m-diphosphonates (skull, ribs, pelvis, and right proximal femur), consistent with bone metastases. Subsequent ^{123}I-MIBG scintigraphy was performed and whole-body in anterior (**c**) and posterior (**d**) projections confirmed a stage IV neuroblastoma

Table 1. Patterns of tracer distribution usually observed on three-phase bone scintigraphy in musculosekletal disorders in children

Pathology	Vascular phase	Blood-pool phase	Late phase
Inflammation/infection			
Cellulitis	++	+/++	– (normal)
Transient synovitis	+/++	+	–/+ (diffuse)
Septic arthrits	++	++	+ (diffuse)
Osteomyelitis	++/+++	++/+++	+++ (focal)
Trauma/related disorders			
Recent fracture	++/+++	++	+++ (linear, spiroid)
Sympathetic reflex neurodystrophy	Diffusely decreased	Diffusely decreased	Diffusely decreased
Primary bone tumors			
Benign			
– Osteoid osteoma	+++	+++	+++ (focal)
– Osteochondrom	–/+	–/+	–/+
– Fibrous dysplasia	+++	+++	+++
– Langerhans cell hystiocytosis	–/+	–/+	–/++ (photopenic central area)
Malignant			
– Osteosarcoma	+++	+++	+++
– Ewing sarcoma	+/++	+/++	+/++
Metastases			
– Neuroblastoma	++	++/+++	++/+++ (focal or diffuse)
– Hodgkin's disease	NA	NA	+/++ (focal or diffuse)
– Alveolar rhabdomyosarcoma	–/+	–/+	++ (diffuse)

NA, Not available; –, similar to normal bone; +, slight increase; ++, moderate increase; +++, marked increase

In this case, the tracer cannot reach the site of infection, which therefore appears as a photopenic area. False-positive findings can be observed after joint aspiration or bone biopsy. The overall accuracy of BS for the diagnosis of AHO is close to 90% [1, 2].

An inflammatory/infectious process induces hyperemia in the early vascular and blood-pool phases of the bone scan. BS has to be interpreted with knowledge of the radiographs and ultrasound because it lacks specificity. The differential diagnosis of a positive lesion on BS includes AHO, histiocytosis, trauma, and tumor. In AHO, a radiograph usually remains normal until 7-10 days after the onset of symptoms, whereas tumors and histiocytosis are generally diagnosed on radiographs. The location of the abnormality observed on a BS is helpful for the diagnosis of AHO: osteoarticular infection affects predominantly the metaphysis of long bones (75% of cases), the lower limbs being more frequently involved than the upper limbs [9]. Typically, AHO produces an intense and focal hyperemia and eventually involves the metaphyseal bone near the growing plate, whereas arthritis induces a diffuse hyperemia involving both sides of the joint with no or minimal late changes. A challenging situation for scintigraphy is the hip area, where bladder activity can hide a hyperemic focus. A bladder that is full of non-radioactive urine before injection of the radiopharmaceutical may allow better visualization of a localized hyperemia in the pelvis during the early phase of the bone scan. An empty bladder is mandatory for late acquisition because urinary activity may prevent correct identification of a lesion (Fig. 2). Transient synovitis and cellulitis induce only minimal hyperemia persisting in the blood-pool phase but no significantly increased bone activity on late images (Fig. 3). When joint effusion is present in the hip, the increased intra-articular pressure may

cause a tamponade of the intracapsular vessels and lead to ischemia of the femoral head [10, 11].

Back pain is uncommon in children and a three-phase BS, including SPECT or SPECT/CT of the spine may help to localize the abnormality and guide further imaging with CT or MRI. The differential diagnosis of back pain includes discitis in children and spondylolysis in adolescents. All these disorders can be missed on planar images whereas SPECT increases both the sensitivity and the specificity of BS by picking up the increased tracer uptake and demonstrating the precise localization in the vertebra.

Chronic recurrent multifocal osteomyelitis (CRMO) is a distinct variant of osteomyelitis that occurs in children and adolescents. Clinical presentation includes recurrent attacks of bone pain at multiple sites, with or without fever. Symptoms may evolve for weeks or months and resolve spontaneously in an unpredictable clinical course. Antibiotics are ineffective. Typical sites are the metaphyseal regions of the long bones, medial portion of the clavicules, the face, spine, pelvis, and upper extremities. Radiography may show mixed lesions, purely sclerotic le-

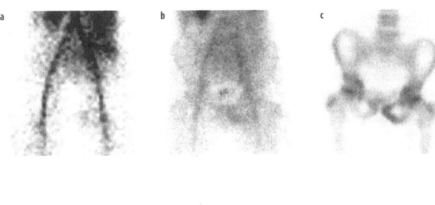

Fig. 2 a-c. Three-phase bone scintigraphy was performed in an 8-year old girl presenting with high fever and pain of the left hip for a period of one week. She was first treated with nonsteroidal anti-inflammatory drugs over 5 days based on clinical suspicion of transient synovitis of the left hip. Bone scintigraphy demonstrated an intense and focal hyperemia in the region of the left obturator rim (a). The anterior blood-pool and delayed images (b, c) showed increased tracer uptake in the inferior ramus and body of the pubis, with a diffuse hyperactivity of the left hip. MRI revealed a soft-tissue abscess near the inferior ramus of the pubis and confirmed osteomyelitis

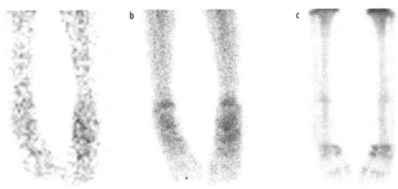

Fig. 3 a-c. Three-phase bone scintigraphy was performed 24 h after the onset of symptoms in a 4-year-old boy based on clinical suspicion of osteomyelitis. The vascular phase (a) demonstrated diffuse hyperemia of the left foot, affecting predominantly the dorsal and medial part of the hindfoot and midfoot, and persisting in the blood-pool phase (b). The delayed anterior view, performed 3 h after tracer injection (c), showed a diffuse increase of activity in the left foot but no focal bone abnormality. The final diagnosis was cellulitis

sions, and bone destruction. BS has the advantage of demonstrating multifocal lesions, both symptomatic and asymptomatic ones.

The use of other tracers more specific for infection/inflammation, such as Tc-99m-labeled leukocytes or Tc-99-murine monoclonal antigranulocyte antibodies, is not recommended in children [1, 2]. The role of ^{18}F-FDG PET and PETCT in osteomyelitis and arthritis has been investigated in adults but few reports are available in children so far [12]. These imaging modalities may provide useful information in special clinical conditions or in the investigation of fever of unknown origin.

Trauma and Related Disorders

Bone scan is indicated in case of equivocal radiographs, persistent symptoms despite normal radiographs, suspicion of post-traumatic sympathetic reflex neurodystrophy, and suspicion of child abuse. In toddlers, the most commonly affected bone is the tibia, and trauma is generally diagnosed on radiographs [2, 3, 9, 10]. If radiographs are equivocal or the fibula or small bones of the feet are affected, BS may diagnose fracture in a child presenting acute pain and limping and no signs or symptoms suggesting infection. Another issue is the correct diagnosis of scaphoid fracture, which may be difficult to assess even on repeated radiographs. Here, BS has been proven to be helpful when the diagnosis is uncertain [13]. In non-communicative children, BS may help to identify the source of persistent pain and to guide further imaging [14]. The role of scintigraphy in suspected child abuse is to provide a quick characterization of the trauma and its extent [15, 16]. The advantages of BS are its sensitivity to detect soft-tissue and subtle bony lesions that may remain undetected on radiographs and to provide a whole-body survey. Typical sites of abuse are the ribs, the diaphyses of the long bones, and the metaphyses of the upper limbs. Positioning is essential for the correct diagnosis of trauma, but also to assess a normal study [17] (Fig. 4). It is mandatory to obtain at least two different projections of the same region and to have the limbs positioned symmetrically, to avoid false-positive diagnosis of a lesion due to overlapping of small bones of the hands or feet.

Reflex sympathetic dystrophy (RSD) is frequently associated with trauma but may reflect malignancy, infection, or psychological stress [2, 3]. It is a clinical diagnosis that is often delayed in children because typical trophic changes are less prominent than in adults and symptoms may lead to the misdiagnosis of arthritis. BS can play an important role in diagnosing RSD because radiographs may be normal or show non-specific diffuse osteopenia with or without soft-tissue swelling. In adults, the typical appearances of RSD include increased periarticular activity on the late phase, associated with an intense hyperemia and increased blood-pool activity in a similar distribution. In children, however, RSD is most often observed in its "cold variant" and may therefore be difficult to differentiate from a "dis-

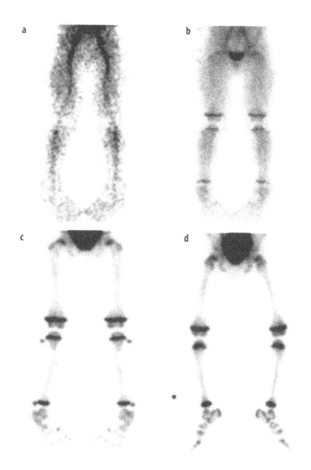

Fig. 4 a-d. Three-phase bone scintigraphy was performed in this 18-month-old girl presenting with intermittent limping on the right leg. A radiograph showed an equivocal photopenic lesion of the proximal tibia. Biological parameters were normal except for an increased sedimentation rate. Anterior views in vascular (**a**), blood-pool (**b**), and delayed (**c**) phases were normal. All metaphyseal regions of the long bones and small bones of the feet are clearly demonstrated and appear symmetric. On the posterior view (**d**), the bones of the hindfoot are well-delineated and of normal appearance. The child did not receive any treatment and the symptoms resolved spontaneously

use dystrophy." Girls are more affected than boys, and the lower limb is involved in up to 70% of cases.

Tumors

Benign Bone Tumors

Benign bone tumors include Langerhans cell histiocytosis, osteochondroma, fibrous dysplasia, and osteoid osteoma. They are generally first diagnosed on plain radiographs, with BS performed to assess the degree of activity of the lesion and to look for possible multiple localizations. The peak incidence and frequent sites of bone tumors are summarized in Table 2. Osteochodroma is the

Table 2. Peak incidence and common localizations of benign and malignant primary bone tumors in children. (Modified from [18])

	Peak incidence	Frequent sites	Usual localization in bone
Benign tumors			
Osteoid osteoma	>10 years	Femur, tibia	Diaphysis (tibia), femoral neck
Langerhans cell histiocytosis (eosinophil granuloma)	5-10 years	Pelvis, femur, tibia, vertebra, humerus, skull, ribs	Diaphysis
Osteochondrom (exostosis)	>10 years	Knee (femur, tibia), humerus	Metaphysis
Enchondrom (solitary)	>15 years	Hand and foot, femur, humerus	Diaphysis, metaphysis
Enchondrom (multiple, Morbus Ollier)	>10 years	Upper and lower limbs, ilac bone	Diaphysis, metaphysis
Non-ossifying fibroma	2-20 years	Femur, tibia	Metaphysis
Fibrous dysplasia (monostotic)	>10 years	Tibia, femoral neck, ribs	Diaphysis (tibia)
Fibrous dysplasia (polyostotic)	2-30 years	Iliac bone, femur, tibia, skull, mandible, ribs, humerus	Diaphysis, metaphysis
Malignant tumors			
Primary bone tumors			
– Osteogenic sarcoma	10-20 years	Knee (femur, tibia), humerus	Metaphysis
– Ewing sarcoma	5-25 years	Iliac bone, ribs, scapula, femur, tibia, humerus	Diaphyis
Metastases			
– Neuroblastoma	1-4 years	Skull, periorbital	–
– Hodgkin's disease	15 years	Axial skeleton	–
– Rhabdomyosarcoma (alveolar type)	3-6 years	Diffuse infiltration	–

most frequent benign bone tumor and accounts for 45% of benign tumors and 12% of all bone tumors [18]. Other lesions, such as aneurysmal cyst, simple bone cyst, and fibrous dysplasia, may remain undiagnosed until complication (fracture) occurs. These lesions can demonstrate variable hyperemia on the early phase of BS and marked delayed increase of tracer uptake. Cartilaginous tumors generally show no significant increase in the vascular and delayed phases, but increased tracer uptake during follow-up may indicate malignant degeneration. BS can demonstrate unsuspected multiple localizations of enchondroma and osteochondroma, which are often asymptomatic lesions, malignant degeneration being more frequent in multicentric than in unicentric forms.

Osteoid osteoma is generally diagnosed by radiographs and a clinical history of recurrent localized pain occurring predominantly at night. The size of the lesion and mild osteoporosis rather than osteosclerosis in small spongious bones may lead to misdiagnosis on CT and MRI if the study is not perfectly targeted to the lesion. On BS, osteoid osteoma is characterized by an intense focal hyperemia and high tracer uptake on delayed phase [19, 20]. BS together with SPECT (SPECT/CT) has a high sensitivity for the detection and localization of the lesion. A negative study excludes the presence of an osteoid osteoma.

Langerhans cell histiocytosis (LCH) may involve a single system, such as bone or skin, or multiple systems, including lungs, liver and the central nervous system (CNS). Its clinical course is unpredictable and varies from spontaneous resolution to rapid progression and death. Ninety percent of children with LCH will have bone lesions. BS is routinely used to assess the extent of the disease, to monitor the response to therapy, and to detect reactivation after treatment. Recently, ^{18}F-FDG PETCT was found to be useful in monitoring the early response to treatment

and was able to detect new lesions or reactivation before BS [21]. A limitation to the systematic use of ^{18}F-FDG PETCT in children is the radiation burden and the need for sedation. In another study, it was observed that benign nonossifying tumors may show high uptake of ^{18}F-FDG and non-increased uptake of ^{99m}Tc-DPD, and thus may be misdiagnosed as malignancies [22]. In such cases, the correlation of PET with CT and/or radiography enables the benign nature of the lesions to be assessed. ^{18}F-fluoride PET and PETCT had a higher sensitivity and specificity than BS for the diagnosis of various bone disorders, including benign tumors [23]. These procedures are not widely used because of the limited availability of the tracer and the limited availability of PET/PETCT systems, but they could replace BS in the future. Imaging is carried out 30 min after tracer injection and the radiation burden is similar to that delivered by ^{99m}Tc-DPD.

Malignant Tumors

Primary malignant bone tumors in the pediatric population are relatively rare, being sixth in incidence behind leukemia, CNS tumors, lymphoma, neuroblastoma, and Wilm's tumor [19, 20]. Osteosarcoma accounts for 60% of malignant bone tumors, the remainder being Ewing's sarcoma or Ewing's-like tumors (peripheral neuroectodermal tumors). The diagnosis of these tumors is often delayed because of their rarity and non-specific symptoms. A history of trauma is quite frequent and in patients with persistent non-mechanical pain a high degree of suspicion of tumor must be retained. Multimodality imaging is mandatory to provide accurate staging before treatment and must include radiographs, BS, CT scan, and MRI. Osteosarcoma and Ewing's sarcoma are unusual in infants and are generally observed in the second decade of life. Approximately 20%

of children will have detectable metastases at diagnosis, mostly in the lungs, followed by bone [24]. On BS, osteosarcoma appears as a highly vascularized lesion marked by intense tracer uptake on late images, sometimes heterogeneous or with a central photopenic area indicating central necrosis (Fig. 5). Occasionally, a skip lesion may be diagnosed on BS. Ewing's sarcoma may also be visualized as an intense hyperemic lesion but its appearance on delayed images is more variable (Fig. 6). ^{18}F-FDG PET seems to be more sensitive than BS for the detection of bone metastases in children with Ewing's sarcoma and is therefore recommended for staging by the Children's Oncology Group Bone Tumor Committee [24]. In osteosarcoma, ^{18}F-FDG has not yet proven to be superior to BS but studies are limited and the technique may become useful for monitoring response to treatment and to detect recurrence [25].

Bone metastases are frequently observed in children with neuroblastoma (NBL), less commonly in children presenting with rhabdomyosarcoma or lymphoma [26, 27]. NBL is the most frequent extracranial solid tumor in children. It is rarely diagnosed after the age of 5 years. Bone metastases are present at diagnosis in up to 70% of children with NBL and BS is usually indicated to assess disseminated disease. A previously unknown disseminated stage IV NBL is typically diagnosed on a three-phase

BS performed for suspicion of osteomyelitis in a child presenting with pain and limping. ^{123}I-MIBG is the tracer of choice for imaging NBL in children. It is routinely used to stage the disease, monitor the response to chemotherapy, and for follow-up after treatment completion. The current primary role of ^{18}F-FDG PET in NBL is the evaluation of tumors that do not concentrate MIBG. Rhabdomyosarcoma can develop in any tissue or organ; the most common sites are the head (orbit and paranasal sinuses), the neck, and the genitourinary system. Metastases may occur in the lungs and bones. BS is indicated to search for cortical bone lesions and/or diffuse infiltration of the skeleton, which may be observed in alveolar rhabdomyosarcoma. The degree of ^{18}F-FDG uptake in rhabdomyosarcoma is variable and the role of PET has not yet been established in these patients. Hodgkin's disease is the most frequent lymphoma in children and accounts for about 6% of all childhood cancers. Bone metastases occur in 5-20% of patients (Fig. 7). ^{18}F-FDG PET has recently replaced ^{67}Ga citrate scintigraphy in the workup of patients with Hodgkin's and non-Hodgkin's lymphoma. ^{18}F-FDG PET has been reported to change tumor staging in 10-26% of children at initial evaluation. It is particularly accurate in the prediction of clinical outcome after treatment completion. The absence of FDG uptake in a residual mass is pre-

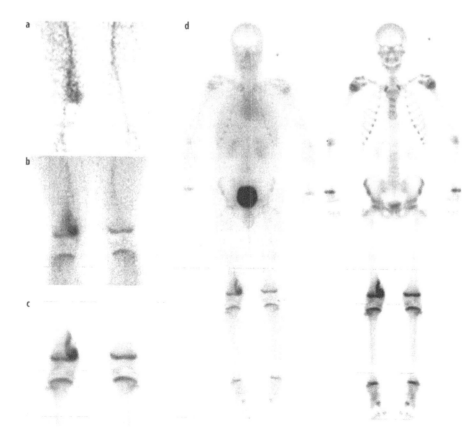

Fig. 5 a-c. Three-phase bone scintigraphy was performed for initial staging of an osteogenic sarcoma of the right distal femur diagnosed in a 14-year-old boy who presented with recurrent pain of the right knee of 3 months duration. The tumor is highly vascularized and appears as a focus of intense hyperemia on the vascular phase of the bone scan (**a**). On the blood-pool image (**b**), the tumor demonstrated variable intensity of tracer uptake, the more intense area being in contact with the medial part of the growth plate of the distal femur. The late image (**c**) showed a heterogeneous lesion of the distal and medial metaphyseal regions of the right femur, with intensely increased tracer uptake surrounding a "photopenic" area corresponding to central necrosis

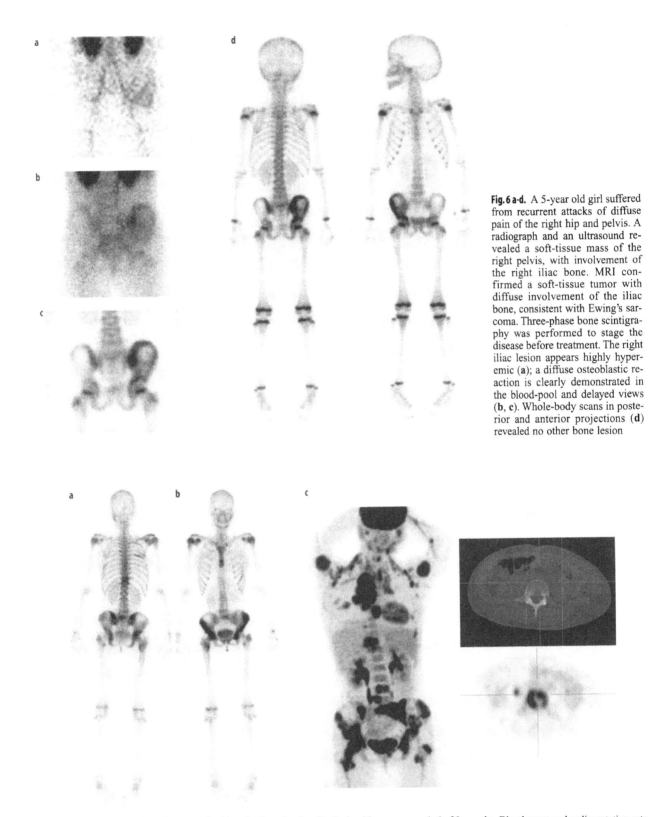

Fig. 6 a-d. A 5-year old girl suffered from recurrent attacks of diffuse pain of the right hip and pelvis. A radiograph and an ultrasound revealed a soft-tissue mass of the right pelvis, with involvement of the right iliac bone. MRI confirmed a soft-tissue tumor with diffuse involvement of the iliac bone, consistent with Ewing's sarcoma. Three-phase bone scintigraphy was performed to stage the disease before treatment. The right iliac lesion appears highly hyperemic (**a**); a diffuse osteoblastic reaction is clearly demonstrated in the blood-pool and delayed views (**b, c**). Whole-body scans in posterior and anterior projections (**d**) revealed no other bone lesion

Fig. 7 a-c. This 14-year old girl presented with asthenia and pain of both shoulders over a period of 2 months. Blood count and sedimentation rate were normal, and C-reactive protein was elevated. CT scan revealed a mediastinal mass and lymphadenopathies of the axillae. Whole-body scintigraphy in posterior (**a**) and anterior (**b**) projections showed multiple foci of increased tracer uptake (shoulders, ribs, vertebrae, pelvis, proximal femurs), indicating bone metastases. Hodgkin's disease was diagnosed by lymph node biopsy. F-18-FDG PETCT was performed before the initiation of chemotherapy (**c**) and confirmed stage IV disease with multiple sites of bone involvement

dictive of remission, even if minimal residual disease can be missed, whereas high uptake indicates persistent or recurrent tumor.

Conclusions

Nuclear medicine procedures are helpful for the diagnosis and management of children presenting with various disorders affecting the musculoskeletal system. Despite the growing interest and increased availability of ^{18}F-FDG and PET/PETCT systems, BS with ^{99m}Tc-diphosphonates remains a useful and non-invasive "first-line" diagnostic tool for the diagnosis of infection, trauma, primary tumors, and bone metastases. In the future, PET/PETCT studies will probably replace conventional nuclear medicine procedure in specific situations. For each child who presents with symptoms and signs of musculoskeletal disease, the best nuclear medicine procedure has to be chosen based on clinical history, biology and/or histology, and results of all available radiological examinations. Each examination should address the individual child in order to minimize the radiation burden in the pediatric population.

References

1. Hahn K, Fischer S, Colarhina P et al (2001) Guidelines for bone scintigraphy in children. Eur J Nucl Med 28:BP42-47
2. Nadel HR, Stilwell ME (2001) Nuclear medicine topics in pediatric musculoskeletal disease. Radiol Clin North Am 39:619-651
3. Nadel HR (2007) Bone scan update. Semin Nucl Med 37:332-339
4. Connolly LP, Treves ST, Connolly SA et al (1998) Pediatric skeletal scintigraphy: applications of pinhole magnification. Radiographics 18:341-354
5. Ferroni A (2007) Epidemiology and bacteriological diagnosis of paediatric acute osteoarticular infections. Arch Pediatr 14:S91-96
6. Frank G, Mahoney HM, Eppes SC (2005) Musculoskeletal infections in children. Pediatr Clin North Am 52:1083-1106
7. Rasmont Q, Yombi JC, van der Linden D, Docquier P (2008) Osteoarticular infections in Belgian children: a survey of clinical, biological, radiological and microbiological data. Acta Orthop Belg 74:374-385
8. Riise ØR, Kirkhus E, Handeland KS et al (2008) Childhood osteomyelitis-incidence and differentiation from other acute onset musculoskeletal features in a population-based study. BMC Pediatr 20:8-45
9. Azoulay R, Alison M, Sekkal A et al (2007) Imaging of child osteoarticular infections. Arch Pediatr 14:S113-121
10. Connolly LP, Connolly SA (2003) Skeletal scintigraphy in the multimodality assessment of young children with acute skeletal symptoms. Clin Nucl Med 28:746-754
11. Do TT (2000) Transient synovitis as a cause of painful limps in children. Curr Opin Pediatr 12:48-51
12. Stumpe KDM, Strobel K (2009) Osteomyelitis and arthritis. Semin Nucl Med 39:27-35
13. Cheow HK, Set P, Robinson S et al (2008) The role of bone scan in the diagnosis of carpal fracture in children. J Pediatr Orthop 17:165-170
14. Bajelidze G, Belthur MV, Littleton AG, Dabney KW, Miller F (2008) Diagnostic evaluation using whole-body technetium bone scan in children with cerebral palsy. J Pediatr Orthop 28:112-117
15. Mandelstam SA, Cook D, Fitzgerald M, Ditchfield MR (2003) Complementary use of radiological skeletal survey and bone scintigraphy in detection of bony injuries in suspected child abuse. Arch Dis Child 88:387-390
16. Kemp AM, Dunstan F, Harison S, Morris S, Mann M, Rolfe K, et al (2008) Patterns of skeletal fractures in child abuse: systematic review. BMJ 337:859-862
17. Van der Wall H, Storey G, Frater C, Murray P (2001) Importance of positioning and technical factors in anatomic localization of sporting injuries in scintigraphic imaging. Semin Nucl Med 31:17-27
18. Greenspan A, Remagen W. Knochentumoren. Differential-diagnose in Radiologie und Pathologie (2000). Georg Thieme Verlag, Stuttgart New York
19. Davies AM (2001) Imaging in skeletal paediatric oncology. Eur J Radiol 37:79-94
20. Focacci C, Lattanzi R, Iadeluca ML, Campioni P (1998) Nuclear medicine in primary bone tumors. Eur J Radiol 27:S123-S131
21. Kaste SC, Rodriguez-Galindo C, McCarville ME, Shulkin BL (2007) PET-CT in pediatric Langerhans cell histiocytosis. Pediatr Radiol 37:615-622
22. Goodin GS, Shulkin BL, Kaufman RA, McCarville MB (2006) PET/CT characterisation of fibroosseous defects in children: 18F-FDG uptake can mimic metastatic disease. AJR Am J Roentgenol 187:1124-1128
23. Even-Sapir E, Mishani E, Flusser G, Metser U (2007) 18F-fluoride positron emission tomography and positron emission tomography/computed tomography. Semin Nucl Med 37:462-469
24. Meyer JS, Nadel HR, Marina N et al (2008) Imaging guidelines for children with Ewing sarcoma and osteosarcoma: a report from the Children's Oncology Group bone tumor committee. Pediatr Blood Cancer 51:163-170
25. Jadvar H, Alavi A, Mavi A, Shulkin B (2005) PET in pediatric disease. Radiol Clin N Am 43:135-152
26. Jadvar H, Connolly LP, Fahey FH, Shulkin B (2007) PET and PET/CT in pediatric oncology. Semin Nucl Med 37:316-331

Nuclear Medicine in the Diagnosis and Treatment of Hyperparathyroidism

Maria Cristina Marzola, Gaia Grassetto, Domenico Rubello

Department of Nuclear Medicine – PET Centre, Santa Maria della Misericordia Hospital, Rovigo, Italy

Anatomy of the Parathyroid Glands

The parathyroid glands arise from the pharyngeal pouches; usually, there are four such glands but the incidence of a supernumerous gland is 2-5% [1, 2]. The parathyroid glands are usually localized behind the thyroid gland. The two behind the upper lobe are also called the superior glands or P4 (originating from the fourth pouch), and the two behind/beyond the lower lobe are also referred to as the inferior glands or P3 (originating from the third pouch) [1, 2]. It is worth noting that the location of normal inferior parathyroid glands is more variable than that of the superior glands, probably due to their longer developmental pathway and more difficult developmental migration process. Consequently, the P3 glands can be intrathyroidal, within the thyrothymic ligament, within the thymus, or in the mediastinum. The parathyroid glands are generally found in the peri-thyroid sheath but may also occur outside the thyroid capsule or, very rarely, in a subcapsular site [1-5].

Supernumerary or accessory glands derive from the numerous dorsal and ventral wings of the pouches and can have various locations, from the cricoid cartilage to as far as the lower mediastinum [2]. The most probable location of accessory glands is the thymic region [1-3]. In some individuals, fewer than four parathyroid glands may be present, or the parathyroid glands may be completely absent. The latter is the result of abnormalities in genes encoding transcription factors required for parathyroid tissue development, such as *Gcm2*, or of immunological disorders, such as Digeorge syndrome.

The normal gland differs considerably in shape and size between individuals and within the same individual. Usually, the parathyroids are ovoid or bean-shaped but they may be elongated, leaf-like, or multi-lobulated. Their diameter is variable, although it should not be >7 mm, and the weight of an individual gland ranges from 20 to 45 mg [2, 4].

The parathyroid gland has two main components: parenchymal cells and fat cells. There are relatively few fat cells until adolescence after which the number increases gradually, such that by the age of 30 years these cells account for 10-25% of the glandular volume [2].

In the normal gland, parenchymal cells are predominantly chief cells. These are active endocrine cells that produce parathyroid hormone (PTH) and have a slightly eosinophilic cytoplasm with few mitochondria. Minor cellular components of the parathyroid gland include oxyphilic and transitional-oxyphilic cells, which increase in number with age and may produce PTH. Parathyroid clear cells are fundamentally inactive but their true function is as yet unknown [2]. Finally, vascular and nervous cells are also present in the parathyroid tissue.

Physiology of PTH

The parathyroid glands produce PTH, a key hormone in the maintenance of calcium, phosphate, and vitamin D homeostasis. PTH is produced by chief cells in the form of pre-pro-PTH (115 amino acids), which in subsequent steps is converted first into pro-PTH (90 amino acids) and then into PTH. This final form is stored in cytosolic granules that, in response to a suitable stimulus, release PTH into the blood flow [2, 3, 5].

The major stimulus to PTH secretion is the level of ionized calcium in the blood, such that a reduction stimulates PTH production and secretion. The surface of parathyroid cells is equipped with a cation-sensitive receptor mechanism through which the cytosolic calcium concentration and PTH secretion are regulated [2-4]. Calcium homeostasis is maintained by four different mechanisms: (1) increased calcium absorption from the gastrointestinal tract; (2) stimulation of osteoclastic activity, resulting in the reabsorption of calcium and phosphate from bone; (3) inhibition of phosphate reabsorption by the proximal renal tubules; and (4) enhancement of renal tubular calcium reabsorption [1, 2, 4].

The majority of PTH's actions on its target organs are mediated by the binding of the hormone to a specific PTH type I receptor, which results in the stimulation of the second messenger cyclic AMP (cAMP). In primary hyperparathyroidism, urinary cAMP levels are increased. The functions of PTH, especially in the intestine, are also mediated by active vitamin D, whose production is stimulated by PTH acting on the kidney, again mediated by cAMP. Vitamin D also increases the skeletal effects of PTH [5].

Hyperparathyroidism

The pathologically increased production and secretion of PTH result in hyperparathyroidism, which may be a primary, secondary, or tertiary disease [1, 2].

Primary hyperparathyroidism, the most frequent pathological condition of the parathyroid glands, results in a lack of calcium homeostasis: increased blood and urine calcium levels, decreased blood phosphate levels, and increased urinary phosphate [2-4]. Clinically, hyperparathyroidism is characterized by nephrocalcinosis, urolithiasis, bone disease, neuropsychiatric disorders, gastrointestinal disturbances, and neuromuscular manifestation [3]; however, as most new cases of primary hyperparathyroidism are diagnosed in the subclinical stage, these features are rarely seen [1, 2, 4].

In about 80% of patients, primary hyperparathyroidism is caused by a solitary adenoma of the parathyroid glands [2-4, 6]. This is a benign tumor that can vary in weight from less then 100 mg to more than 100 g, with some correlation between the size of the adenoma and the degree of hypercalcemia [2, 4]. In about 5% of patients, "double-adenomas", affecting more than one gland, are present.

Parathyroid hyperplasia accounts for less than 15% of the cases of primary hyperparathyroidism [2, 4], with chief-cell hyperplasia being the most common type. In primary hyperparathyroidism, hyperplasia affects the glands asymmetrically and to varying degrees, such that one or two glands may be of normal size albeit with microscopic signs of endocrine hyperfunction [2].

Carcinoma of the parathyroid glands represents less than 1% of cases of primary hyperparathyroidism and can arise in any gland. It usually occurs in patients 30-60 years of age and is generally accompanied by overt clinical signs of hyperparathyroidism [2, 7].

Primary hyperparathyroidism can be sporadic or familial. The familial form can affect the parathyroid glands exclusively or, more often, can be part of a multi-endocrine syndrome (MEN). MEN1, the more common type, consists of hyperparathyroidism and pituitary and pancreatic neuroendocrine tumors. In the less-common MEN2, hyperparathyroidism is accompanied by medullary thyroid cancer and pheochromocytoma. The parathyroid disease of MEN usually involves more than one gland (parathyroid hyperplasia). In a patient with recurrent hyperparathyroidism, MEN syndrome must be suspected.

Secondary hyperparathyroidism is consequent to a chronic hypocalcemic condition, which in turn is caused by renal failure, gastrointestinal malabsorption, dietary rickets, or the ingestion of drugs (phenytoin, phenobarbital and laxatives) that lead to decreased intestinal absorption of calcium. In chronic hypocalcemia, there is a continuous stimulus for the parathyroids to produce and secrete PTH. This results in a form of parathyroid gland hyperplasia that generally involves all of the glands symmetrically [2, 4]. Secondary hyperparathyroidism is a frequent and serious complication in hemodialysis patients.

Tertiary hyperparathyroidism is a condition in which parathyroid hyperplasia secondary to chronic hypocalcemia becomes autonomous, with the subsequent development of hypercalcemia. This condition generally does not regress after correction of the cause underlying the chronic hypocalcemia. In tertiary hyperparathyroidism, there is usually asymmetrical hyperplasia of the parathyroid gland [2, 4]. Tertiary hyperparathyroidism also refers to hyperparathyroidism that persists or develops after renal transplantation.

Nuclear Medicine in Hyperparathyroidism

Nuclear medicine offers several very useful imaging modalities in the diagnosis of parathyroid disease, including both conventional nuclear medicine and positron emission tomography (PET). However, of utmost importance is the fact that nuclear medicine, or any other imaging modality, does not diagnose hyperparathyroidism, which is instead established by measuring calcium and PTH plasma levels. Imaging serves as a localization technique that is useful when hyperparathyroidism has already been diagnosed. It reveals abnormal parathyroid glands but does not identify normal parathyroid glands, which are too small (20-50 mg) to be seen. The correct localization of diseased parathyroid gland(s) is the basis of a definitive treatment of hyperparathyroidism.

Before the advent of tracers labeled with ^{99m}Tc, surgery of the parathyroid glands was carried out without pre-operative localization imaging. Indeed, in 1986, Doppman stated that the best way to localize a diseased parathyroid gland(s) was to localize an experienced surgeon [4, 8]. However, recently, the ability to minimize the aggressiveness of surgery through minimally invasive surgery of the neck (endoscopic, video-assisted, and radio-guided) has yielded increased interest in pre-operative localization imaging and its use in treatment planning for primary hyperparathyroidism [9-13].

Conventional nuclear medicine techniques remain the first choice for localizing hyperfunctional parathyroid glands in patients with known primary hyperparathyroidism and in those with secondary, tertiary, and recurrent hyperparathyroidism. There are many different protocols to perform this kind of scintigraphy, the most important being double-tracer subtraction scintigraphy and dual-phase scintigraphy.

Double-Tracer Subtraction Scintigraphy

The rationale of double-tracer parathyroid scintigraphy derives from the fact that a specific tracer for parathyroid tissue does not exist. In fact, the tracers used in routine parathyroid nuclear medicine imaging, e.g., ^{201}Tl-chloride, but above all ^{99m}Tc-sestamibi, and also ^{99m}Tc-tetrofosmin, known myocardial perfusion tracers, are taken-up not only by the hyperfunctioning parathyroid glands but also by thyroid tissue. This necessitates comparison of the results with those obtained using a second tracer, one that is taken-up by the thyroid only, such as ^{99m}Tc-pertechnetate ([99m]TcO4-) or [123]iodine, and then digital subtraction of the thyroid scan from the parathyroid scan to remove the thyroid activity and enhance visualization of the parathyroid tissue.

Many double-tracer subtraction protocols have been developed, the first, involving sestamibi, was described by Coakley and colleagues. In this protocol, sequential acquisition of ^{99m}Tc-sestamibi and [123]iodine images is followed by image realignment and image subtraction [14, 15]. A prospective evaluation confirmed the superiority of this method over the thallium-technetium subtraction scan [16], the first subtraction technique, introduced by Ferlin and co-workers in the 1980s [17]. The lower sensitivity of [201]thallium and its higher radiation dose compared to ^{99m}Tc-sestamibi has made its use for parathyroid scanning obsolete.

[99m]Tc-tetrofosmin is an alternative to sestamibi for parathyroid scanning, but it is an appropriate tracer only for double-tracer scanning and not for dual-phase scintigraphy because, unlike sestamibi, it does not have a differential wash-out in the thyroid vs. the parathyroid tissue [18].

Two thyroid tracers can be combined with sestamibi (and also with ^{99m}Tc-tetrofosmin even if the reported experience is smaller), [123]iodine or ^{99m}Tc-pertechnetate, both of which can be used in many different ways [12]. As a general rule, ^{123}I requires at least 2 h for adequate uptake by the thyroid and is more expensive than ^{99m}Tc-pertechnetate. Its use is reasonable if the nuclear medicine department has a routine I[123] protocol for thyroid scans or if multiple parathyroid scans are done on the same day (37 MBq of ^{123}I currently costs approximately 125 euros in Europe and suffices for imaging studies in three patients). However ^{123}I has a selective advantage in that images of ^{99m}Tc-sestamibi and of ^{123}I can be recorded simultaneously [19, 20]. This is a substantial gain in gamma-camera imaging time. Moreover, because the two images are acquired simultaneously, image realignment is not necessary and there are no motion artifacts on the subtraction image.

Nonetheless, the principal subtraction scan protocols are based on sequential image acquisition with the most commonly used tracers, sestamibi and 99mTcO4- [21-23]:
1. [99m]TcO4-/^{99m}Tc-sestamibi: The patient is injected i.v. with 185 MBq [99m]TcO4-; after 20 min, the thyroid image is acquired. At the end of imaging, with the patient remaining in the same position, 300 MBq of ^{99m}Tc-Sestamibi are administered i.v. and a 20-min dynamic acquisition is performed. This protocol has good sensitivity and specificity but its drawback is that the high counts from the thyroid gland do not allow, after sub-

traction, the identification of a small hyperfunctioning parathyroid gland located behind the thyroid [4, 24].
2. [99m]TcO4-/^{99m}Tc-sestamibi, modified by Geatti and co-workers [23]: In this approach, the 99mTcO4- activity is reduced and the ^{99m}Tc-sestamibi dose increased. Twenty min after injection of 40-60 MBq of ^{99m}Tc-pertechnetate, a 10-min image of the neck is obtained. Then, without moving the patient, 600 MBq of ^{99m}Tc-sestamibi are injected and the corresponding scan performed.
3. [99m]TcO4- + potassium perchlorate (KClO4-)/^{99m}Tc-sestamibi: This is a variant of the technique described above, suggested by Rubello and colleagues. Here, 400 mg of potassium perchlorate are orally administered immediately before starting acquisition of the thyroid scan. The aim is to induce rapid [99m]TcO4- wash-out from the thyroid and reduce its interference with the ^{99m}Tc-sestamibi image [22]. The doses in this protocol are 150-200 MBq of [99m]TcO4- and 550-600 MBq of sestamibi.

It is worth noting that investigations should be done in the absence of iodine saturation. Thus, before the start of the scan, the nuclear medicine physician must be sure that the patient has not recently (at least 30-40 days) undergone radiological studies with iodine contrast medium and has stopped thyroid hormone replacement therapy (for at least 40 days) or treatment with methimazole or propylthiouracil (for at least 1 week). If these prerequisites cannot be fulfilled, the alternative is to use the dual-phase protocol. However, this protocol has lower sensitivity and specificity than the double-tracer subtraction scan, which is the preferred method [1, 3, 4].

Dual-Phase Protocol

The rationale behind dual-phase parathyroid scintigraphy is the exploitation of the different wash-out times of some radiotracers in thyroid and parathyroid tissues. To identify hyperfunctioning parathyroid tissue, the wash-out time of a radiotracer in the parathyroid must be slower than in thyroid tissue. This type of parathyroid scintigraphy is a simplification of the double-tracer scan and was first introduced by Taillefer and colleagues [25].

For dual-phase parathyroid scintigraphy ^{99m}Tc sestamibi is the agent of choice, at a recommended dose of 740-900 MBq (20-24 mCi) injected intravenously. Sestamibi is taken up in both normal thyroid tissue and hyperfunctioning parathyroid glands but wash-out from normal thyroid tissue is faster. In this protocol, early images, acquired 10 min after tracer injection, are visually compared with a second group of delayed images, acquired 2 h after injection. In some patients, especially those with thyroid disease, after the dual-phase scan a thyroid scan with [99m]TcO4- may be helpful to differentiate between thyroid nodules and pathological parathyroid tissue, since sestamibi uptake by a thyroid nodule resembles that by a hyperfunctioning parathyroid. This "hybrid technique" is recommended above all in regions where goiter is endemic, but it is necessary to be sure that the patient is not iodine-saturated and is not receiving thyroid hormones, methimazole, or propylthiouracil. This technique increases the specificity of the simple dual-phase scan but does not reach the specificity and sensitivity of the double-tracer scan [1, 3].

As mentioned above, ^{99m}Tc-tetrofosmin is not an alternative to sestamibi for dual-phase scintigraphy because it has a slower wash-out at the thyroid level [3, 18], thereby prohibiting an effective differential wash-out [3].

With double-tracer and dual-phase protocols, an image that includes the entire mediastinal space is needed to evaluate the presence of ectopic parathyroid gland(s). For this purpose, a SPECT scan of the neck and thorax is very useful because it better localizes ectopic foci; it is thus routinely obtained by some clinicians [1, 26, 27]. Moreover, hybrid SPECT/CT yields a more accurate localization. It is worth noting that with the dual-phase protocol tomographic acquisition must be done after the planar early images are obtained, while with the double-tracer scan SPECT is done at the end of the investigation. There is also evidence that pin-hole SPECT provides better-quality images than parallel-hole SPECT.

Positron Emission Tomography

Neither PET nor related tracer studies are the methods of choice to study hyperparathyroidism. Initial PET studies of parathyroid disease were carried out with FDG, the most widely used PET radiopharmaceutical, but the results obtained were conflicting. In some cases, its sensitivity was too low for routine use in the pre-operative detection and localization of the parathyroid glands. Moreover, in patients with an inflammatory condition who are scheduled for imaging of the head and neck, non-specific uptake of FDG that mimics or obscures an active parathyroid gland is very frequent [4]. Other authors tried to use ^{18}F-DOPA to detect parathyroid adenomas but none of their patients with histologically proven cases of the tumor showed significant uptake of ^{18}F-DOPA in their diseased parathyroid glands [4, 28].

Currently, the only PET tracer that seems to have a role in the study of parathyroid disease is ^{11}C-methionine, but it is not still possible to compare ^{11}C-methionine PET and classical scintigraphic techniques (especially those using sestamibi). This is due to the fact that the reported studies have consisted of highly pre-selected patient populations in whom conventional scintigraphy and ultrasound failed. Nonetheless, ^{11}C-methionine PET seems to yield accurate technical imaging, and some authors have found that in primary hyperparathyroidism (adenoma) patients the results are more accurate than those obtained with sestamibi [4]. ^{11}C-methionine PET is also a reliable approach in patients with recurrent primary hyperparathyroidism and in those with secondary hyperparathyroidism when classical sestamibi scintigraphy has failed [4]. Moreover, compared with sestamibi, ^{11}C-methionine PET has the advantage of better resolu-

tion. It was estimated that in parathyroid adenoma the lower limit of detection by ^{11}C-methioine is about 200 mg [4] vs. 500 mg with sestamibi [4]. Moreover, while PET is already established as a tomographic technique, with good localization of the parathyroids, it has been substantially improved in hybrid systems such as PET/CT. One limitation is that ^{11}C has a short half-life (about 20 min) and ^{11}C-methionine production requires close proximity to the source of the isotope and the ability to rapidly conjugate ^{11}C with the amino acid. These conditions restrict the use of this tracer, such that it is available only in a few centers. Thus, ^{11}C-methionine offers a good imaging alternative when standard scintigraphic techniques are not diagnostic.

Radio-Guided Surgery

The therapy of hyperparathyroidism is surgery. Based on the success of pre-operative imaging in patients with hyperparathyroidism, particularly sestamibi scintigraphy and ultrasonography, minimally invasive parathyroidectomy, employing a shorter (<2-3 cm) incision, has become the preferred operative strategy [29]. This approach, which can be video-assisted, endoscopic with gas insufflation, or radio-guided, often substitutes for aggressive types of surgery, such as bilateral and unilateral neck exploration. Minimally invasive radio-guided surgery uses a gamma-detecting intra-operative probe (a hand-held radiation detector device which gives both auditory signals and digitals counts) to guide the surgeon in the dissection of radioactive parathyroid target tissue. This technique is recommended in patients without a history of familial hyperparathyroidism, MEN, or previous neck irradiation in whom sestamibi scintigraphy indicates a high probability of a solitary parathyroid adenoma with significant uptake and no concomitant thyroid nodules showing uptake of the tracer [1]. Radio-guided parathyroidectomy is also indicated in re-operation for persistent or recurrent hyperparathyroidism and ectopic adenomas.

The advantages of radio-guided surgery are manifold: reduction of surgery time, a less aggressive surgical incision, less need of anesthesia, and the ability to evaluate the correctness of the removed tissue through "ex-vivo" radioactivity counting. The success of radio-guided surgery is dependent on the differential kinetics of sestamibi in the thyroid and parathyroid glands [30]. This technique is most helpful when there is a significant difference between the thyroid and parathyroid count rates, which generally occurs within a window of 2-3 h after injection. To optimize the parathyroid-thyroid count ratio, different protocols have been introduced:

1. Norman and Chheda's [31] protocol consists of dual-phase sestamibi scintigraphy on the day of surgery, beginning at the completion of scintigraphy, about 2.5-3 h after the injection of radioactivity. The standard activity of dual-phase scintigraphy that must be used is about 740 MBq.

2. In the protocol of Casara et al. [32], radio-guided surgery and parathyroid scan are done on separate days. Sestamibi diagnostic imaging, preferably following a double-tracer protocol, is performed a few days before surgery. On the day of surgery, the patient is administered a smaller activity of sestamibi (about 37 MBq) in the operating room just before the operation. This protocol reduces the radiation dose to the surgical team and allows localization of parathyroid tissue with rapid wash-out timing (<2.5-3 h). Moreover, if after double tracer scintigraphy doubt remains about the correct localization of the hyperfunctioning gland(s), there is time to acquire SPECT (or SPET/CT) images and to further explore the neck using ultrasound.

3. The protocol of Bozkurt et al. [33] is based on their conclusion that the optimal time to surgery is patient-specific. Dual-phase MIBI scintigraphy is performed on a day before surgery and includes a dynamic MIBI acquisition to obtain a time-activity-curve showing the differential parathyroid/thyroid ratio, which is then used to determine the optimum time to surgery. The authors reported a different optimal time to surgery for each patient, with a mean time of 136±43 min.

When bilateral neck exploration is the surgery method of choice, even if the pre-surgical scintigraphy seems to be negative, the use of a gamma-probe preceded by sestamibi injection has several benefits. In fact, the probability to correctly localize diseased parathyroid tissue increases as both the surgeon's experience and the amount of radio-guided data obtained increase.

References

1. Mariani G, Seza A Gulec, Rubello D et al (2003) Preoperative localization and radioguided parathyroid surgery. J Nucl Med 44:1443-1458
2. Elgazzar A (2001) Parathyroid gland. In: Elgazzar A (ed) The pathophysiologic basis of nuclear medicine. Springer-Verlag, Berlin Heidelberg New York, pp 141-146
3. Giordano A, Rubello D (2003) Le Paratiroidi – sez. endocrinologia. In: Dondi M, Giubbini R (ed) Medicina nucleare nella pratica clinica. Patron, Bologna, pp 171-183
4. Grassetto G, Alavi A, Rubello D (2008) PET and parathyroid. PET Clinics 2:385-393
5. Guyton A (1995) Ormone paratiroideo. Calcitonina. Metabolismo de' calcio e del fosforo. Vitamina D. Osso e denti. In: Guyton A (ed) Trattato di fisiologia medica. Piccin, Padova, pp 948-966
6. DeLellis RA, Mazzaglia P, Mangray (2008) Primary hyperparathyroidism: a current perspective. Arch Pathol Lab Med 132(8):1251-1262
7. DeLellis RA (2005) Parathyroid carcinoma: an overview. Adv Anat Pathol 12(2):53-61
8. Doppman J (1986) Reoperative parathyroid surgery: localization procedures, parathyroid surgery. Prog Surg 18:117-136
9. O'Doherty MJ, Kettle AG (2003) Parathyroid imaging: preoperative localisation. Nucl Med Commun 24:125-131
10. Beggs AD, Hain SF (2005) Localization of parathyroid adenomas using 11Cmethionine positron emission tomography. Nucl Med Commun 26: 133-136
11. Otto D, Boerne AR, Hofmann M et al (2004) Pre-operative localization of hyperfunctional parathyroid tissue with 11C-methionine PET. Eur J Nucl Med Mol Imaging 31:1405-1412
12. Giordano A, Rubello D, Casara D (2001) New trends in parathyroid scintigraphy. Eur J Nucl Med 28:1409-1420
13. Rubello D (2006) How should the "optimal" pre-operative localizing imaging work-up in hyperparathyroid patients be? J Endocrinol Invest 29(9):854-856
14. Coakley AJ, Kettle AG, Wells CP et al (1989) Tc-99m-sestamibi: a new agent for parathyroid imaging. Nucl Med Commun 10: 791-794
15. O'Doherty M J, Kettle A G, Wells PC et al (1992) Parathyroid imaging with technetium-99m-sestamibi: preoperative localisation and tissue uptake studies. J Nucl Med 33: 313-318
16. Hindié E, Melliere D, Simon D et al (1995) Primary hyperparathyroidism: is technetium 99m-Sestamibi/iodine-123 subtraction scanning the best procedure to locate enlarged glands before surgery? J Clin Endocrinol Metab 80:302-307
17. Ferlin G, Borsato N, Camerani M et al (1983) New perspectives in localising enlarged parathyroids by technetium-thallium subtraction scan. J Nucl Med 24:438-431
18. Fjeld J G, Erichson K, Pfeffer PF (1997) Tc-99m-tetrofosmin for parathyroid imaging: comparison with sestamibi. J Nucl Med 38:831-834
19. Hindié E, Mellière D, Jeanguillaume C et al (1996) Acquisition double-fenêtre 99mTc-MIBI/123I vs 99mTc-MIBI seul dans l'hyperparathyroïdie primitive. Communication Orale, XXXVe Colloque de Médecine Nucléaire, Lille, pp 15-18
20. Hindié E, Mellière D, Jeanguillaume C et al (1998) Parathyroid imaging using simultaneous double-window recording of technetium-99m-sestamibi and iodine-123. J Nucl Med 39:1100-1105
21. Johnston LB, Carroll MJ, Britton KE et al (1996) The accuracy of parathyroid gland localization in primary hyperparathyroidism using sestamibi radionuclide imaging. J Clin Endocrinol Metab 81:346-352
22. Rubello D, Saladini G, Casara D et al (2000) Parathyroid imaging with pertechnetate plus perchlorate/MIBI subtraction scintigraphy: a fast and effective technique. Clin Nucl Med 25:527-531
23. Geatti O, Shapiro B, Orsolon PG et al (1994) Localization of parathyroid enlargement: experience with technetium-99m methoxyisobutylisonitrile and thallium-201 scintigraphy, ultrasonography and computed tomography. Eur J Nucl Med 21:17-22
24. Casara D, Rubello D, Saladini G et al (1992) Imaging procedures in evaluation of hyperparathyroidism: the role of scintigraphy with 99mTc-MIBI. In: Ravelli E, Samori G (ed) Primary and secondary hyperparathyroidism. Wichtig, Milan, pp 133-136
25. Taillefer R, Boucher Y, Potvin C et al (1992) Detection and localization of parathyroid adenomas in patients with hyperparathyroidism using a single radionuclide imaging procedure with Technetium-99m-Sestamibi (double-phase study). J Nucl Med 33:1801-1807
26. Torregrosa JV, Fernandez-Cruz L, Canaleyo A et al (2000) 99mTc-sestamibi scintigraphy and cell cycle in parathyroid glands of secondary hyperparathyroidism. World J Surg 24:1386-1390
27. Billotey C, Sarfati E, Aurengo A et al (1996) Advantages of SPECT in technetium-99m-Sestamibi parathyroid scintigraphy J Nucl Med 37:1773-1778
28. Lange-Nolde A, Zajic T, Slawik M et al (2006) PET with 18F-DOPA in the imaging of parathyroid adenoma in patients with primary hyperparathyroidism. A pilot study. Nucklearmedizin 45:193-196
29. AACE/AAES Task force on primary hyperparathyroidism (2005) The American Association of Clinical Endocrinologists and the American Association of Endocrine Surgeons position

statement on the diagnosis and management of primary hyperparathyroidism. Endocr Pract 11:49-54

30. Ugur O, Bozkurt MF, Rubello D (2008) Nuclear medicine techniques for radioguided surgery of hyperparathyroidism. Minerva Endocrinol 33:1-10

31. Norman J, Chheda H (1997) Minimally invasive parathyroidectomy facilitated by intraoperative nuclear mapping. Surgery 122:998-1004

32. Casara D, Rubello D, Piotto A et al (2000) Tc99m-MIBI radioguided minimally invasive parathyroid surgery planned on the basis of a preoperative combined Tc99m-pertechnetate/Tc-99m MIBI and ultrasound imaging protocol. Eur J Nucl Med 27:1300-1304

33. Bozkurt MF, Ugur O, Hamaloglu E et al (2003) Optimization of the gamma probe-guided parathyroidectomy. Am Surg 69:720-725

PEDIATRIC SATELLITE COURSE "KANGAROO"

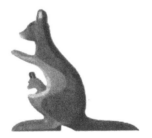

The Spectrum of Non-accidental Injuries (Child Abuse) and Its Imitators

Paul K. Kleinman

Department of Radiology, Children's Hospital Boston, Boston, MA, USA

Introduction

Skeletal injuries are the most common findings noted on imaging studies in cases of child abuse. In infants (<1 year), they result from manual assault that may include shaking. In contrast to central nervous system and other visceral injuries, they are rarely life-threatening. However, documentation of skeletal trauma is often central to the diagnosis of abuse. In infants, certain lesions are sufficiently characteristic to point strongly to the diagnosis of inflicted trauma (Table 1). Other fractures are less specific for abuse, but when correlated with other imaging findings and clinical information their presence may add strong support for the diagnosis.

Since Caffey's original description in 1946, radiologists have become familiar with the imaging features of commonly encountered inflicted skeletal injuries [1]. In recent years, increasing attention has been given to those conditions that are viewed as simulators of inflicted injury. A variety of normal variants, naturally occurring diseases, and accidental skeletal injuries may be confused with the findings of child abuse (Table 2). Sophisticated attorneys charged with the defense against allegations of abuse are often well versed in the differential diagnosis of inflicted injury. It is therefore essential that diagnostic imaging specialists involved with cases of alleged abuse conduct their studies in a thorough and conscientious fashion that will provide the greatest likelihood of a correct diagnosis in the clinical setting – one that can also be sustained in a highly adversarial legal arena.

Classic Metaphyseal Lesion (CML)

The corner-fracture and bucket-handle lesions described in 1957 by Caffey are frequent findings in young abused infants [2]. Pathologically, the fracture extends in a planar fashion through the primary spongiosa. Centrally, the fracture abuts the chondro-osseous junction; peripherally, it

Table 1. Specificity of radiologic findings

High specificity[a]
    Classic metaphyseal lesions
    Rib fractures, especially posteromedial
    Scapular fractures
    Spinous process fractures
    Sternal fractures

Moderate specificity
    Multiple fractures, especially bilateral
    Fractures of different ages
    Epiphyseal separations
    Vertebral body fractures and subluxations
    Digital fractures
    Complex skull fractures

Common but low specificity
    Subperiosteal new bone formation
    Clavicular fractures
    Long-bone shaft fractures
    Linear skull fractures

[a] Highest specificity applies in infants

Table 2. Differential diagnosis of inflicted skeletal injury

Accidents
Developmental variants
Syndromes, dysplasias and metabolic disorders
    Menkes' disease
    Chondrometaphyseal dysplasia, Schmid type
    Spondylometaphyseal dysplasia, corner fracture type
    Osteogenesis imperfecta, types 1 and 4
    Rickets
    Scurvy
    Copper deficiency
    Congenital indifference to pain
    Caffey's disease

Iatrogenic
    Obstetric
    Cardiopulmonary resuscitation
    Orthopedic manipulation
    Physical therapy
    Medications

Miscellaneous
    Osteomyelitis
    Congenital syphilis
    Leukemia
    Metastatic neuroblastoma

veers from the physis to undercut a larger segment encompassing the subperiosteal bone collar. The fracture may extend partially or completely across the metaphysis (Fig. 1). Such fractures are most common in the distal femur, proximal and distal tibia/fibula, and proximal humerus; they are much less frequent at the elbow, wrist, and proximal femur (Fig. 2). The fractures occur with torsion and traction of the extremities as the infant is grabbed by the arm or leg. They may also occur following sudden acceleration and deceleration of the extremities as the infant is shaken violently while grabbed by the thorax. When present in an otherwise normal infant, these findings point strongly to inflicted injury [3]. However, there are a variety of differential considerations for CML [3, 4].

Developmental Variants

The subperiosteal bone collar, an osseous ring that surrounds the primary spongiosa of the metaphysis and to a variable extent the physis, can produce a variety of imaging appearances that may simulate metaphyseal fractures [3].

The subperiosteal collar can result in an abrupt step-off of the metaphyseal cortex as it approaches the physis (Fig. 2a). The collar may extend beyond the metaphysis, forming a discrete mineralized spur at the periphery of the physis.

Physical Therapy and Orthopedic Manipulation

When the bones are poorly mineralized and/or underdeveloped due to underlying neuromuscular disorders, fractures may occur in response to forces less than those required in the normal skeleton. Fractures resembling CMLs and Salter-Harris injuries have been described in young children with myelodysplasia undergoing physical therapy [3]. Grayev et al. noted metaphyseal fractures, some of which resembled CMLs, in infants undergoing orthopedic manipulation for club-foot deformity [5].

Rickets

Metaphyseal irregularity, cupping, physeal widening, and bony demineralization are the hallmarks of rickets (Fig. 3).

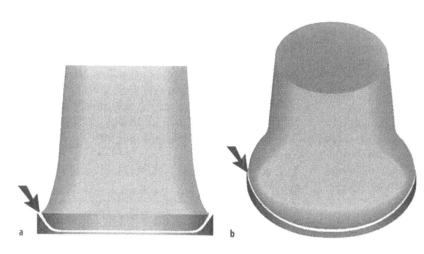

Fig. 1. Corner-fracture and bucket-handle patterns of the classic metaphyseal lesion (CML). Fractures (*arrows*) extend adjacent to the chondro-osseous junction and then veer toward the diaphysis to undercut the large peripheral segment that encompasses the subperiosteal bone collar. When the physis is viewed tangentially (**a**), the CML appears as a corner-fracture pattern. When a view is obtained with beam angulation (**b**), a bucket-handle pattern appears

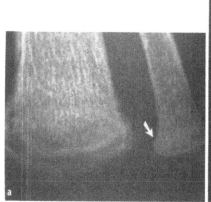

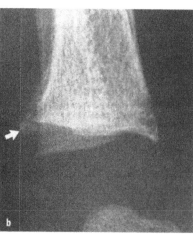

Fig. 2. Distal tibial CML showing the evolution of healing. (**a**) Anteroposterior (AP) view of the distal tibia in a 5-month-old abused infant. A bucket-handle pattern is noted. (**b**) The lateral view shows a corner-fracture pattern (*arrow*)

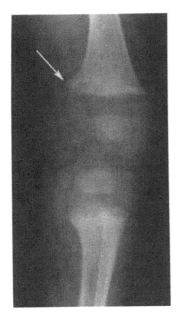

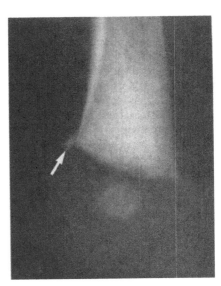

Fig. 3. Rickets. Frontal film of the left knee in an 18-month-old exclusively milk-fed boy who never received vitamin D supplementation. There is demineralization, metaphyseal fragmentation and widening of the physes

Fig. 4. Obstetric CML. A corner-fracture pattern is present in this newborn (*arrow*)

On occasion, discrete osseous fragments resembling corner fractures may be identified in the absence of more dramatic signs of the disease. The diagnosis may be particularly difficult if the metabolic disturbance is partially treated, because demineralization may be modest and the density of the zone of provisional calcification may be relatively normal. The small premature infant may demonstrate metaphyseal fractures indistinguishable from those of a CML, and infants with rickets undergoing vigorous passive range of motion exercises may develop these lesions [3].

Nutritional vitamin D deficiency is a world-wide problem, and a small proportion of young children may develop laboratory and radiographic features indicative of rickets (Fig. 3) [6]. This may have clinical consequences to bone heath in infants and toddlers. It has been suggested that maternal vitamin D deficiency may lead to congenital rickets, the features of which can simulate those of classic cases of child abuse [7], but the assertion has been severely criticized on scientific grounds [8, 9].

Birth Injury

Caffey noted that metaphyseal injuries identical to those occurring with abuse can result from birth injury [1]. Vigorous extraction from a breech or armling presentation can result in forces similar to those occurring in abusive situations [10]. The tractional and torsional forces can produce metaphyseal lesions, particularly in the lower extremities (Fig. 4) [11]. Such injuries can be overlooked at birth but may be identified within the first few weeks of life. However, these fractures are uncommon in the modern obstetrical era and can be readily excluded by a detailed birth history. A recent report describing a 22-year experience at a busy obstetric service found three cases of CML-like fractures in neonates born by cesarean section [12].

Inherited Bone Dysplasias

Although metaphyseal irregularity and fragmentation are seen in a variety of skeletal dysplasias, the presence of an underlying disease is usually apparent on clinical and/or radiologic grounds. Certain bone dysplasias, however, may manifest only modest osseous changes in early infancy, and the bony metaphyseal fragments in these cases may raise strong concerns of inflicted injury. Metaphyseal chondrodysplasia, Schmid type, may present in an infant of normal stature, with metaphyseal fragments indistinguishable from those occurring due to abuse [13]. Similar findings have been described in spondylometaphyseal dysplasia, corner-fracture type [13]. A thorough skeletal survey will generally point to the diagnosis. A follow-up skeletal survey performed several weeks later will show no change in the metaphyseal fragments, in contrast to features of healing noted with the CML.

Osteogenesis Imperfecta

Most cases of osteogenesis imperfecta are accompanied by blue sclera, frank bony demineralization, and other typical clinical and radiologic features (type I). Rarely, blue sclera may be absent (type IV). Most long-bone fractures involve the shafts or metadiaphyseal regions [13]. However, on rare occasions, small metaphyseal fragments with a corner-fracture pattern may be encountered [3]. The presence of demineralization and other radiologic features of osteogenesis imperfecta confirm the diagnosis. Paterson and colleagues described a group of children with metaphyseal lesions as well as other osseous injuries characteristic of abuse [14]. They coined the term "temporary brittle bone disease" to explain these injuries. The lack of rigorous scientific methodology in their publications makes it impossible to draw any meaningful conclusions from the work [15, 16]. More recently Miller proposed that "temporary brittle bone disease" is due to diminished intrauterine movement [17, 18]. His work has been strongly criticized on methodologic grounds [19].

Rib Fractures

Rib fractures are strong predictors of child abuse and are the most common fractures noted in infants dying from inflicted injury [3, 20, 21]. Fractures can occur anywhere along the rib arc but are most common near the costovertebral articulations. These fractures, as well as fractures near the costochondral junction are the most difficult to identify radiographically (Fig. 5a) and are optimally visualized on CT (Fig. 5b). Fractures at the costovertebral junctions will become more visible on follow-up studies at two weeks; fractures at the costochondral junctions tend to heal with little subperiosteal new bone and to become less distinct with time. Most fractures occur with thoracic compression. There is evidence that excessive leverage of the ribs over the transverse processes with anteroposterior compression of the chest results in fractures of the rib head and neck [3].

Birth Injury

Rib fractures with birth injury are rare, but several reports have suggested that obstetrical rib fractures are more common than generally believed [22]. Typically, the fractures occur in the mid-posterior rib arc in large infants delivered by vacuum extraction and/or with shoulder dystocia (Fig. 6). The absence of this history weighs strongly against birth injury. The absence of radiographic signs of healing by ten days of age on high-quality radiographs helps to exclude obstetrical injury.

Cardiopulmonary Resuscitation

Although cardiopulmonary resuscitation (CPR) occasionally results in rib fractures in older children, documented cases of CPR-induced fractures in infants are rare. Large studies of infants undergoing long periods of CPR administered by inexperienced individuals failed to reveal radiographic or autopsy evidence of rib fracture [3]. When fractures are noted with CPR, they are typically situated anterolaterally. The excessive levering forces occurring with inflicted rib fractures do not appear to occur with one-handed CPR [23].

Physical Therapy

It is well-recognized that physical therapy may cause rib fractures in a poorly mineralized rib cage, but fractures are rare in healthy infants. Chalumeau et al. described rib fractures in infants receiving chest physiotherapy for bronchiolitis or pneumonia. Interestingly, the technique entailed a two-handed maneuver similar to the one involved in abusive events [24].

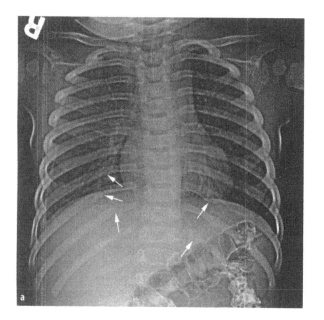

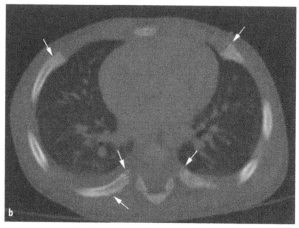

Fig. 5. Inflicted rib fractures in an 8-month-old abused infant. **a** AP radiograph of the thorax with high-detail technique shows multiple rib fractures (*arrows*). **b** Other fractures, particularly those involving the costovertebral articulations and costochondral junctions, are seen to advantage on CT (*arrows*)

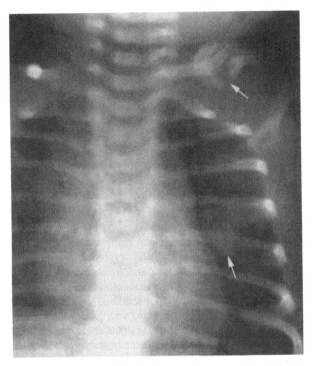

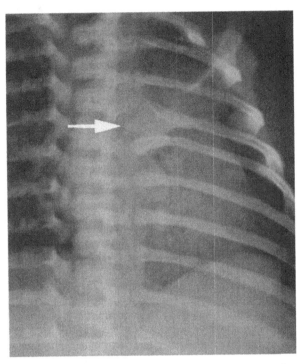

Fig. 6. Obstetric rib and clavicle fractures (presumed) in a 3-week-old neonate with a history of a difficult delivery. There are healing fractures with similar exuberant callus involving the mid-posterior arc of the left 6th rib and left clavicle (*arrows*)

Fig. 7. Rib fusion anomaly. AP radiograph in a 1-month-old infant shows a fusion anomaly of the posteromedial ribs (*arrow*) that was initially thought to be a healing injury

Accidental Rib Fractures

Rib fractures are rarely noted in normal infants and young children sustaining mild to moderate traumatic injury. Accidental rib fractures near the costovertebral articulations have been described in infants involved in motor vehicle accidents in which there is severe anteroposterior compression of the chest, presumably associated with levering forces similar to those resulting from abusive assaults [23].

Developmental Variants

Developmental variants and other misleading imaging findings may suggest rib fractures (Fig. 7). High-detail radiography, and CT if needed, will usually resolve any confusion.

Skull Fractures

Linear skull fractures are common accidental injuries in young infants. Clinical and laboratory studies indicate that a fall from several feet can result in a nondiastatic linear fracture in a young infant. In these cases, the diagnosis of abuse must rest on other imaging and clinical

findings. The 3D rendering of axial CT data can be quite helpful in defining fractures and differentiating them from normal variants.

Long-Bone Fractures

Although long-bone fractures are commonly identified in abused children and are the most common fracture beyond one year of age, they must be viewed in conjunction with other clinical and imaging findings. The early literature suggested that an oblique or spiral fracture pattern was a strong indicator of abuse, but it is now clear that the pattern of shaft fracture has little correlation with the presence or absence of abuse. Patient age appears to be the most important factor in predicting whether a shaft fracture is accidental or inflicted.

Most femoral fractures in infants under one year of age are inflicted (Fig. 8). The percentage of fractures due to abuse declines dramatically in toddlers and older children. It is now well-recognized that the running child may twist and fall, generating sufficient torsional forces to result in a spiral femoral shaft fracture. Femoral fractures may occur in infants who fall downstairs while being held by a caretaker.

As with the femur, most humeral fractures in infants are inflicted. This association diminishes beyond one year

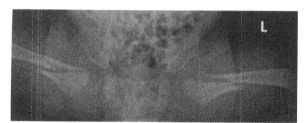

Fig. 8. Bilateral femur fractures. AP view of the pelvis in a 3-month-old boy with swollen thighs reveals bilateral oblique femoral fractures. There were also posteromedial rib fractures and a CML, indicating abuse

Table 3. The skeletal survey

AP skull	AP humeri
Lateral skull	AP forearms
Lateral cervical spine	Oblique hands
AP thorax	AP femurs
Lateral thorax	AP tibias
AP pelvis	AP feet
Lateral lumbar spine	

AP, Anteroposterior. Oblique views of the ribs are recommended. If head injury is suspected, Towne's and both lateral views of the skull are advised

of age particularly with regard to supracondylar fractures, which are usually accidental. Rarely, a humeral shaft fracture can occur if an infant is held by one arm and forcefully turned from a prone to a supine position, trapping the other arm beneath the baby [25].

The toddler's fracture, an oblique or spiral fracture of the mid/distal tibial shaft, is a common accidental injury in infants who have begun to bear weight [26]. As is generally the case with abuse, specific trauma is minimal or absent. Although toddler-type fractures do occur with abuse, an isolated nondisplaced oblique or spiral fracture of the distal tibia in a weight-bearing infant or toddler has a strong correlation with accidental injury.

In infants and toddlers, developmental variants may mimic inflicted long-bone injuries. Physiologic subperiosteal new bone formation is common in infants between one and five months of age, particularly in the lower extremities, and may be unilateral. Symmetric cortical irregularity of the shaft of the radius is common in young infants and should not be confused with a remote fracture (Fig. 9).

Imaging Approach

The skeletal survey remains the preferred approach for imaging of suspected abuse in infants and toddlers [27-32]. The American College of Radiology (ACR) and the British

Society of Pediatric Radiologists have published standards for the performance of skeletal surveys in cases of suspected abuse [33, 34]. The ACR protocol is outlined in Table 3. Film-screen images should be obtained with a high-detail system using a spatial resolution of at least 10 line pairs per millimeter and a speed no greater than 200. When digital radiography is employed, departments should carefully select their imaging systems and optimize technical factors/processing parameters suitable to the detection of subtle indicators of infant abuse, such as CMLs and rib fractures [35]. Since multiple projections of the thorax increase the yield of rib fractures, oblique views are advisable [36, 37]. Thoracic CT increases the detection of rib fractures compared to radiography, but this comes at a substantial increase in radiation dose [38, 39]; therefore, only selective use of this technique is currently advisable. When extremity fractures are identified, at least two projections should be obtained. When head trauma is suspected, a full skull series should be performed. A follow-up examination in two weeks may increase the diagnostic yield [40, 41]. Skeletal scintigraphy plays a complementary role to radiography, and fluorine-18 PET bone scans may provide improved performance over traditional imaging with technetium-based radiopharmaceuticals [42, 43].

Conclusions

Child maltreatment constitutes a major public health problem, a fact evidenced by the recent creation of the board-certified subspecialty in the USA of Child Abuse Pediatrics [44].

The fundamental role of diagnostic imaging in cases of suspected abuse is much the same as with other medical conditions. The diagnostic process is characterized by gathering facts through appropriate imaging studies, integrating these findings with clinical and laboratory data, consultation with colleagues, and formulating a diagnosis based on one's knowledge and expertise. This process is predicated on a thorough understanding of the varied manifestations of child abuse and its imitators on modern diagnostic imaging studies. Imaging strategies for suspected abuse are therefore formulated to minimize the

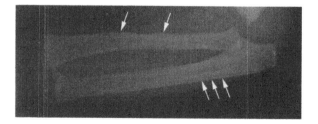

Fig. 9. Developmental long-bone variants. Frontal view of the right forearm in a 3-month-old infant shows cortical irregularity of the shaft of the radius, and the suggestion of subperiosteal new bone formation involving the ulna. These normal patterns were also present on the opposite side

risk of a missed diagnosis. Overzealous efforts by professionals who are ill-prepared to differentiate child abuse from other conditions can have a profoundly negative impact on children and their families [3].

References

1. Caffey J (1946) Multiple fractures in the long bones of infants suffering from chronic subdural hematoma. AJR Am J Roentgenol 56:163-173
2. Caffey J (1957) Some traumatic lesions in growing bones other than fractures and dislocations: clinical and radiological features. Br J Radiol 30:225-238
3. Kleinman P (1998) Diagnostic imaging of child abuse, 2nd edn. Mosby-Year Book, St. Louis, MO
4. Kleinman PK (2008) Problems in the diagnosis of metaphyseal fractures. Pediatr Radiol 38(Suppl 3):S388-S394
5. Grayev A, Boal D, Wallach D et al (2001) Metaphyseal fractures mimicking abuse during treatment for clubfoot. Pediatr Radiol 31:559-563
6. Gordon CM, Feldman HA, Sinclair L et al (2008) Prevalence of vitamin D deficiency among healthy infants and toddlers. Arch Pediatr Adolesc Med 162:505-512
7. Keller KA, Barnes PD (2008) Rickets vs. abuse: a national and international epidemic. Pediatr Radiol 38:1210-1216
8. Jenny C (2008) Rickets or abuse? Pediatr Radiol 38:1219-1220
9. Slovis TL, Chapman S (2008) Evaluating the data concerning vitamin D insufficiency/deficiency and child abuse. Pediatr Radiol 38:1221-1224
10. Ekengren K, Bergdahl S, Ekstrom G (1978) Birth injuries to the epiphyseal cartilage. Acta Radiol Diagn (Stockh) 19:197-204
11. Snedecor S, Wilson H (1949) Some obstetrical injuries to the long bones. J Bone Joint Surg 31A:378-384
12. O'Connell AM, Donoghue VB (2008) Classic metaphyseal lesions follow uncomplicated caesarean section NOT brittle bone disease. Pediatr Radiol 38:600
13. Taybi H, Lachman R (1996) Radiology of syndromes, metabolic disorders and skeletal dysplasias, 4th edn. Mosby-Year Book, St. Louis, MO
14. Paterson CR, Burns J, McAllion SJ (1993) Osteogenesis imperfecta: the distinction from child abuse and the recognition of a variant form. Am J Med Genet 45:187-192
15. Ablin DS, Sane SM (1997) Non-accidental injury: confusion with temporary brittle bone disease and mild osteogenesis imperfecta. Pediatr Radiol 27:111-113
16. Chapman S, Hall CM (1997) Non-accidental injury or brittle bones. Pediatr Radiol 27:106-110
17. Miller M, Hangartner TN (1999) Temporary brittle bone disease: associated with decreased fetal movement and osteopenia. Calcif Tissue Int 64:137-143
18. Miller ME (1999) Temporary brittle bone disease: a true entity? Semin Perinatol 23:174-182
19. Spivack B (2000) Contributing editor's note. Child Abuse Quarterly Medical Update 8:20
20. Barsness KA, Cha ES, Bensard DD et al (2003) The positive predictive value of rib fractures as an indicator of nonaccidental trauma in children. J Trauma 54:1107-1110
21. Bulloch B, Schubert CJ, Brophy PD et al (2000) Cause and clinical characteristics of rib fractures in infants. Pediatrics 105:E48
22. van Rijn RR, Bilo RA, Robben SG (2009) Birth-related midposterior rib fractures in neonates: a report of three cases (and a possible fourth case) and a review of the literature. Pediatr Radiol 39:30-34
23. Kleinman PK, Schlesinger AE (1997) Mechanical factors associated with posterior rib fractures: laboratory and case studies. Pediatr Radiol 27:87-91
24. Chalumeau M, Foix-L'Helias L, Scheinmann P et al (2002) Rib fractures after chest physiotherapy for bronchiolitis or pneumonia in infants. Pediatr Radiol 32:644-647
25. Hymel KP, Jenny C (1996) Abusive spiral fractures of the humerus: a videotaped exception. Arch Pediatr Adolesc Med 150:226-227
26. Dunbar J, Owen H, Nogrady M et al (1964) Obscure tibial fracture of infants – the toddler's fracture. J Can Assoc Radiol 15:136-144
27. Belfer RA, Klein BL, Orr L (2001) Use of the skeletal survey in the evaluation of child maltreatment. Am J Emerg Med 19:122-124
28. Kemp AM, Butler A, Morris S et al (2006) Which radiological investigations should be performed to identify fractures in suspected child abuse? Clin Radiol 61:723-736
29. Kleinman PL, Kleinman PK, Savageau JA (2004) Suspected infant abuse: radiographic skeletal survey practices in pediatric health care facilities. Radiology 233:477-485
30. Offiah AC, Hall CM (2003) Observational study of skeletal surveys in suspected non-accidental injury. Clin Radiol 58:702-705
31. Schmit P (2007) Inflicted injuries in children: variability of imaging practice among pediatric radiologists. Pediatr Radiol 37:S49
32. Slovis TL, Smith W, Kushner DC et al (2000) Imaging the child with suspected physical abuse. American College of Radiology. ACR Appropriateness Criteria. Radiology (215 Suppl):805-809
33. Anonymous (2006) ACR Practice Guideline for Skeletal Surveys in Children (Res. 47, 17, 35) In: American College of Radiology: ACR Standards. American College of Radiology, Reston, VA, pp 145-149
34. The British Society of Paediatric Radiology (2008) Standard for skeletal surveys in suspected non-accidental injury (NAI) in children. Retrieved February 25, 2008 from http://www.bspr.org.uk/nai.htm
35. Kleinman PL, Zurakowski D, Strauss KJ et al (2008) Detection of simulated inflicted metaphyseal fractures in a fetal pig model: image optimization and dose reduction with computed radiography. Radiology 247:381-390
36. Hansen KK, Prince JS, Nixon GW (2008) Oblique chest views as a routine part of skeletal surveys performed for possible physical abuse – is this practice worthwhile? Child Abuse Negl 32:155-159
37. Ingram J, Connell J, Hay T et al (2000) Oblique radiographs of the chest in nonaccidental trauma. Emerg Radiol 7:42-46
38. Renton J, Kincaid S, Ehrlich PF (2003) Should helical CT scanning of the thoracic cavity replace the conventional chest x-ray as a primary assessment tool in pediatric trauma? An efficacy and cost analysis. J Pediatr Surg 38:793-797
39. Traub M, Stevenson M, McEvoy S et al (2007) The use of chest computed tomography versus chest X-ray in patients with major blunt trauma. Injury 38:43-47
40. Kleinman PK, Nimkin K, Spevak MR et al (1996) Follow-up skeletal surveys in suspected child abuse. AJR Am J Roentgenol 167:893-896
41. Zimmerman S, Makoroff K, Care M, et al (2005) Utility of follow-up skeletal surveys in suspected child physical abuse evaluations. Child Abuse Negl 29:1075-1083
42. Drubach LA, Sapp MV, Laffin S et al (2008) Fluorine-18 NaF PET imaging of child abuse. Pediatr Radiol 38:776-779
43. Mandelstam SA, Cook D, Fitzgerald M et al (2003) Complementary use of radiological skeletal survey and bone scintigraphy in detection of bony injuries in suspected child abuse. Arch Dis Child 88:387-390; discussion 387-390
44. Block RW, Palusci VJ (2006) Child abuse pediatrics: a new pediatric subspecialty. J Pediatr 148:711-712

The Imaging of Injuries to the Immature Skeleton

Diego Jaramillo

Department of Radiology, The Children's Hospital of Philadelphia, Philadelphia, PA, USA

Introduction

In children, the types of traumatic accidents, the patterns of injury, and the imaging findings change dramatically with age. The types of injuries change as the activities become more complex as children grow older: infants have mostly inflicted injuries, toddlers have fractures related to early walking, young children are either involved in car vs. pedestrian accidents or suffer injuries while playing, and older children and adolescents frequently have sports-related injuries. Musculoskeletal trauma can be acute or may be the result of repetitive trauma to the growing skeleton, as in the case of sports injuries. This chapter reviews the most important type of injuries and their imaging manifestations, as well as those imaging characteristics that are unique to injuries of the immature skeleton.

Peculiarities and Signal Characteristics of the Immature Skeleton

In the growing skeleton, transitions between bone and cartilage or between different types of bone are the areas most vulnerable to injury. Most physeal injuries and epiphyseal separations occur at the zone of provisional calcification [1]. The junction between the dense lamellar bone of the diaphysis and the more porous bone of the metaphysis is the site of most distal radial fractures. Although trauma is usually accidental, it appears that decreased bone density as a consequence of inactivity may be a contributing factor.

Physeal cartilage signal intensity is homogeneous and very high on spin echo or gradient-recalled echo intermediate and T2-weighted images and on T1-weighted gradient-recalled echo images. It is intermediate on spin echo on T1-weighted images [2]. Three-dimensional (3D) gradient echo images allow reconstructions in all planes. Maximal physeal conspicuity is obtained by suppressing the signal from adjacent bone by fat saturation (for proton density-weighted and T1-weighted gradient echo images). On gradient-recalled echo images, increased conspicuity of cartilage can also be achieved by increasing its signal

intensity using water excitation (Fig. 1), decreasing the signal intensity of the adjacent bone by lengthening the echo times, or by obtaining images when water and fat are out of phase [3]. The zone of provisional calcification has low signal intensity on practically all sequences. Epiphyseal cartilage has a short T2 relaxation time and is of very low signal intensity on T2-weighted images. Differentiation between epiphyseal and physeal cartilage is best on T2-weighted images, where the epiphysis is of lower signal intensity than the physis. The epiphyseal cartilage changes with development. In newborns, most of the epiphyses show homogeneous signal intensity in the epiphyseal cartilage. With weight-bearing, there is a decrease in the signal intensity of the cartilage along the weight-bearing region. Ossifying cartilage shows an increase in signal intensity on T2-weighted images [4].

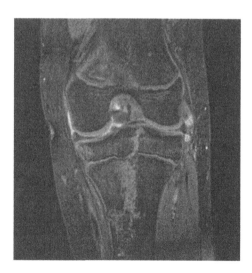

Fig. 1. A 12-year-old boy who fell during a basketball game. Coronal 3D gradient recalled echo image using water excitation shows that a fracture extends from the metaphysis through the physeal cartilage and into the epiphysis. There is intra-articular extension in the region of the tibial spine. There is also marked edema at the tibial insertion of the medial collateral ligament, with separation between the ligament and the bone, indicating an avulsive injury

Acute Physeal Injury

Physeal fractures are common, accounting for nearly 10% of all fractures in childhood. The main significance of these fractures is that they can result in growth arrest. The frequency of complications varies depending on the specific physis that is injured. The incidence of growth arrest after a physeal fracture is approximately 40% in the distal femur and 20% in the distal tibia. In fractures of these higher risk regions, magnetic resonance imaging (MRI) may help define the prognosis and detect associated cartilaginous injury before growth arrest, angular deformity, and shortening have occurred. In most of these injuries, MRI is also required to evaluate injury to the articular cartilage, ligaments, and menisci. MRI can depict the pathway of the injury within the cartilage, which may serve as a prognostic indicator. Injuries along the main axis of the bone ("vertical") involve all layers of the physis (Figs. 1, 2) while transverse fractures propagate along the zones of the growth plate. Vertical fractures more often lead to growth arrest, presumably because they allow communication between epiphyseal and metaphyseal vessels and the formation of a bony bridge. On MRI, fractures extending through the germinal zone, immediately adjacent to the epiphysis, presumably have a worse prognosis than those extending through the zone of provisional calcification, near the metaphysis.

Trauma during sports may injure the physis of older children and young adolescents (Fig. 3). In gymnasts, repeated wrist trauma may injure the distal radial physis, producing focal areas of physeal widening and sometimes transphyseal bridging, as well as associated tears of the triangular fibrocartilage complex.

Growth Arrest

Among all fractures of the physis, 2-5% cause the physis to fuse prematurely. Growth arrest can result from the formation of a bridge of bone or fibrous tissue across the physis or from distortion of the cytoarchitecture of the physis. Resection of a transphyseal bony bridge can restore normal physeal function. Best results are obtained when lesions involve less than one-fourth of the physis and when bridges are peripheral.

The goal of MRI in growth arrest is to define the size and location of the bridge as well as the percentage of the cartilage affected by the abnormality. A 3D gradient recalled echo image, in which the cartilage is of high signal intensity and the adjacent bone of low signal intensity, provides most, if not all, of the information related to assess growth arrest [5]. The image is usually acquired in the coronal plane, with very thin slices to allow isometric reconstructions. Sagittal reconstructions and an axial maximal intensity projection map of the physis can be generated. The ratio of physeal abnormality (between the area of the bridge and the area of the physis) aids in determining the resectability of the bridge. On coronal T1-weighted images, coronal gradient-recalled echo images, and sagittal fat-suppressed conventional spin echo proton density and T2-weighted images, a bony bridge (focal closure of the physis) is seen as interruption of the high signal from the cartilage. If the interruption is sufficiently large, hyperintense fatty marrow will be noted on T1-weighted images [6]. Growth recovery lines (or Parks-Harris lines) confirm abnormal physeal function. The distance between the physis and the line indicates the amount of growth since the injury.

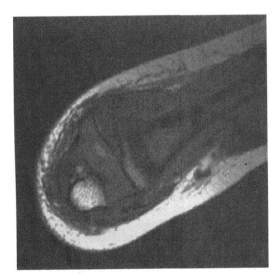

Fig. 2. A 2-year-old girl who fell from a wall. Coronal T1-weighted image shows a lateral condylar fracture extending from the lateral humeral metaphysis to the articular surface. The epiphyseal fragment is displaced

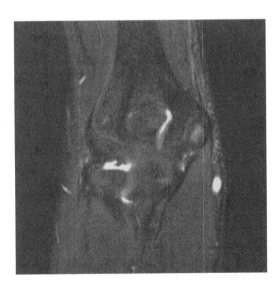

Fig. 3. An 8-year-old baseball player with pain while pitching. Coronal fat suppressed T2-weighted image shows increased signal in the marrow of the medial epicondyle and the adjacent physis

If there is tethering of growth by a bony bridge, the growth recovery line and the physis will converge in the area of the bridge. Growth recovery lines are of low signal intensity on all pulse sequences. Disruption of the hypointense zone of provisional calcification is also seen in the area of bridging.

Epiphyseal Injuries

Separation of the unossified epiphysis results from birth trauma or child abuse and involves most often the proximal and distal humerus, proximal femur, or the cartilaginous radial head. MRI can be helpful by showing a gap between the epiphysis and metaphysis and by excluding dislocation. In a lateral or medial condylar fracture of the distal humerus, MRI shows the extension of the fracture into the unossified epiphysis. The lateral condylar fracture, the second most common elbow injury in children, involves a small fragment of the lateral humeral metaphysis, the physis, and part of the epiphysis. Whether the injury extends into the articular surface (and is thus potentially unstable), or stops within the substance of the epiphyseal cartilage, and is stable, can be determined by MRI (Fig. 3).

Articular Cartilage Injuries

Two osteochondral injuries are common in the pediatric population. In the acute setting, osteochondral injuries can involve the articular cartilage alone or they can extend into the subchondral bone [7] (Fig. 4). Larger osteochondral

fragments can be seen within the joint and can result in significant symptoms (Fig. 4c). The juvenile form of osteochondritis dissecans is the more chronic variety of osteochondral injury and is probably due to repetitive microtrauma. It is most frequent in young boys 10-15 years of age. In the knee, osteochondritis dissecans most often affects the lateral aspect of the medial femoral condyle and the posterior portion of either femoral condyle. Other common locations include the talus and the capitellum. MRI can determine the status of the articular cartilage overlying the osteochondral injury (intact or ruptured), the size of the osteochondral fragment, the stability of the fragment, and the presence of loose bodies [8]. High-resolution intermediate-weighted images (with TE of 35-40 ms) or spoiled gradient-recalled echo images result in excellent contrast between the articular fluid and the adjacent cartilage [9]. T2-weighted images evaluate whether there is fluid of high signal intensity between the parent bone and the fragment, a sign that the fragment is unstable even if the overlying cartilage appears to be intact. More severe lesions result in a disruption of the overlying cartilage, and ultimately in a separation of the fragment from the native bone. MRI is insensitive for detection of small loose osteochondral fragments. Outcome is favorable with an open physis, a small lesion, and evidence of stability on serial MRI, but it is poor when there is cartilage fracture or an articular defect [8].

Injuries to the Menisci and Ligaments

Normal developmental variants constitute potential pitfalls when evaluating meniscal and ligamentous injuries

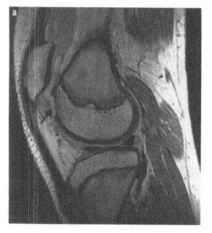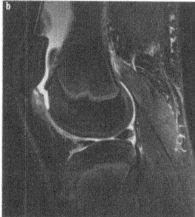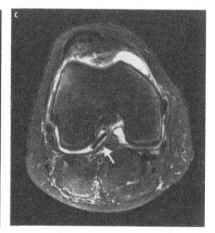

Fig. 4 a-c. A 14-year-old boy who fell while playing soccer. **a** Sagittal intermediate-weighted image of the distal femur shows a 9-mm defect in the articular cartilage (*arrow*) of the anterior lateral femoral condyle. There is also prominence and irregularity of the tibial tubercle and thickening of the tibial insertion of the patellar tendon, suggestive of Osgood-Schlatter disease. **b** Sagittal T2-weighted imaging shows that although the subchondral bone is not broken, there is bruising adjacent to the articular cartilage defect. There is no soft edema in the vicinity of the tibial tubercle, indicating that the Osgood-Schlatter lesion has healed. **c** Axial T2-weighted image shows that the cartilage fragment is lodged in the intercondylar notch just posterior to the lateral femoral condyle (*arrow*)

with MRI. The posterior cruciate ligament is more horizontal in young children [10]. The menisci, richly vascularized during the first years of life, can have areas of increased signal intensity that may resemble tears. Specifically, in children under the age of 12 years, a central, horizontal, linear area of increased signal intensity that originates from the capsular attachment of the meniscus is most likely a nutrient vessel. Meniscal tears in children are usually vertical [11]. In children and young adolescents, stress along the anterior cruciate ligament (ACL) that would have resulted in an ACL tear in an adult may instead avulse the tibial eminence [12]. In general, however, the MRI characteristics and distribution of meniscal and ligamentous injuries in children are similar to those of adults although in skeletally immature patients ACL tears are more frequent in boys [13] and have associated meniscal lesions in 60-79% of cases and collateral ligament injuries in 26% of cases.

Injury to the Marrow

Diagnosis of subtle marrow injuries in children and adolescents is difficult because a history of trauma or change in activity is sometimes difficult to elicit and initial radiographs may be normal. T1-weighted images, short inversion time inversion recovery (STIR) sequences, and fat-suppressed gadolinium-enhanced T1-weighted images readily demonstrate marrow edema and, in stress fractures, the fracture line. Young children learning to walk can present with fatigue stress fractures in the tibia, calcaneus, and cuboid bone. In the growing athlete, overuse despite pain may also lead to stress injuries in the tibia, fibula, and pars interarticularis. Diffuse, poorly defined marrow edema is seen most frequently. In adolescents who become active, stress fractures can occur in the tibia, femoral neck, and sacrum. Insufficiency stress fractures (normal activity on an abnormal bone) occur less frequently in children.

Injury to the Bone

Computed tomography (CT) provides exquisite detail of the extent of complex fractures. Multidetector-row CT allows simple multiplanar and 3D multiplanar reconstructions (Fig. 5). Strict attention to dose reduction techniques, including automatic dose modulation and shielding, are important to minimize exposure. For complex fractures in which the main goal is to assess the relationships of the bony fragments, CT has considerable advantage over MRI. In triplane fractures (Fig. 5) and juvenile Tillaux fractures, the separation of the epiphyseal fragments is the determinant of whether treatment will require internal fixation. These two injuries occur when the tibia begins to fuse medially, such that the fracture extends vertically across the epiphysis and horizontally around the physis [14].

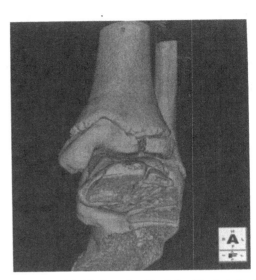

Fig. 5. A 13-year-old girl who twisted her left ankle. Anterior shaded surface display 3D reconstruction of the distal tibia shows a vertical epiphyseal fracture that extends from the articular surface into the physis and then propagates along the lateral physis, which is slightly wide. The sagittal images showed a coronal extension of the fracture into the metaphysis, defining it as a triplane fracture

Conclusions

The patterns of skeletal injury change with age, and their imaging characteristics change as skeletal structures mature. Cross-sectional images, particularly those obtained with MRI (and ultrasound), play an increasingly important role in the imaging of pediatric musculoskeletal injury because of their capacity to image unossified structures and to depict the lesions in multiple planes.

References

1. Peterson HA (1996) Physeal and apophyseal injuries. In: Rockwood Jr CA, Wilkins KE, Beaty JH (eds) Fractures in children. Lippincott-Raven, Philadelphia, pp 103-165
2. Laor T, Jaramillo D (2009) MR imaging insights into skeletal maturation: what is normal? Radiology 250:28-38
3. Jaramillo D, Laor T (2008) Pediatric musculoskeletal MRI: basic principles to optimize success. Pediatr Radiol 38:379-391
4. Varich LJ, Laor T, Jaramillo D (2000) Normal maturation of the distal femoral epiphyseal cartilage: age-related changes at MR imaging. Radiology 214:705-709
5. Craig JG, Cody DD, Van Holsbeeck M (2004) The distal femoral and proximal tibial growth plates: MR imaging, three-dimensional modeling and estimation of area and volume. Skeletal Radiol 33:337-344
6. Ecklund K, Jaramillo D (2001) Imaging of growth disturbance in children. Radiol Clin North Am 39:823-841
7. Oeppen RS, Connolly SA, Bencardino JT, Jaramillo D (2004) Acute injury of the articular cartilage and subchondral bone: a common but unrecognized lesion in the immature knee. AJR Am J Roentgenol 182:111-117
8. Kijowski R, Blankenbaker DG, Shinki K et al (2008) Juvenile versus adult osteochondritis dissecans of the knee: appropriate MR imaging criteria for instability. Radiology 248:571-578

9. Potter HG, Linklater JM, Allen AA et al (1998) Magnetic resonance imaging of articular cartilage in the knee. An evaluation with use of fast-spin-echo imaging. J Bone Joint Surg Am 80:1276-1284

10. Kim HK, Laor T, Shire NJ et al (2008) Anterior and posterior cruciate ligaments at different patient ages: MR imaging findings. Radiology 247:826-835

11. Major NM, Beard LN, Jr, Helms CA (2003) Accuracy of MR imaging of the knee in adolescents. AJR Am J Roentgenol 180:17-19

12. Cassas KJ, Cassettari-Wayhs A (2006) Childhood and adolescent sports-related overuse injuries. Am Fam Phys 73:1014-1022

13. Prince JS, Laor T, Bean JA (2005) MRI of anterior cruciate ligament injuries and associated findings in the pediatric knee: changes with skeletal maturation. AJR Am J Roentgenol 185:756-762

14. Brown SD, Kasser JR, Zurakowski D, Jaramillo D (2004) Analysis of 51 tibial triplane fractures using CT with multiplanar reconstruction. AJR Am J Roentgenol 183:1489-1495

Peculiarities and Pitfalls in the Imaging of Pediatric Musculoskeletal Infections

Simon G.F. Robben

Department of Radiology, Maastricht University Medical Centre, Maastricht, The Netherlands

Introduction

This chapter addresses the role of imaging in the diagnosis of various "trivial" infectious diseases in childhood, including cellulitis, subcutaneous abscess, necrotizing fasciitis, pyomyositis, infectious bursitis and arthritis, osteomyelitis, foreign bodies, infectious lymphadenitis, as well as some "peculiar" pediatric infectious diseases.

The child's musculoskeletal system differs from the adult musculoskeletal system in many ways. These differences account for many pitfalls and peculiarities in pediatric musculoskeletal imaging.

Anatomical Differences

Growth plates, epiphyses, and metaphyses are unique to the pediatric skeleton, and thus diseases involving these structures are seen only in the pediatric population.

Acute hematogeneous osteomyelitis primarily affects the metaphyses. The microorganisms flourish in the large, slow-flowing venous sinusoids, facilitated by a decreased phagocytic function of macrophages [1].

Growth plates in children act as cartilaginous, nonvascularized barriers against the infectious spread of microorganisms from metaphysis to epiphysis. However, these barriers can also facilitate disease because the epiphyseal feeding vessels course through the joint capsule to reach the epiphysis. These vessels are extremely vulnerable to increased joint pressure due to joint effusion, e.g., septic arthritis, causing avascular necrosis. Spontaneous avascular necrosis occurs in epiphyses, as is the case with Perthes' disease in the hip and Kohler's disease in the navicular bone of the foot. Moreover, growth plates are vulnerable to acute (Salter Harris fractures) and chronic (slipped capital femoral epiphysis) stress. Premature closure of a growth plate can be caused by infectious, traumatic, and ischemic events and will result in growth arrest and deformity. The younger the child, the more severe the final deformity.

Physiological Differences

Their increased metabolism causes the metaphyses to appear as hot spots on isotope bone scans, which can either simulate or obscure an infection or trauma. Adults lack metaphyses. The distribution between red and yellow bone marrow differs significantly from that in children, especially very young ones. Also, because the composition of red bone marrow differs from yellow bone marrow, pathology manifests differently.

Congenital and Hereditary Differences

Many, if not all, inborn errors of metabolism manifest themselves in childhood. Some of these conditions simulate osteomyelitis, by subperiosteal new bone formation (gangliosidosis). In some patients, they are associated with an increased risk of developing infections, such as the diseases associated with neutropenia and congenital immunodeficiency diseases. Sickle cell disease and chronic granulomatous disease may cause multiple foci of osteomyelitis.

Psychological Differences

If children have pain, they experience the uncomfortable sensation but they are not worried by it, and do not seek medical attention themselves. Instead they try to relieve the pain by limping or disuse, which is noted by the parents. Moreover, "referred pain" is more often seen in children than in adults: It is important to remember that knee pain may be the result of referred pain from a nearby site of pathology, such as the hip. Pneumonia, appendicitis, and pyelonephritis are a few common causes of referred back pain in children.

These differences between the pediatric and adult musculoskeletal system can cause differences in clinical and radiological presentation. For instance, vitamin D deficiency has an age-dependent clinical and radiological presentation.

In children, it causes rickets, with its classical radiological metaphyseal abnormalities. In adults, vitamin D deficiency causes osteomalacia, with radiologically nonspecific osteopenia and, occasionally, characteristic Looser's zones. Thus, the same disease but two different presentations.

Imaging Techniques

Scintigraphy and cross-sectional imaging techniques such as ultrasonography (US), computed tomography (CT) and magnetic resonance imaging (MRI) have dramatically improved the ability to evaluate infectious and non-infectious inflammatory diseases. Selection of the optimal techniques for each individual patient is essential, and factors such as cost, radiation exposure, and need for sedation all must be considered. US is an important initial modality in the evaluation of musculoskeletal infections in children because it is rapid, non-ionizing, and very sensitive to the presence of (infectious) fluid collections and joint effusions. Moreover, the images are not degraded by metallic or motion artifacts, in contrast to CT and MRI, Finally, US offers the possibility of fine-needle aspiration to confirm the infectious nature of a fluid collection without unnecessary contamination of adjacent anatomical compartments. US should be combined with radiography, with which it is complimentary. Along with conventional radiography, US is a very valuable modality for the early diagnosis and follow-up of musculoskeletal infections in children.

Scintigraphy (three-phase bone scan with technetium 99m) has a high sensitivity for bone disease but a low specificity. In bone scintigraphy, the combined use of gallium-67 and indium-111 can improve diagnostic performance [2].

MRI and CT are not screening methods but are very useful in detailing osseous and soft-tissue changes. CT allows good definition of cortical bone changes and deep soft-tissue abscesses that can not be seen with US. The major drawback of CT is the radiation load. MRI is superior in diagnosing soft-tissue abnormalities, bone-marrow changes, cartilage destruction and involvement of the growth plate by an infectious process. The major drawback of MRI is the need for sedation in children 6 years of age or younger.

"Trivial" Pediatric Musculoskeletal Infections

Cellulitis

Cellulitis is defined as an infection of the skin and subcutaneous tissues. In children, there is a predilection for the extremities [3]. *Staphylococcus aureus* and *Streptococcus pyogenes* account for the majority of these infections. Depending on the type of infection and the patient's immune system, cellulitis may spread or remain localized to form an abscess. Patients present with soft-tissue swelling, erythema, and fever.

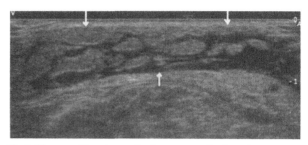

Fig. 1. Non-specific edema of subcutaneous fat (area between *arrowheads*). Hypoechoic strands surround small islands of hyperechoic fat

Conventional radiographs often show nonspecific soft-tissue swelling. The US appearance resembles edema of the subcutaneous fat, showing swelling, increased echogenicity of the subcutaneous fat with decreased acoustic transmission, blurring of tissue planes, and progression to hypoechoic strands between hyperechoic fatty lobules (Fig. 1). This appearance is non-specific and cannot be distinguished from non-infectious causes of soft-tissue edema [4]. Increased vascularity at color or power Doppler US may suggest an infectious cause [5].

Cellulitis is usually a clinical diagnosis; the additional value of imaging techniques lies in the detection of underlying abscesses. Therefore, when the initial US examination shows only cellulitis but the symptoms persist, the US examination should be repeated because the characteristic US features of an abscess and liquefaction may become more apparent over time [6]. Moreover, cellulitis, especially in the vicinity of bone, can be simulated by early stages of osteomyelitis. Once a suspicious fluid collection in the soft tissues is identified, US-guided puncture should be performed for diagnostic purposes.

The CT findings of cellulitis include skin thickening, increased attenuation of the subcutaneous fat to more than -90 HU, loss of distinction between tissue planes, heterogeneous enhancement, and normal deep fascial and muscle compartments [7, 8].

MRI shows an ill-defined linear or dome-shaped area of low T1 and high T2 signal intensity, with an interspersed network-like appearance of the subcutaneous fat. Underlying bones and muscles are normal [7].

Necrotizing Fasciitis

Necrotizing fasciitis is a rare, rapidly progressive, and often fatal infection of the subcutaneous tissues, fascia, and surrounding soft-tissue structures. Early diagnosis is mandatory because the disease may have a fatal course if adequate therapy (extensive surgical debridement and antibiotics) is not instituted promptly. The causative organisms are *S. aureus* and group A streptococcus.

Necrotizing fasciitis in its early phase can mimic cellulitis but usually can be distinguished based on the imaging features. The sonographic features of necrotizing fasciitis are: (a) fascial thickening and accumulation of fluid, (b) cloudy fluid or loculated abscess in the fascial plane, allowing US-guided diagnostic aspiration, (c) subcutaneous soft-tissue swelling, and (d) sometimes, gas in soft tissues [5, 9]. On CT, there is decreased attenuation of the superficial fascia compatible with necrosis and relative sparing of the muscular compartment. Additionally, gas, dissecting along fascial planes, and deeper fluid collections may be seen [8].

On MRI, necrotizing fasciitis resembles infectious cellulitis to a certain extent; however, there is also involvement of the deep fascia and intramuscular spaces. Abnormal gadolinium enhancement is caused by contrast extravasation from damaged capillaries in areas of necrosis. The depth of the soft-tissue involvement does not seem to be a reliable parameter to differentiate between cellulitis and necrotizing fasciitis [7, 10].

Soft-Tissue Abscess

An abscess is defined as a collection of necrotic tissue, neutrophils, inflammatory cells, and bacteria walled off by highly vascular connective tissue [8]. In the majority of cases, the causative organism is by *Staphylococcus aureus*. Superficial abscesses begin as cellulitis but subsequently liquefy to form a localized pus collection. Deep abscesses, such as subperiosteal abscesses and pyomyositis, are discussed later in the text.

Conventional radiographs may show nonspecific soft-tissue swelling and. occasionally, gas in the soft tissues.

The US appearance of abscesses is highly variable, as they may be present with or without mass effect and the liquefied contents may be anechoic, hypoechoic, hyperechoic, or even isoechoic to surrounding tissues. The margins may be relatively sharp, blend in with the surrounding cellulitis, or outlined by an echogenic rim [6, 11]. Because of the variable US appearance, many diseases

may simulate abscesses on US: seromas, hematomas, ganglion, synovial cysts, and cystic tumors (anechoic contents); hematomas and solid masses (hypoechoic contents); solid and necrotic tumors (hyperechoic contents); and cellulitis or edema (isoechoic contents) [4, 6]. To confirm the liquid nature of a non-anechoic mass, the presence of "ultrasonographic fluctuation" should be looked for. This sign implies the motion of particles induced by gentle pressure of either the transducer or the sonographer's finger [6, 11, 12]. This technique is especially effective in the detection of small sinus tracts.

Another important tool in the characterization of soft-tissue masses is color or power Doppler US [4, 5, 11, 13-15]. An abscess shows the absence of flow within its contents and hyperemia in its direct surroundings. Therefore, Doppler US helps to discriminate inflammatory and infectious fluid collections from noninflammatory collections, but it is not possible to discriminate between infectious and noninfectious inflammatory fluid collections [15]. Finally, US is extremely valuable in detecting fluid collections and abscesses around orthopedic hardware (Fig. 2) [5]. The value of CT and MRI is limited by artifacts, especially when the imaged area is next to an orthopedic device. Also, isotope studies may show non-specific findings in patients who have recently undergone surgery of the affected site.

CT demonstrates a focal fluid collection (HU >20) whose density varies with the relative amounts of proteinaceous fluid, debris, and necrosis. The central cavity is surrounded by a thick irregular rim that enhances after contrast injection. These imaging findings are better seen on MRI [16]; the fluid's low signal intensity on T1 and high signal intensity on T2 contrast nicely with the enhancing rim. The presence of an enhancing rim on post-gadolinium images has a high sensitivity and specificity for the diagnosis of soft-tissue abscess. The abscess fluid itself does not enhance.

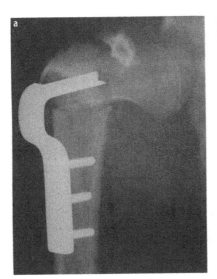
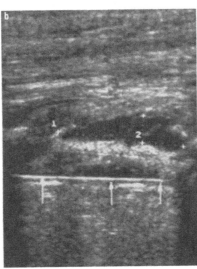

Fig. 2 a, b. An 8-year-old boy with progressive pain and fever after proximal femur osteotomy. Clinical inspection showed minor swelling but normal aspect of the skin. **a** Lucency around the proximal part of the orthopedic hardware and extreme varus deformity of the femoral neck suggest loosening. **b** Turbid fluid has collected (between calipers) along the orthopedic material (arrows) and is sealed from the subcutaneous compartment by the fascia of the tensor lata muscle. Culture showed *S. aureus*

Osteomyelitis

Osteomyelitis is defined as an infection of the bone marrow, usually by *Staphylococcus aureus*. Less frequently, *Streptococcus*, *Escherichia coli*, and *Pseudomonas aeruginosa* are cultured from blood or aspirates [8]. The incidence of osteomyelitis caused by *Haemophilus influenzae* has decreased dramatically since the introduction of HIB vaccination [17]. The manifestation of osteomyelitis in children is age-dependent. In infants, diaphyseal vessels penetrate the growth plate to reach the epiphysis, facilitating epiphyseal and joint infections in this age group [18].

In older children, the growth plate constitutes a barrier for the diaphyseal vessels. Vessels at the metaphysis terminate in slow-flow venous sinusoidal lakes, predisposing the metaphysis as the starting point for acute hematogenous osteomyelitis.

The increased pressure within the medullary cavity causes the infection to spread via the Haversian and Volkmann's canals into the subperiosteal space. Because the periosteum is less firmly attached to the cortex in in-

fants and children than in adults, pressure elevation will be more pronounced in childhood osteomyelitis. In contrast, sequestration is rare in neonatal osteomyelitis [8].

Conventional radiography is usually the initial modality used to demonstrate deep soft-tissue swelling in early disease. Bone destruction and periosteal reaction become obvious but only 7-10 days after the onset of disease. Conventional radiography is a screening method that may suggest the diagnosis and exclude other pathologies. The findings can be correlated with those of other imaging modalities.

Recently, several reports have recommended the use of US for the early diagnosis of osteomyelitis, especially in children [19-23]. The spectrum of initial changes on US comprises deep edema, thickening of the periosteum, intra-articular fluid collection, and subperiosteal abscess formation (elevation of the periosteum by more than 2 mm) [20]. These findings precede radiographic changes by several days [22-25]. In addition, US can detect cortical defects that may develop over the course of the disease (Figs. 3, 4). The detection of subperiosteal abscesses is especially im-

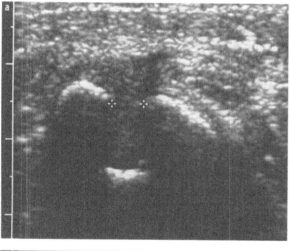

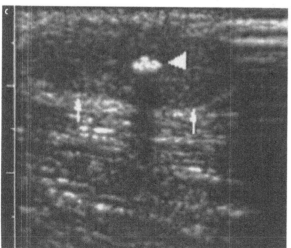

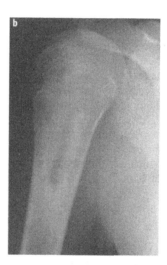

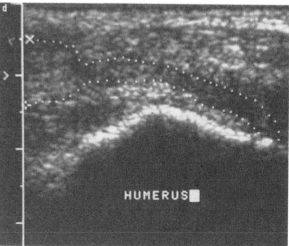

Fig. 3 a-d. Chronic osteomyelitis. A 13-year-old girl presented with complaints of episodes of low-grade fever and a progressive swelling of the proximal humerus, 4 years after treatment for acute osteomyelitis of the same humerus. **a,b** A metaphyseal defect was demonstrated with ultrasonography and radiography. **c** At the site of the swelling, a subcutaneous abscess (*arrows*) is visible, containing a sequestrated bony fragment (*arrowhead*). **d** The abscess (*A*) is in continuity with the cortical defect (*D*) via a long fistula (marked with *dots*)

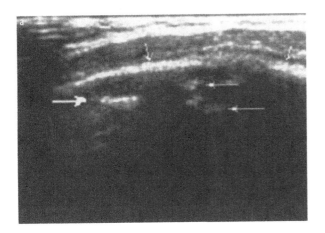 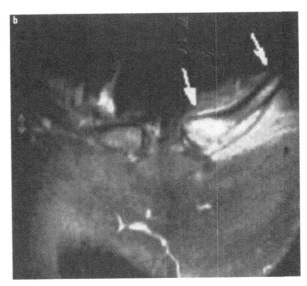

Fig. 4 a, b. Chronic osteomyelitis. A 9-year-old girl with a 7-month history of arthralgia presented with a 3-week history of a swelling at the left sternoclavicular joint. **a** Ultrasonography of the left proximal clavicle showed that, although the cortex (*vertical arrows*) appears to be intact, there are echoes from the medulla (*curved arrows*), suggesting subtle permeating changes of the cortex that facilitated the passage of sound waves into the bone marrow. **b** Coronal T2 weighted MRI with fat suppression (SPIR). The proximal left clavicle (*arrows*) shows increased signal intensity of the medulla, cortex, and surrounding soft tissues. Note the normal right clavicle. A diagnosis of cat-scratch osteitis was made by the detection of *Bartonella henselae* DNA by PCR analysis of bone aspirate. Active infection was confirmed with serological tests

portant because in such patients ultrasonographically guided aspiration or surgical drainage has to be considered, whereas patients with osteomyelitis without abscesses can be treated with antibiotics only. In animal studies, subperiosteal abscesses were visualized with US as a band of decreased echogenicity, bordered by a line of increased echogenicity representing subperiosteal fluid and periosteal reaction, respectively [25, 26]. In children, subperiosteal abscesses are spindle-shaped fluid collections along the cortex of a bone, either with increased or decreased echogenicity. In equivocal cases, the use of color Doppler US is mandatory; pus collections with increased or decreased echogenicity will present as avascular periosteal masses with peripheral hyperemia [27]. However, one should realize that color Doppler flow is detectable not before 4 days after the onset of symptoms [27].

CT demonstrates osseous abnormalities earlier then conventional radiographs, but at the expense of a higher radiation dose. It is superior to MRI for visualizing bony destruction, gas in the bone, and a bony sequestration.

Analogous to CT, MRI is not a screening method but is invaluable in demonstrating the intra- and extraosseous extent of osteomyelitis. Predictors of early osteomyelitis are ill-defined low T1 and high T2 signal intensities, poorly defined soft tissue planes, lack of cortical thickening, and poor interface between normal and abnormal marrow. In chronic osteomyelitis, there is good differentiation between diseased marrow and soft-tissue abnormalities [2]. The sensitivity and specificity of Gd-enhanced MRI for osteomyelitis is reported as 97 and 92%, respectively [16].

Pyomyositis

Pyomyositis is suppurative bacterial infection in striated muscle. It is rare because striated muscle is relatively resistant to bacterial infection and is encountered most frequently in tropical regions. All striated muscles of the skeleton can be involved, but there is a predilection for those in the thigh and pelvis [28]. Contributing factors are trauma, diabetes mellitus, chronic steroid use, connective tissue disorders, and immunosuppression (HIV, malnutrition, and chemotherapy) [4, 8]. Children are affected in one-third of the cases, both in tropical and nontropical regions [28-30]. The most frequent causative organism is *Staphylococcus aureus*. Pyomyositis can be difficult to diagnose because initially the infection is confined to the muscular compartment, causing myalgia, general malaise, and fever. It is often difficult for the child to localize the pain, particularly when pyomyositis involves the hips or pelvis. Also, a lack of familiarity of the disease, especially in non-tropical settings, may cause diagnostic delay.

The findings on US depend on the stage of the disease [12, 31]. Stage 1 (phlegmonous) consists of localized muscle edema and distortion of the filamentous planes with ill-defined areas of decreased echogenicity. In stage 2 (suppurative), liquefaction corresponds with abscess formation. The echogenicity of the pus may be increased, decreased, or the same as that in surrounding tissues. Doppler US and gentle compression with the transducer to visualize motion of particles can be useful in equivo-

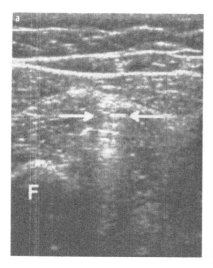
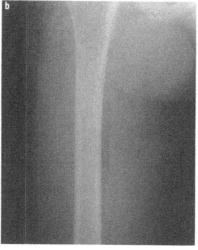
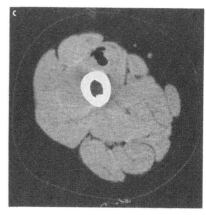

Fig. 5 a-c. A 9-year-old boy with fever and pain of the right thigh occurring 6 months after surgery for an adenocarcinoma of the left kidney. **a** Ultrasonography shows reflections in the quadriceps muscle, with bright acoustic shadowing (arrows) suggestive of intramuscular gas. *F* Femur. **b,c** Conventional radiograph and CT confirm the presence of intramuscular gas. Blood cultures revealed gram-negative bacteria

cal cases (see the sections on osteomyelitis and soft-tissue abscesses). The presence of gas within an inflamed muscle is very suggestive of abscess formation caused by anaerobic organisms (Fig. 5) [32].

The detection of an abscess in myositis is important because it requires drainage for complete resolution, whereas stage 1 disease can be treated with antibiotic therapy alone. US has the advantage over other modalities in that it can be used to guide percutaneous aspiration and drainage.

CT demonstrates enlargement and heterogeneous attenuation of the affected muscle, with a focal fluid collection. Associated findings of cellulitis are always seen, including soft-tissue inflammatory stranding, skin thickening, and a loss of delineation between tissue planes.

Abscesses and co-existing areas of osteomyelitis and septic arthritis can be seen on MRI. In stage 1 disease, a heterogeneous T2 signal intensity is present in the enlarged muscle. In stage 2, abscess formation is seen as a focus of high signal intensity on T2 and low signal intensity on T1. Gadolinium demonstrates peripheral rim enhancement.

Septic Arthritis

The hip joint is the most frequent location of septic arthritis in childhood, but the knee, shoulder, and elbow are also common sites [8, 33]. Early diagnosis is mandatory to prevent cartilage destruction, joint deformity, growth disturbance, and premature arthrosis. Most commonly, septic arthritis is caused by hematogenous seeding; less frequently, it is an extension into the joint space of osteomyelitis. Etiologic organisms are S. *aureus* (most common), group A streptococcus, and S. *pneumoniae*. In neonates, group B streptococcus and *E. coli* are impor-

tant causes whereas *Neisseria gonorrhoeae* is frequently to blame in adolescents [8]. The incidence of H. *influenzae* has declined following the introduction of large vaccination programs [17]. The presenting symptoms are fever, intolerance of weight bearing, erythrocyte sedimentation rate >40, and a peripheral white blood count of >12,000. If all these symptoms are present, the likelihood of septic arthritis is 99% [34]. Unfortunately, many children do not show such an obvious clinical picture and imaging techniques are important tools to obtain additional information concerning the suspected joint.

Conventional radiographs may be normal or demonstrate joint-space widening with adjacent soft-tissue swelling. However, the sensitivity and specificity of this imaging technique for septic arthritis is low.

US is very sensitive for the detection of joint effusion, especially in the pediatric population, and small amounts of fluid (up to 1 ml) can be detected. However, the specificity of the diagnosis is poor [35]. The absence of joint effusion virtually excludes septic arthritis [36], although Gordon et al. recently described two patients with septic arthritis of the hip with symptoms at <24 h that showed no effusion on the initial US examination [37]. Neither the size nor the echogenicity of the effusion can distinguish infectious from non-infectious effusion [36, 38-40] (Fig. 6). Physiological synovial fluid in asymptomatic joints can be visualized during specific maneuvers (endorotation of the hip) and multiple small reflections, even more numerous than in pathological effusions, can be demonstrated (Fig. 7).

In adults, power Doppler US helps to differentiate non-inflammatory fluid collections from those that are inflammatory and infectious, because the latter shows an increased adjacent soft-tissue perfusion. However, this approach does not reliably distinguish inflammatory col-

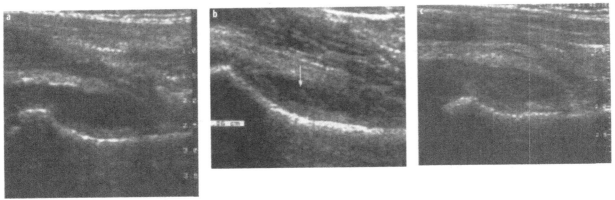

Fig. 6 a-c. Three patients with noninfectious hip-joint effusion. **a** A 6-year-old boy with transient synovitis of 1-day duration. The effusion is clear. **b** A 7-year-old girl with transient synovitis of 7 days duration. Small particles (*arrow*) can be seen floating in the effusion. **c** A 3-year-old girl with postviral reactive arthritis of 20 days duration shows cloudy effusion

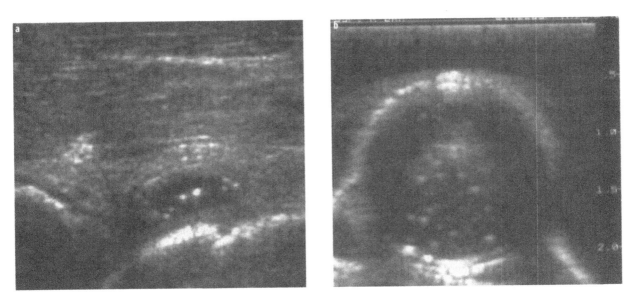

Fig. 7 a, b. Normal synovial fluid in asymptomatic children. **a** A small amount of synovial fluid containing many bright reflections is seen in the superior articular recess of the hip joint during forced endorotation. **b** In vitro study shows normal synovial fluid (diluted with saline) in a test tube containing identical reflections as in (**a**)

lections of infectious and noninfectious origin, because they show the same degree of hyperemia [15]. In a study of children with hip-joint effusion, Strouse et al. showed that increased flow has a sensitivity of 27% and a specificity of 100% for the diagnosis of septic arthritis [41]. Therefore, power Doppler US does not allow exclusion of septic arthritis of the hip. Despite the technical innovations in US, joint aspiration is still necessary in equivocal cases [35].

CT is less sensitive than other imaging modalities for the detection of joint effusion but may identify areas of adjacent osteomyelitis. MRI is very sensitive for the detection of small amounts of fluid. Initially, MRI reveals distention of the joint capsule by fluid of nonspecific

high intensity on T2-weighted images. In later stages, the joint effusion tends to have a more intermediate signal intensity and seems heterogeneous. Importantly, MRI can demonstrate cartilage destruction and adjacent cellulitis [42]. When used with gadolinium injection and fat suppression techniques, MRI has a sensitivity of 100% and a specificity of 77% [43].

Infectious Bursitis

Infectious bursitis in childhood is rare. Indeed, in the past 25 years, only two series, of 10 children each, have specifically addressed pediatric infectious bursitis [44, 45]. As in adults, local trauma is the most common risk factor in childhood cases of the disease [45, 46]. Causative organisms are *S. aureus* in the majority of cases, or group A streptococcus. The prepatellar bursa is most commonly affected; less frequently the olecranon bursa is involved. The affected bursa is distended because of fluid accumulation and/or synovial thickening. The fluid may be clear or turbid, with or without septations [4, 5, 11]. As in infectious arthritis, it is not possible to differentiate between infectious and noninfectious inflammatory bursitis (post-traumatic and rheumatoid bursitis). To confirm the diagnosis, aspiration of fluid is necessary. The advantage of ultrasonographically guided aspiration is twofold: (a) the needle tip can be guided away from the synovial hypertrophy and towards small fluid collections within the bursa, and (b) when infectious bursitis is confused with infectious arthritis, US will identify the bursa as the causative structure, preventing contamination of a normal joint when the needle tip is inadvertently placed into the joint space after passing the infected bursa. Once infectious bursitis is diagnosed and adequately treated, recovery is usually rapid.

On CT, an infected bursa resembles an abscess. The central fluid collection may appear heterogeneous due to debris or hemorrhage. With MRI, the fluid in the bursa is of low T1 and high T2 signal intensity. Large amounts of debris will increase the T1 signal intensity. Adjacent soft tissues may demonstrate feathery edema; after the intravenous injection of gadolinium, the margins of the bursa will show enhancement. Occasionally, adjacent bone shows some edema on fat-suppressed images.

Foreign Bodies

Chronic recurrent infection resistant to antibiotic therapy suggests the presence of a foreign body at the site of infection. US has a sensitivity of 83% for foreign bodies (93% for wooden foreign bodies and 73% for plastic ones). Specificity is rather low (59%) [47]. The ultrasonographic aspect depends on the material involved and the reaction of the surrounding tissues to it. Metal and glass result in posterior reverberation artifacts whereas wood demonstrates posterior acoustic shadowing [48]. Secondary infection causes a suppurative or granulomatous reaction around the foreign body, facilitating its detection (Fig. 8).

"Peculiar" Pediatric Musculoskeletal Infections

Rubella

Antenatal rubella infection is the most common transplacentally acquired viral infection producing skeletal abnormalities (20-50%) [49]. It also causes intrauterine growth retardation, cataract, deafness, hepatosplenomegaly, and cardiovascular lesions. Conventional radiographs demonstrate irregular fraying of the metaphyses of long bones, with alternating longitudinal radiodense lines ("celery stalk" appearance) and delayed skeletal maturation. These changes are considered as secondary nonspecific trophic changes rather than focal viral disease. Periosteal reaction is rare. When these changes are present all TORCH infections (toxoplasmosis, rubella, cytomegaly, and herpes) should be considered [49].

Syphilis

Congenital syphylis is caused by transplacental spread of *Treponema pallidum* in the second or third trimester of pregnancy. Clinical features are a skin rash, anemia, hepatosplenomegaly, ascites, and nephrotic syndrome [49]. The skeletal system is also involved, with the first radiological changes noted in the metaphyses as nonspecific lucent bands, followed by fragmentation and destruction. Other changes include periosteal new bone formation along the diaphyses, lytic lesions in the diaphyses, and Wimberger sign (bone destruction at the medial proximal

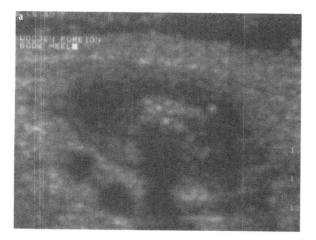 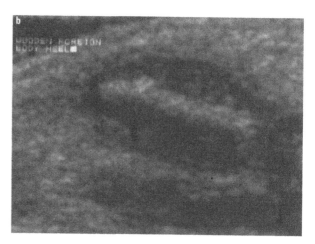

Fig. 8 a, b. Wooden splinter in the subcutaneous tissues of the heel. Transverse (**a**) and sagittal (**b**) images. The acoustic shadowing is caused by the foreign body itself, the surrounding hypoechoic halo is probably due to chronic inflammatory tissue

tibial metaphysis). Thickening of the anterior tibial cortex during healing leads to the "saber-shin" deformity [49]. The bone changes mimic non-accidental injury.

Pyomyositis in Varicella

Pyomyositis is an uncommon but life-threatening complication of chickenpox, particularly in otherwise healthy infants. Necrotizing fasciitis and osteomyelitis also may complicate chickenpox. These diseases are usually caused by group A β-hemolytic streptococcus and *Staphylococcus aureus* [50, 51]. Pyomyositis due to invasive group A β-hemolytic streptococcal complications appears to be increasing [52]. Presenting clinical features may consist of continuous or recurrent fevers, localized redness and swelling, and refusal to bear weight on the involved limb. A delayed diagnosis can result in toxic shock syndrome and acute renal failure. The best imaging technique is MRI, especially in complex regions such as the shoulder and pelvis.

Chronic Recurrent Multifocal Osteomyelitis

Chronic recurrent multifocal osteomyelitis (CRMO) is most likely the pediatric variant of SAPHO syndrome, which is a combination of synovitis, acne, pustulosis, hyperostosis, and osteitis [53-55]. CRMO is considered to be rare but may be underdiagnosed because of the absence of specific clinical, laboratory, or radiological findings. The etiology is unknown. It affects children and adolescents. The presenting symptom is inflammatory pain, whereas fever is not a common finding. Virtually all patients have an increased erythrocyte sedimentation rate and raised levels of C-reactive protein, while some also have mildly elevated WBC counts. Radiological examination demonstrates focal lysis and reactive hyperostosis with periosteal reaction. MRI shows nonspecific bone marrow signal intensity changes (T1 hypointense and T2 hyperintense) but is useful to demonstrate the extent of the disease. Isotope bone scans show a mean number of foci of five per patient. The lower limbs are most frequently affected, followed by the pelvis, spine, and anterior chest wall (including claviculae) [55].

While CRMO is a self-limiting disease, flares occur at variable intervals and the disease can remain active into adulthood.

(Spondylo)discitis

Spondylitis, spondylodiscitis, and discitis in children are perhaps different manifestations of the same disease – a low-grade infection affecting the vertebral body and intervertebral disc [56]. Many organisms cause spondylodiscitis, and even low-grade viral infection has been postulated in patients without positive cultures (50%) [1]. The clinical symptoms may be subtle, varying from the inability to stand or sit upright to frank back pain. The first radiological sign is intervertebral disc space narrow-

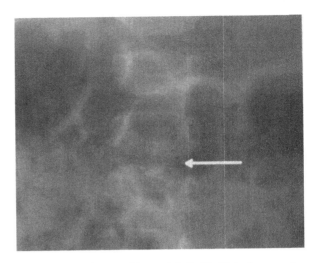

Fig. 9. A 1-year old boy with spondylodiscitis. Note the narrowing of the L2-L3 disc space as the sole radiological sign of early spondylodiscitis (*white arrow*)

ing (Fig. 9) with indistinctness of the endplates on either sides and, eventually, destruction of the endplates. The best imaging technique is MRI, which shows abnormalities in signal intensity in the intervertebral disc and adjacent vertebral bodies.

Pitfalls

Some pediatric "diseases" feature early or abundant periosteal new bone formation, simulating osteomyelitis. Examples are: several storage diseases, prolonged prostaglandin E2 medication, osteoid osteoma, congenital indifference to pain, Caffey's disease, and osteoarthropathy (Pierre Marie syndrome).

Conclusions

Diagnosis of musculoskeletal infectious and noninfectious inflammatory disease in children is difficult and challenging. Imaging studies, initially with conventional radiography and ultrasonography, play an important role.

The most important additional value of US in pediatric musculoskeletal infections over other imaging modalities is the capability to detect fluid and the possibility to perform ultrasonographically guided aspiration. The value of gray-scale and Doppler imaging should not be underestimated, as these techniques provide important information on localization, architecture, relation to surrounding tissues, vascularity, and the behavior of a lesion over time. Each of these items alone contributes to the definitive diagnosis. The diagnostic capacity of US adds to its other unrivaled advantages, such as portability, availability, speed, and patient comfort. An important limitation of US for visualizing deeper structures, such as pelvic, paravertebral, and mediastinal lesions, is its restricted acoustic window, limited penetration depth, and lack of penetration through bone and air. In such cases, CT and MRI are valuable additional techniques to evaluate the suspected anatomical region.

It is important to bear in mind that there are many differences between the pediatric and adult musculoskeletal system. Knowledge of these differences will aid in recognizing the pitfalls and peculiarities of pediatric musculoskeletal infectious diseases and thus prevent unnecessary delays in their diagnosis and treatment.

References

1. Blickman JG, van Die CE, de Rooy JW (2004) Current imaging concepts in pediatric osteomyelitis. Eur Radiol 14(Suppl 4):L55-L64
2. Oudjhane K, Ażouz EM (2001) Imaging of osteomyelitis in children. Radiol Clin North Am 39:251-266
3. Choa H, Lin S, Huang Y, Lin T (2000) Sonographic evaluation of cellulitis in children. J Ultrasound Med 19:743-749
4. Struk DW, Munk PL, Lee MJ et al (2001) Imaging of soft tissue infections. Radiol Clin North Am 39:277-303
5. Cardinal E, Bureau N, Aubin B, Chhem R (2001) Role of ultrasound in musculoskeletal infection. Radiol Clin North Am 39:191-201
6. Loyer EM, DuBrow RA, David CL et al (1996) Imaging of superficial soft-tissue infections: sonographic findings in cases of cellulitis and abscess. AJR Am J Roentgenol 166:149-152
7. Rahmouni A, Chosidow O, Mathieu D et al (1994) MR imaging in acute infectious cellulitis. Radiology 192:493-496
8. Kothari NA, Pelchovitz DJ, Meyer JS (2001) Imaging of musculoskeletal infections. Radiol Clin North Am 39:653-671
9. Chao HC, Kong MS, Lin TY (1999) Diagnosis of necrotizing fasciitis in children. J Ultrasound Med 18:277-281
10. Loh NN, Ch'en IY, Cheung LP, Li KC (1997) Deep fascial hyperintensity in soft-tissue abnormalities as revealed by T2-weighted MR imaging. AJR Am J Roentgenol 168:1301-1304
11. Bureau N, Ry C, Cardinal E (1999) Musculoskeletal infections: US manifestations. Radiographics 19:1585-1592
12. Loyer EM, Kaur H, David CL et al (1995) Importance of dynamic assessment of the soft tissues in the sonographic diagnosis of echogenic superficial abscesses. J Ultrasound Med 14:669-671
13. Sofka CM, Collins AJ, Adler RS (2001) Use of ultrasonographic guidance in interventional musculoskeletal procedures. J Ultrasound Med 20:21-26
14. Newman JS, Adler RS, Bude RO, Rubin JM (1994) Detection of soft-tissue hyperemia: value of power Doppler sonography. AJR Am J Roentgenol 163:385-389
15. Breidahl WH, Newman JS, Taljanovic MS, Adler RS (1996) Power Doppler sonography in the assessment of musculoskeletal fluid collections. AJR Am J Roentgenol 166:1443-1446
16. Mazur JM, Ross G, Cummings J et al (1995) Usefulness of magnetic resonance imaging for the diagnosis of acute musculoskeletal infections in children. J Pediatr Orthop 15:144-147
17. Bowerman SG, Green NE, Mencio GA (1997) Decline of bone and joint infections attributable to haemophilus influenzae type b. Clin Orthop 341:128-133
18. Asmar BI (1992) Osteomyelitis in the neonate. Infect Dis Clin North Am 6:117-132
19. Bar-Ziv J, Barki Y, Maroko A, Mares AJ (1985) Rib osteomyelitis in children. Early radiologic and ultrasonic findings. Pediatr Radiol 15:315-318
20. Howard CB, Einhorn M, Dagan R, Nyska M (1993) Ultrasound in diagnosis and management of acute haematogenous osteomyelitis in children. J Bone Joint Surg Br 75:79-82
21. Kaiser S, Rosenborg M (1994) Early detection of subperiosteal abscesses by ultrasonography. A means for further successful treatment in pediatric osteomyelitis. Pediatr Radiol 24:336-339
22. Abernethy LJ, Lee YC, Cole WG (1993) Ultrasound localization of subperiosteal abscesses in children with late-acute osteomyelitis. J Pediatr Orthop 13:766-768
23. Riebel TW, Nasir R, Nazarenko O (1996) The value of sonography in the detection of osteomyelitis. Pediatr Radiol 26:291-297
24. Mah ET, LeQuesne GW, Gent RJ, Paterson DC (1994) Ultrasonic features of acute osteomyelitis in children. J Bone Joint Surg Br 76:969-974
25. Cheon JE, Chung HW, Hong SH et al (2001) Sonography of acute osteomyelitis in rabbits with pathologic correlation. Acad Radiol 8:243-249
26. Abiri MM, DeAngelis GA, Kirpekar M et al (1992) Ultrasonic detection of osteomyelitis. Pathologic correlation in an animal model. Invest Radiol 27:111-113
27. Chao HC, Lin SJ, Huang YC, Lin TY (1999) Color Doppler ultrasonographic evaluation of osteomyelitis in children. J Ultrasound Med 18:729-734
28. Spiegel DA, Meyer JS, Dormans JP et al (1999) Pyomyositis in children and adolescents: report of 12 cases and review of the literature. J Pediatr Orthop 19:143-150
29. Christin L, Sarosi GA (1992) Pyomyositis in North America: case reports and review. Clin Infect Dis 15:668-677
30. Chiedozi LC (1979) Pyomyositis. Review of 205 cases in 112 patients. Am J Surg 137:255-259
31. Belli L, Reggiori A, Cocozza E, Riboldi L (1992) Ultrasound in tropical pyomyositis. Skeletal Radiol 21:107-109
32. Brook I (1996) Pyomyositis in children, caused by anaerobic bacteria. J Pediatr Surg 31:394-396
33. Lim-Dunham JE, Ben-Ami TE, Yousefzadeh DK (1995) Septic arthritis of the elbow in children: the role of sonography. Pediatr Radiol 25:556-559
34. Kocher MS, Zurakowski D, Kasser JR (1999) Differentiating between septic arthritis and transient synovitis of the hip in children: an evidence-based clinical prediction algorithm. J Bone Joint Surg Am 81:1662-1670
35. van Holsbeeck M, Introcaso JH (1992) Musculoskeletal ultrasonography. Radiol Clin North Am 30:907-925
36. Zawin JK, Hoffer FA, Rand FF, Teele RL (1993) Joint effusion in children with an irritable hip: US diagnosis and aspiration. Radiology 187:459-463
37. Gordon JE, Huang M, Dobbs M et al (2002) Causes of false-negative ultrasound scans in the diagnosis of septic arthritis of the hip in children. J Pediatr Orthop 22:312-316
38. Dorr U, Zieger M, Hauke H (1988) Ultrasonography of the painful hip. Prospective studies in 204 patients. Pediatr Radiol 19:36-40
39. Robben SG, Lequin MH, Diepstraten AF et al (1999) Anterior joint capsule of the normal hip and in children with transient synovitis: US study with anatomic and histologic correlation. Radiology 210:499-507
40. Marchal GJ, Van Holsbeeck MT, Raes M et al (1987) Transient synovitis of the hip in children: role of US. Radiology 162:825-828
41. Strouse PJ, DiPietro MA, Adler RS (1998) Pediatric hip effusions: evaluation with power Doppler sonography. Radiology 206:731-735
42. Greenspan A, Tehranzadeh J (2001) Imaging of infectious arthritis. Radiol Clin North Am 39:267-276
43. Hopkins KL, Li KC, Bergman G (1995) Gadolinium-DTPA-enhanced magnetic resonance imaging of musculoskeletal infectious processes. Skeletal Radiol 24:325-330
44. Paisley JW (1982) Septic bursitis in childhood. J Pediatr Orthop 2:57-61

45. Harwell JI, Fisher D (2001) Pediatric septic bursitis: case report of retrocalcaneal infection and review of the literature. Clin Infect Dis 32 E102-104
46. Garcia-Porrua C, Gonzalez-Gay MA, Ibanez D, Garcia-Pais MJ (1999) The clinical spectrum of severe septic bursitis in northwestern Spain: a 10 year study. J Rheumatol 26:663-667
47. Hill R, Conron R, Greissinger P, Heller M (1997) Ultrasound for the detection of foreign bodies in human tissue. Ann Emerg Med 29:353-356
48. Roberts CS, Beck DJ Jr, Heinsen J, Seligson D (2002) Review article: diagnostic ultrasonography: applications in orthopaedic surgery. Clin Orthop 401:248-264
49. Laor T, Jaramillo D, Oestreich AE (1998) Transplacentally acquired infections. In: Kirks DR, Griscom NT (eds) Practical pediatric imaging, 3rd edn. Lippincot-Raven, Philadelphia, p 381
50. Aebi C, Ahmed A, Ramilo O (1996) Bacterial complications of primary varicella in children. Clin Infect Dis 23:698-705
51. Cowan MR, Primm PA, Scott SM et al (1994) Serious group A beta-hemolytic streptococcal infections complicating varicella. Ann Emerg Med 23:818-822
52. Mills WJ, Mosca VS, Nizet V (1996) Orthopaedic manifestations of invasive group A streptococcal infections complicating primary varicella. J Pediatr Orthop 16:522-528
53. Brown T, Wilkinson RH (1988) Chronic recurrent multifocal osteomyelitis. Radiology 166:493-496
54. Giedion A, Holthusen W, Masel LF, Vischer D (1972) Subacute and chronic "symmetrical" osteomyelitis. Ann Radiol (Paris) 15:329-342 [French]
55. Job-Deslandre C, Krebs S, Kahan A (2001) Chronic recurrent multifocal osteomyelitis: five-year outcomes in 14 pediatric cases. Joint Bone Spine 68:245-251
56. Swischuk E (1997) Infections of the spine and spinal cord. In: Imaging of the newborn, infant, and young child. 4th edn. Williams & Wilkins, Baltimore, p 1044

Imaging of Pediatric Musculoskeletal Neoplasms

Philippe Petit[1], Michel Panue[2]

[1] Service de Radiopediatrie, Hôpital Timone-Enfants, Marseille, France
[2] Service d'Imagerie, Hôpital Nord, Marseille, France

Introduction

Information regarding the frequency, location, imaging criteria, and diagnostic clues of pediatric bone and soft-tissue lesions, either benign or malignant, are described in several excellent radiology text books [1, 2]. Ideally, this information is sufficiently known to radiologist such that these pathologies can be diagnosed quickly and confidently. In current practice, the radiologist's job can be described as comprising three essential responsibilities.

The Choice of the Proper Imaging Modality

The choice of the proper imaging modality depends on the initial clinical signs.

Cases Involving Trauma and/or Pain

In patients who have suffered trauma or experience pain, plain-film X-rays constitute the first diagnostic step, as they guide the radiologist's decision to subsequently perform an imaging exploration or other procedures.

First, it will identify the presence of a bony or soft-tissue lesion. Here, the radiologist's role is to describe the aggressiveness, location (longitudinal and transverse for long bones), degree of mineralization of a bony lesion, and the density and its relationships with the underlying bone of a soft-tissue mass. The next step is to decide whether the lesion is actually a normal variant (Fig. 1) [3, 4] or an incidental finding, definitely benign and not requiring treatment (Figs. 2, 3).

Second, if the lesion needs further imaging exploration, i.e., it is of unknown origin or exhibits marked aggressiveness, the most appropriate modality must be chosen. The endpoint of imaging is not employ the entire armamentarium of imaging modalities but the one that will yield the greatest degree of diagnostic accuracy, with minimal radiation exposure of the patient and the lowest cost, while affording surgeons and clinicians information essential to the child's management. Depending on the initial imaging suspicion, the strategy generally proceeds as follows:

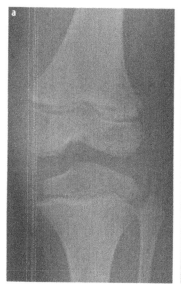
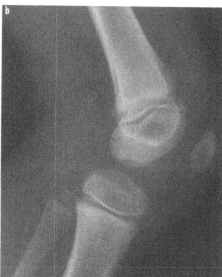

Fig. 1 a, b. Anteroposterior (**a**) and lateral (**b**) views of the left knee in a 6-year-old boy: normal irregular ossification of the lateral aspect of the distal femoral epiphysis

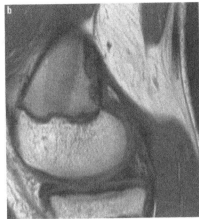
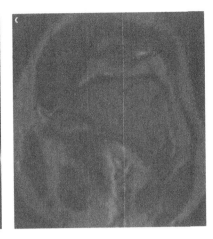

Fig. 2 a-c. Posterior cortical defect of the medial condyle created by chronic avulsions of the medial gastrocnemius; (**a**) lateral view, (**b**) sagittal T1-weighted image, (**c**) axial T2-weighted image

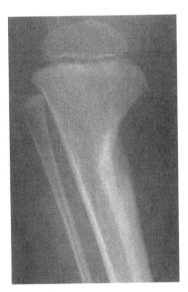

Fig. 3. Congenital tibia vara

- Stress fracture: In the acute phase magnetic resonance imaging (MRI) is preferred over computed tomography (CT); in the delayed phase (>10 days after the first X ray): the plain-film X-ray should be repeated (Fig. 4).
- Osteoid ostema, osteoblastoma, myositis ossificans/para- and peri-osteal sarcomas: CT is recommended to analyze mineralization, position of the calcification (central or peripheral), and the relationship with the underlying bone (Fig. 5). In osteoid osteoma, this step precedes percutaneous treatment [5].
- Other lesions: MRI is the method of choice to evaluate the signal of the lesion and its extension either in the medulla and/or the soft tissues [6].

- Metastatic disease (rare) or a potentially diffuse process (fibrous dysplasia): While bone scintigraphy Tc-99 was previously recommended in these cases, it has largely been replaced by 3D whole-body MR (STIR or diffusion) [7].

Third, if the lesion needs to be biopsied, it must be preceded by a thorough imaging work-up, ideally discussed during a multidisciplinary meeting (pathologist, oncologist, orthopedic surgeon, radiologist) [8]. The margins of the lesion, as seen on MRI, will be greatly increased due to the trauma of biopsy, leading to unnecessary bone and soft-tissue resection if a surgical procedure is planned. MRI and positron emission tomography (PET)-CT are the two most important examinations for, respectively, local and general assessment of the nature of a lesion. Both techniques are used not only in the initial work-up but also in the follow-up of patients with malignant tumors, to assess the response to chemotherapy [9-11].

However, it may be that a lesion is not visible on plain X-ray. Assuming that the patient's symptoms have been correctly assessed, the appropriate clinician prescriptions chosen, and the X-ray images (or those obtained with other imaging technique) are of adequate quality, then several different sceneries are possible: (1) if there is no lesion and the patient has become asymptomatic; a clinical follow-up, but not further imaging, is required. (2) If a lesion should be visible (Fig. 6), the discrepancy with the clinical status indicates the need for a repeat X-ray or a more sensitive imaging mode (bone scintigraphy or MRI). (3) It may be the case that the clinical signs persist but that the lesion is not yet visible on X-ray; in this case, the recommendations of step (2) should be followed.

Cases Involving a Soft-Tissue Mass

The first imaging exam carried out in our department is ultrasound-Doppler examination [12-14]. Nonetheless,

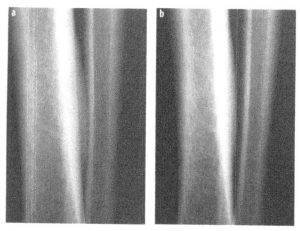

Fig. 4 a, b. Plain-film follow-up of a cortical stress fracture

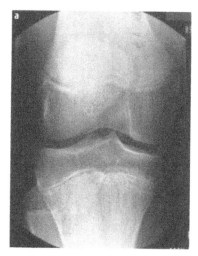

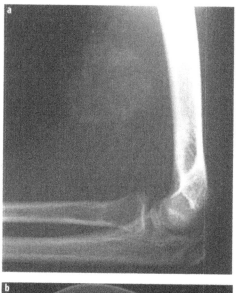

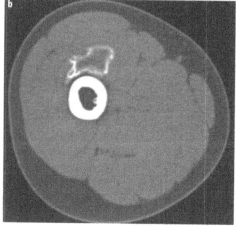

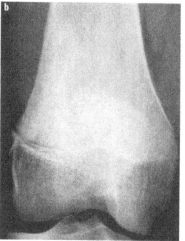

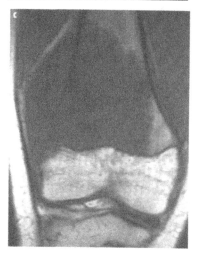

Fig. 5 a, b. Myositis ossificans, typical appearance on plain film X-ray (**a**) and CT scan (**b**)

Fig. 6 a-c. Post traumatic right knee pain. The initial AP view (**a**) was much too localized to the joint. Repeat X-rays obtained 15 days later cover the metaphyseal-diaphyseal junction (**b**) and show loss of cortical contour as well as a thin periostal reaction, revealing an aggressive process that was subsequently evaluated by MRI, which revealed (**c**) osteosarcoma

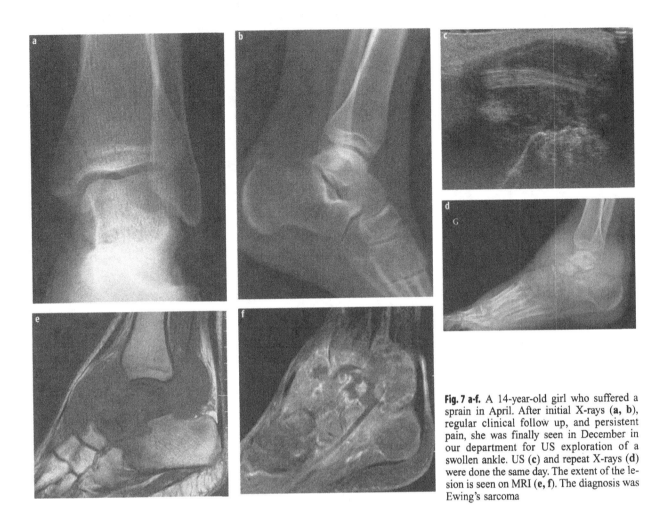

Fig. 7 a-f. A 14-year-old girl who suffered a sprain in April. After initial X-rays (**a**, **b**), regular clinical follow up, and persistent pain, she was finally seen in December in our department for US exploration of a swollen ankle. US (**c**) and repeat X-rays (**d**) were done the same day. The extent of the lesion is seen on MRI (**e, f**). The diagnosis was Ewing's sarcoma

all explorations of a soft-tissue mass located close to the skeleton must include a plain-film X-ray (Fig. 7). The goal is to look for: (1) the underlying bone, which could be either the origin of the soft tissue mass or involved by the process, and (2) elements frequently characteristic of a soft-tissue mass (fat, calcification).

Ultrasound can describe the parameters of the mass, including echo texture, borders, size, relationship with the adjacent bone or joint, and vascularization. However, it should be noted that ultrasound, especially Doppler study, is of limited value in agitated infants and newborns.

Depending on these results and the clinical data, either the diagnosis is established and there is no need for surgery (Fig. 8) or the diagnosis remains uncertain and biopsy or surgery are required, in which case MRI is the examination of choice (Fig. 7), as it will aid in characterization of the lesion, its extent, and its relationship with major structures (i.e., nerves, vessels) [15-17].

Correlating the Imaging Findings and Clinical Data to Propose a Diagnosis

Based on the results obtained with the chosen imaging strategy, the second part of the radiologist's job is to associate the imaging findings with the clinical data and to propose a diagnosis. The diagnostic possibilities can be reduced by considering several clinical parameters, foremost being the patient's age as it is one of the most important clues as to whether the diagnosis will involve a bony or soft-tissue mass.

- In the differential diagnosis of an aggressive bony lesion in a child less than 5 years of age, histiocytosis > infection > neuroblastoma metastasis >> Ewing's sarcoma.
- An aggressive lesion in a child older than 5 years of age is most likely an osteosarcoma or an Ewing's sarcoma.
- A hypervascular soft-tissue lesion that appeared and grew a few days after birth is most likely an immature hemangioma.

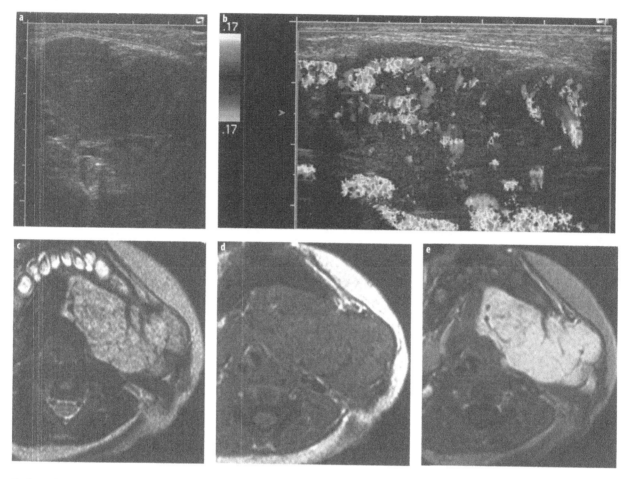

Fig. 8 a-e. Two-month-old-baby with a deep immature hemangioma. Ultrasound shows (**a**) a homogeneous hypoechoic mass and (**b**) arterial hypervascularization. (**c, d**) T2- and T1-weighted magnetic resonance images revealed a homogenous mass with flow voids. (**e**) T1-weighted gadolinium-enahnced MRI shows homogenous enhancement

- A vascular lesion present at birth suggests a tumor (congenital hemangioma) or a vascular malformation.

The second point to consider is the evolution of the lesion. A long-standing process of more than 6 months duration favors the diagnosis of a benign tumor. Nonetheless, it must be kept in mind that malignant tumors are often revealed during the examination of a minor trauma, in which case the diagnosis may be delayed by several months. Furthermore, the patient should be asked whether he or she experiences pain at night, since a "wake-up" lesion is a sign of aggressiveness.

Therapy and Follow-Up

Lastly, it is the job of the radiologist to ensure imaging follow-up of these lesions as needed, with the aim of assessing therapeutic efficiency and absence of recurrence. In these situations, MRI and PET-CT are the modalities of choice [15, 18].

References

1. Resnick D (1989) Tumors and tumor-like lesion of bone: radiographics principles. In: Resnick D (ed) Bone and joint imaging. Saunders, Philadelphia, pp 1096-1106
2. Silverman SF (1993) Tumors of the soft tissues of the limbs and bone. In: Caffey's pediatric X-ray diagnosis: an integrated imaging approach, 9th edn. Mosby, St-Louis, pp 1869-1911
3. Keats TE, Anderson MW (2007) Atlas of normal roentgen variants that may simulate disease, 8th edn. Mosby Elsevier, Philadelphia
4. Köhler A, Zimmer EA (1993) Borderlands of normal and early pathologic findings in skeletal radiology, 4th edn. Thieme, New York
5. Aschero A, Gorincour G, Glard Y et al (2008) Percutaneous treatment of osteoid osteoma by laser thermocoagulation under computed tomography guidance in pediatric patients. Eur Radiol (Epub ahead of print)
6. Panuel M, Gentet JC, Scheiner C et al (1993) Physeal and epiphyseal extent of primary malignant bone tumors in childhood. Correlation of preoperative MRI and the pathologic examination. Pediatr Radiol 23(6):421-424

7. Mentzel HJ, Kentouche K, Sauner D et al (2004) Comparison of whole-body STIR-MRI and 99mTc-methylene-diphosphonate scintigraphy in children with suspected multifocal bone lesions. Eur Radiol 14(12):2297-2302

8. Meyer JS, Nadel HR, Marina N et al (2008) Imaging guidelines for children with Ewing sarcoma and osteosarcoma: a report from the Children's Oncology Group Bone Tumor Committee. Pediatr Blood Cancer 51(2):163-167

9. Brisse H, Ollivier L, Edeline V et al (2004) Imaging of malignant tumours of the long bones in children: monitoring response to neoadjuvant chemotherapy and preoperative assessment. Pediatr Radiol 34(8):595-605

10. Uhl M, Saueressig U, Koehler G et al (2006) Evaluation of tumour necrosis during chemotherapy with diffusion-weighted MR. imaging: preliminary results in osteosarcomas. Pediatr Radiol 36(12):1306-1311

11. Hayashida Y, Yakushiji T, Awai K et al (2006) Monitoring therapeutic responses of primary bone tumors by diffusion-weighted image: Initial results. Eur Radiol 16(12):2637-2643

12. Latifi HR, Siegel MJ (1994) Color Doppler flow imaging of pediatric soft tissue masses. J Ultrasound Med 13(3):165-169

13. Dubois J, Garel L, David M, Powell J (2002) Vascular soft-tissue tumors in infancy: distinguishing features on Doppler sonography. AJR Am J Roentgenol 178(6):1541-1545

14. Gorincour G, Kokta V, Rypens F et al (2005) Imaging characteristics of two subtypes of congenital hemangiomas: rapidly involuting congenital hemangiomas and non-involuting congenital hemangiomas. Pediatr Radiol 35(12):1178-1185

15. Brisse H, Orbach D, Klijanienko J et al (2006) Imaging and diagnostic strategy of soft tissue tumors in children. Eur Radiol 16(5):1147-1164

16. Laor T (2004) MR imaging of soft tissue tumors and tumor-like lesions. Pediatr Radiol 34(1):24-37

17. Park K, van Rijn R, McHugh K (2008) The role of radiology in paediatric soft tissue sarcomas. Cancer Imaging 22(8):102-115

18. Völker T, Denecke T, Steffen I et al (2007) Positron emission tomography for staging of pediatric sarcoma patients: results of a prospective multicenter trial. J Clin Oncol 25(34):5435-5441

Printed in March 2009